Medical Terms Simplified

Medical

Terms

Simplified

Wilson Stegeman, M.D., F.A.C.S.

DIPLOMATE, AMERICAN BOARD OF UROLOGY
Santa Rosa, California

WEST PUBLISHING CO. | St. Paul · New York · Boston
Los Angeles · San Francisco

Dedicated to the thousands of nice people who would enjoy a better understanding of medical terms.

Library of Congress Cataloging in Publication Data

Stegeman, Wilson, 1897–
    Medical Terms Simplified.
    Includes Index.

        1. Medicine—Terminology.   I.   Title.
DNLM: 1.   Nomenclature.   W15   S817m
R123.S74   610'.3   75–12977
ISBN   0–8299–0062–4
ISBN   0–8299–0118–3
2nd Reprint—1977

Preface

Every medical office has a medical dictionary for the use of the "office family"—the secretary, the nurse, the assistant, even the boss. Unfortunately, the bigger and more complete the dictionary, the harder it is to find a word unless you know exactly how it is spelled, and this problem is frequently compounded by the fact that many doctors' nonchalant enunciation is about on a par with their well publicized penmanship.

Every trade and profession has its own specialized terminology, and the proficient use of the language of medicine is, unfortunately, only laboriously acquired. There are no usable shortcuts. Nonetheless, it seems that a working acquaintance with the more common medical terms should be more easily obtainable, both for the constantly expanding group of paramedical workers, for patients, and for other lay people. This short book devoted to the spelling, pronunciation, and informal—but reliable—definition of less than 6,000 commonly-used medical words is intended to fill that gap.

Of the numerous books available to the medically interested individual without medical schooling, many are too technical to make easy reading; others become too complicated by taking in too much territory. This book tries to avoid the more conspicuous inadequacies and does not expect the reader to be a doctor. Obviously, you can't study a dictionary, with its 125,000 entries, most of them never used. But anyone willing to study this condensed volume should be rewarded by learning most of the common medical words and a lot of the tricks about how they are made.

The writer has a feeling of loyalty and gratitude toward the practice of medicine. His long association with it has brought many varied pleasures and rewards. The expenditure of the effort involved in trying to fill an obvious need has been a pleasure.

It is hoped, then, that this informal book—unorthodox certainly, and maybe even irreverent—will serve its intended purpose. If it manages to take some of the mystery out of medical language, that would be an added bonus.

W.S.

Acknowledgements

Without the help of the consultants this glossary would have been impossible. The time these scholarly colleagues took from their busy lives and the thought they expended in helping with this project were a constant encouragement to me in a time-consuming effort. They helped select the terms most commonly used in their specialties and later assisted in tailoring the definitions into medically acceptable but brief, simplified form. My thanks to them is as sincere as my hope that the finished product will exceed their expectations.

To Dr. John F. Stegeman, my nephew, my special thanks for his prodigious effort in selecting and putting into shape the long list of terms used by internists. Dr. Lewis Etter was most kind in allowing me to borrow from his "Words and Phrases Used in Radiology and Nuclear Medicine." The American Psychiatric Association was equally generous in allowing me to make use of their excellent "Psychiatric Glossary" in phrasing and shortening the definitions of difficult psychiatric terms.

To Mrs. Helen Null my thanks for years of extracurricular typing and intelligent assistance, and for the uncomplaining copying and re-copying of seemingly endless lists. And to Mrs. Patricia Escamillo, my thanks for her enthusiastic help during the early stages of the book.

To my friend James Ransom, Ph.D., editor for Lange Medical Publications, my special thanks for his invaluable suggestions and advice, and for his patience in reviewing copy. His cheerful help has been a source of encouragement, and his wide horizon of knowledge provides continual enjoyment.

To my wife, Peg, my thanks for her years of tolerance and for her many helpful suggestions. Her alert paramedical mind has long ago learned to recognize obsessions, and her patience with this particular one was phenomenal.

W.S.

Consultants

SAMUEL D. AIKEN, M.D.
Diplomate, American Board of Ophthalmology; Former Assistant Clinical Professor, Ophthalmology, University of California Medical Center; Santa Rosa, California

LAWRENCE H. ARNSTEIN, M.D.
Diplomate, American Board of Neurosurgery; Palo Alto, California

WILLIAM H. AUFRANC, M.D.
Diplomate, American Board of Preventive Medicine; Former Regional Director, United States Public Health Service; San Francisco, California

WALTER BIRNBAUM, M.D., F.A.C.S.
Diplomate, American Board of Surgery; Clinical Professor, Surgery, University of California Medical Center; San Francisco, California

MARVIN A. BROWNSTEIN, M.D.
Diplomate, American Board of Pathology; Oakland, California

ROBERT H. BUTLER, M.D.
Diplomate, American Board of Radiology; Associate Professor, Clinical and Ambulatory Medicine, University of California Medical Center; Santa Rosa, California

DOUGLAS W. CARDOZO, M.D., F.A.C.S.
Diplomate, American Board of Surgery; Santa Rosa, California

ROBERT W. CHURCHILL, M.D.
Diplomate, American Board of Anesthesiology; Former Associate Professor, Anesthesiology, Stanford University School of Medicine; Santa Rosa, California

HARDING CLEGG, M.D.
Santa Rosa, California

PAUL M. CROSSLAND, M.D.*
Diplomate, American Board of Dermatology; Former Assistant Professor, Dermatology, Stanford University School of Medicine; Santa Rosa, California

ROBERT L. DENNIS, M.D.
Diplomate, American Board of Pathology; Director, Pathology, San Jose Hospitals and Health Center; San Jose, California

WILLIAM J. DUNN, M.D.
Diplomate, American Board of Obstetrics and Gynecology; Santa Rosa, California

WARREN K. HANSEN, M.D.
Diplomate, American Board of Dermatology; Associate Clinical Professor, Dermatology, Stanford University School of Medicine; San Francisco, California

FRANK HINMAN, JR., M.D., F.A.C.S.
Diplomate, American Board of Urology; Clinical Professor, Urology; University of California Medical Center; San Francisco, California

T. WESLEY HUNTER, M.D., F.A.C.S.
Diplomate, American Board of Orthopedic Surgery; Assistant Clinical Professor, Orthopedics, University of California Medical Center; Santa Rosa, California

ROBERT M. ISAAC, M.D.
Diplomate, American Board of Psychiatry and Neurology (Psychiatry); Santa Rosa, California

FRANKLIN P. JEPPESEN, M.D., F.A.C.S.
Diplomate, American Board of Urology; Boise, Idaho

A. PAUL KELLER, JR., M.D.
Diplomate, American Board of Ophthalmology; Diplomate, American Board of Otolaryngology; Athens, Georgia

LEO H. LaDAGE, M.D., F.A.C.S.*
Diplomate, American Board of Plastic Surgery; Long Beach, California

JOSEPH J. LITTELL, M.D., F.A.C.S.*
Diplomate, American Board of Otolaryngology; Former Assistant Professor, Otolaryngology, University of Indiana College of Medicine, Indianapolis; Santa Rosa, California

STEPHEN S. LOWE, M.D.
Diplomate, American Board of Psychiatry and Neurology (Psychiatry); Santa Rosa, California

DONALD MACRAE, M.D., M.R.C.P., F.R.F.P.S.
Diplomate, American Board of Psychiatry and Neurology (Neurology); Professor and Chairman of Neurology, University of California Medical Center; San Francisco, California

SEDGWICK MEAD, M.D.
Diplomate, American Board of Physical Medicine and Rehabilitation; Chief, Neurology, Kaiser Rehabilitation Center; Vallejo, California

LOUIS W. MENACHOF, M.D.
Diplomate, American Board of Pediatrics; Assistant Clinical Professor, Pediatrics, University of California Medical Center; Santa Rosa, California

SYDNEY M. MILLER, M.D.
Diplomate, American Board of Radiology; Santa Rosa, California

FRANK W. NORMAN, M.D.
Former President, California Academy of General Practice; Santa Rosa, California

JOHN M. OLNEY, JR., M.D.
Diplomate, American Board of Surgery; Santa Rosa, California

FRANK L. PRIOR, M.S.
Director, Empire Medical Laboratory; Santa Rosa, California

H. EDWARD RAITANO, M.D.
Diplomate, American Board of Surgery; Santa Rosa, California

EDWARD B. SHAW, M.D.
Diplomate, American Board of Pediatrics; Emeritus Professor and former Chief, Pediatrics, University of California Medical Center; San Francisco, California

DAVID G. SHEETZ, M.D.
Diplomate, American Board of Neurosurgery; Santa Rosa, California

THEODORE S. STASHAK, M.D., F.A.C.S.
Diplomate, American Board of Obstetrics and Gynecology; Santa Rosa, California

JOHN F. STEGEMAN, M.D., F.A.C.P.
Diplomate, American Board of Internal Medicine; Athens, Georgia.

ROBERT A. TECKEMEYER,
Washington, D.C.

DOUGLAS D. TOFFELMIER, M.D., F.A.C.S.
Diplomate, American Board of Orthopedic Surgery; Oakland, California

CLARENCE E. TOSHACH, M.D., F.A.C.S.*
Diplomate, American Board of Obstetrics and Gynecology; Saginaw, Michigan

ALBERT M. TRUCKER, M.D.
Diplomate, American Board of Plastic Surgery; Santa Rosa, California

ROBERT S. TUTTLE, D.D.S.
President, California Board of Dental Examiners; Santa Rosa, California

JAMES L. WATERS, M.D.
Santa Rosa, California

WALTER E. WEBER, M.D.
Diplomate, American Board of Dermatology; former Associate Clinical Professor, Dermatology, Stanford University School of Medicine; Santa Rosa, California

BRUCE G. WHITAKER, PH.D., M.D.
Diplomate, American Board of Otolaryngology; Assistant Clinical Professor, Otolaryngology, University of California Medical Center; Santa Rosa, California

*deceased

Contents

Contents

Illustrations

GENERAL MATTERS

1 How to Use This Book

RATHER THAN BEING considered authentic or official, this book would much prefer to be regarded as an understanding, helpful ally in your quest for greater familiarity with medical words. It is, hopefully, something any intelligent, interested person can follow and grasp without exercising fierce determination. This book started out to be only a short "Speller and Pronouncer" for doctors' secretaries, but gradually — as logic, obvious necessity, or critics' insistence demanded — other features were added. Regardless, it is still a layman's book; not a doctor's book.

In attempting to fulfill the above qualifications, about 5,200 commonly used words were selected from the usual 125,000 medical dictionary listings and they were divided into general medical terms and those terms limited to specialist practice. Each selected specialty list was sent to two or three scholarly physicians practicing in that field, and these consultants cut out "deadwood" and suggested additional terms. Later they reviewed the informal definitions and indulgently tailored them until they met the demands of official approval. The only stipulation imposed was that the definitions emerge uncomplicated, informal, understandable, and brief.

If you are a secretary and you aren't sure whether tonsillitis has one or two "l's," you need only look in the *INDEX* to check. And for more complex requirements, you can usually begin your search with the *INDEX*. If your dictating belt mumbles the name of an operation and the dictator is a plastic surgeon, you can run down the probabilities in that section's list of terms. If you can detect how the word starts and you know approximately what the doctor is talking about, you will probably recognize the term without much trouble.

Or, if you are a patient and you are wondering what your young obstetrician meant when he kept talking about parturition—and he was too busy to be asked to explain—looking over the "p's" in the Obstetrics list will tell you quickly that parturition is just a fancy name for the (unfancy) business of having a baby.

General Glossary Rules

Here are some rules that have been followed in compiling these glossaries:

1. Defined words and phrases are printed in **bold type.** Some definitions include terms which may be unfamiliar to the reader but which are needed to clarify the definitions. These terms are printed in **bold type.** By referring to the *INDEX*, you can readily locate the pages on which they are defined.
2. A term's pronunciation is indicated by its phonetic respelling, which immediately follows its listing (explained on page 4).
3. The listed term is generally the singular noun form; when the commonly-used word is an adjective, or a verb, or a plural, this is indicated (**premature**—*adj.*; **resect**—*verb*; **steroids**—*plural*).
4. When the term's plural or adjective form is irregular, this is shown (pelvis: *plural*—pelves; fever: *adj.*—febrile).
5. If another word is used interchangeably with the listed word, this is indicated (measles—rubeola; enterobiasis—pin-worm infestation).
6. Procedures, diseases, operations, etc. commonly identified by a proper name (eponym) are listed in the alphabetical position of the eponym (McBurney incision under "M," not under "I"). Commonly accepted vernacular words, phrases or "medical jargon" equivalents or abbreviations are shown in quotation marks (chorea—"St. Vitus dance"; Urology—"G.U.").
7. Proprietary or patented names of common drugs are identified by initial capitals (Butesin) to differentiate them from generic equivalents (penicillin).
8. Helpful root "clues" are shown following the phonetic respelling of some terms. Clues are explained in the chapter *ROOTS AND STEMS* and when they first appear in each chapter; recurring clues are not constantly redefined (CALC = stone).
9. Optional spellings are often indicated. General usage prevails for suggested pronunciation, which may vary in different geographical areas.
10. Medical abbreviations are not listed in the *INDEX* unless they are defined in a specific glossary.

Pronunciation

Let's start out by admitting that the correct pronunciation of medical terms is often difficult; many medical words just don't sound the way they are spelled. Since knowing the sound of a word is helpful and necessary not only in understanding and using it but also in recognizing it subsequently, this gap must be bridged in some manner. Normally this is the function of phonetic respelling.

Because few of us can recall the various diacritical markings we once knew and the subtle sound values they assign to each vowel, it seemed permissible to try to build a simple pronouncing system—the simpler the better. Numerous and varied tests demonstrated that if we built syllables that sounded like the parts of the word, marked only the *long* vowels, and indicated only the *primary* accent, the sound and—more importantly—the "swing" of the word could be fairly well conveyed. Unorthodox, certainly, and unscholarly, probably, but in these days everyone makes his own rules and so shall we, claiming as excuse a desire to be helpful.

There will be some deficiencies in the system, no doubt, but it should suit our purposes well enough. **Olecranon** works out ō-lek′ra-non, and **pterygium** sounds out ter-ij′ē-um. A macron over the vowel makes it a long vowel; if it isn't marked, it's short. If you know the approximate sound of the syllables, know which vowels are long, and where the primary accent falls, you can come fairly close to sensing the swing of the word and you won't miss the pronunciation very far. It would be nice to be able to show the different values of the shorter vowel sounds, but we have been unable to devise a system that isn't complicated; and numerous attempts and trial-checks have shown that for lay people the additional confusion outweighs the advantages.

Definitions

Defining medical terms in simple, nonmedical language is difficult, at best. Trying to keep these definitions not only accurate and inclusive but also brief and uncomplicated makes it doubly difficult—in fact, almost impossible. Additional informative comments are frequently required to make the definitions useful at all. The rule adopted here is that "What you say must be true, but what you don't say can't legitimately be held against you."

****

Small books have natural limitations—inclusions must be decided upon, rejections dutifully carried out. The compiler assumes sole responsibility for (unintentional) omissions, (deplorable) errors, and (apparent) inconsistencies—and firmly expects to hear about them!

One additional word: Although this book started out primarily as a speller, it is *not* a spelling *primer!* It is intended for use by persons who can spell common words unaided, even if those words also happen to relate to medical topics. So phalanx and mandible you will find; finger and jaw, no.

2 Some Everyday Medical Customs

THERE ARE SEVERAL descriptive words and phrases that doctors use continuously, and almost unconsciously, of which you should be aware. Otherwise you are never going to enjoy reading or hearing medical language, and it will continue to be confusing.

To start with, medical descriptions always visualize the body as *facing* you, with both palms turned toward you. This is the so-called *anatomical position,* and terms of external location always refer back to this position. The front side of the body is *always* its **anterior** surface and the back side of the body is its **posterior** surface. The **posterior** side of the body is also called its **dorsal** surface, and the **anterior** side (of the abdomen, particularly) is also the **ventral** surface. Of course, since the patient is always described as if he were facing you, your right is his left, and vice versa. This is why the *anatomical position* is important to remember.

There are several other terms, many of them used in pairs, that identify and designate locations and positions within the body itself. **Medial** and **lateral** are two such paired "position words" that are used constantly. They do not signify the right or left sides of the body, but indicate a position *nearer to* or *farther away from* the **midline,** which separates the right and left halves of the body. They also show positions in relation to each other. This sounds complicated, and a diagram should help. (See Figure 1, page 7.)

In the diagram, anything in the line C is spoken of as being **medial** to A and B, because it is *nearer* to the **midline** of the body. By the same token, since A and B are *farther away* from the **midline** than C, they are both **lateral** to C. And B is **lateral** to C and **medial** to A at the same time.

Similarly, D and E are **medial** to F, and F is **lateral** to both D and

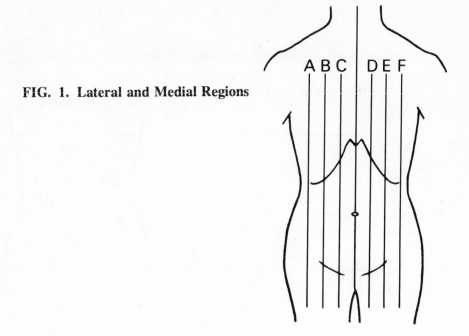

FIG. 1. Lateral and Medial Regions

E. And, again, although E is **medial** to F, it is **lateral** to D. As you see, there is no relationship to right or left, but only to the **midline** of the body, and to each other.

Another pair of location-terms are **proximal** and **distal.** They indicate positions relatively *nearer to* or *farther away from* the *place of origin* of an extremity (or of a nerve or an artery). The closer-in position is said to be **proximal,** and the location farther-out is called **distal.** The knee-joint is **proximal** to the ankle-joint, but it is **distal** to the hip-joint. Although the elbow is **distal** to the shoulder, it is **proximal** to the wrist. Descriptions of other parts follow the same logic. The system is actually an excellent one and offers almost the only possible means of localizing and identifying certain positions definitely and understandably. These are very convenient terms, which are very necessary, and *very commonly used* — as you will discover.

Root and prefix clues are also helpful in remembering the names of the nine anatomical areas into which the abdomen — the region between the chest and the groins — is divided for purposes of identification and localization. Associating the names of these areas with their locations is also aided by mentally superimposing a tic-tac-toe diagram on the abdomen — the squares and the areas coincide fairly closely. (See Figure 2, page 8.)

The center square (A) is the **umbilical** area, for obvious reasons. In

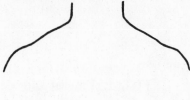

FIG. 2. The Abdominal Areas

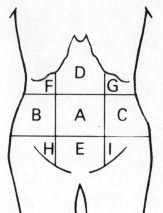

the center horizontal row are the right (B) and left (C) **lumbar** areas. Above and below the middle square are the **epigastric** (D) and the **hypogastric** (E) areas. In the upper corners are the right (F) and left (G) **hypochondriac** areas. And in the lower corners are the right (H) and left (I) **iliac** regions. In surgical dictation the abdomen is frequently just divided into quarters, and each quarter is simply designated as the right or left, upper or lower quadrant, as the case may be.

You should know something about the positions of the body on the operating table or in a hospital bed — or on the floor, for that matter. When the patient is lying flat on his back he is in the **dorsal** or **supine** (   ) position. If he is lying face down he is in the **prone** (   ) position. Halfway between are the **lateral** positions, right and left, depending on which side of his body the patient is lying. And if he is just lying down — any old way — he is in a **recumbent** position.

The **lithotomy** and **Trendelenburg** positions are frequently used during surgical operations. In the **lithotomy** position the patient is lying on his back, with the thighs raised (and secured) at a right (or acute) angle to his upper body. The legs are bent at the knees and the lower legs are generally horizontal (   ). In the **Trendelenburg** position the patient is also lying on his back but the table has been tilted so that his hips are higher than his head. The table may be "broken" beneath the hips and the legs allowed to hang down to any desired extent (   ).

Weights and Measures

Medical weights and measures were once expressed only in terms of the apothecary system. Although the use of the metric (decimal) system has largely replaced it, apothecary system terminology is still used by many doctors. Many drugs are still associated with apothecary system measures, for example, five grains of aspirin, or a half-grain of codeine — seldom 300 milligrams of aspirin, or 30 milligrams of codeine.

The apothecary system uses one set of terms and quantities; the metric system uses another set. To list the factors used in converting apothecary measures to metric system quantities — as pharmacists are constantly required to do in preparing prescriptions — serves little purpose in this book. However, showing the approximate values of the units of both systems in avoirdupois or "household" equivalents may help to orient you. Here, then, are the commonly used units of volume and weight of the apothecary and metric systems, and units of length in the metric system, reduced to common household measures. The apothecary system has no measures of length.

VOLUME — (Liquid Quantity)

Apothecary System	Abbreviations	"Household" Equivalents
pint — 16 fluid ounces	pt. or O	About 2 cupfuls
ounce — 8 fluid drams (drachms), 30 ml. (metric)	fl. oz. or ℥	Approx. 8 teaspoonfuls
fluid dram — 4 ml. (metric)	fl. dr. or f3	Approx. 1 teaspoonful
minim — a drop	ℳ	Approx. a drop

Metric System		
liter — 1000 milliliters (or cc.)	L	Slightly more than a quart; a 4″ cube of liquid. A liter is 1000 ml; a quart is 950 ml.
cubic centimeter	cc.	About 15 drops
milliliter (preferred) Each, 1/1000th of a liter Each, equivalent to 15 minims (apothecary)	ml.	4 ml. — 1 teaspoonful

WEIGHT

Apothecary System	Abbreviations	"Household" Equivalents
ounce — 480 grains	oz.	An ounce
dram — 60 grains	3	Approx. 1/8 of an ounce
scruple — 20 grains, (not used today)	℈	
grain — 65 milligrams (metric), 0.065 grams (metric)	gr.	

Metric System	Abbreviations	"Household" Equivalents
kilogram (or "kilo") — 1000 grams	Kg.	Two and one-quarter pounds (2.2 pounds)
gram — 1/1000th of a kilo	G. or Gm., g. or gm.	30 grams = 1 ounce
milligram — 1/1000th of a gram	mg.	About 10 specks of dust
microgram — 1/1000th of a milligram	mcg. or μg	Practically invisible!
nanogram, picogram, etc. — Parts of micrograms		Infinitesimal!

LENGTH

Metric System	Abbreviations	"Household" Equivalents
meter	M	Slightly more than a yard (39.17 inches)
centimeter — 1/100th of a meter	cm.	Slightly less than 1/2 inch (0.39 inch; 2.5 cm. = 1 inch)
millimeter — 1/1000th of a meter	mm.	About 1/25th of an inch (0.039 in.)
kilometer — 1000 meters	Km.	Hardly a medical measure (0.62 mile)

Doctors

Some information relative to medical practice requirements, licenses, additional degrees (and their meaning), and medical ethics may be appropriate here. Most medical colleges require a Bachelor of Science degree for admission. The degree of Doctor of Medicine (M.D.) is earned after completing four years of medical college work, although many colleges withhold the degree until an approved internship has been satisfactorily completed. A license to practice must then be secured from the State Board of Medical Examiners, generally following a three-day examination and the previous submission of evidence of other suitable qualifications.

Most of the specialties maintain their own "Boards," consisting of seven or more members picked from various organizations connected with that specialty. Board members personally examine applicants for a certificate that indicates competence in the specialty. Previous written examinations must have been passed, and most Boards require three years of approved postgraduate training and two years of actual practice in that specialty. The holder of a certificate issued by the Board is allowed to be referred to as a "Board specialist," or as a "Diplomate" of that Board. Board certification is not a requirement for practicing that specialty, and application for certification is purely a voluntary matter.

The American College of Surgeons may also confer a degree, "Fellow of the American College of Surgeons" (F.A.C.S.) on an applicant from a surgical specialty. The applicant is required to have completed a course of postgraduate training equivalent to "Board requirements" and to have submitted fifty detailed, substantiated case reports of varied surgical procedures in which the applicant has been the chief surgeon during the last three years of his practice prior to application. The American College of Surgeons has been very effective in raising and maintaining the standards of both hospital and surgical practice. The American College of Physicians issues a similar fellowship degree (F.A.C.P.) to certain selected applicants who have completed approved postgraduate training and who have exhibited special interest and competence in one of the nonsurgical specialties.

The ethics of medical practice disapprove of large signs, newspaper advertisements, and the mentioning of a doctor's name in newspaper publicity connected with a patient. You may wonder what prevents a doctor from representing himself as a specialist immediately after completing his internship and obtaining a state license. Actually, he could legally do so, but the disapproval of his colleagues would deter him from such conduct.

Paramedical Personnel

It seems proper at this point to say something about the importance of the work of paramedical personnel. The dependence of medicine upon paramedical assistance is not always recognized or admitted. The increasing diversity and ramifications of medical practice, with their increasing numbers of regulatory restrictions, make the employment of trained paramedical help more and more essential. The preposition *para-* means *at the side of*, or *alongside of*, and that is exactly what a paramedical person is to the doctor — a helper at his side — and, preferably, on his side.

An important development in paramedical education is the recently introduced training of "medical associates," "physicians' assistants," and "nurse associates." These paramedical people who generally hold a college degree are trained to do the "minor" work in physicians' offices. The possible saving of a doctor's time by a conscientious, trained helper can be tremendous. The training includes how to take routine histories and make preliminary (but essential) tests and examinations. Paramedical personnel may even diagnose simple illnesses and prescribe from a limited drug list — all under the doctor's supervision and responsibility. The numbers of Allied Health courses presently available in many junior colleges, colleges, and medical schools attest to the importance and need for such advanced paramedical courses.

In the office, nurses, medical secretaries, and an "associate" seem to satisfy the doctor's needs. But the practice of medicine is becoming more and more institutionalized, and a hospital of 250 beds frequently has a work force of 500 persons. The duties of as many as 300 of these individuals are concerned with or related to the care and comfort of patients. In addition to the floor supervisor and the volunteer workers who bring the patient flowers, there are scores of record librarians, x-ray technicians, registered nurses—many with special training—laboratory technicians and assistants, file clerks, dietitians, vocational and practical nurses, orderlies, pharmacists, various kinds of therapists, floor clerks, nurses' aides, supply room personnel, kitchen helpers, electricians, and front-office clerks. All these people are trained in their special duties and are required, and their services are used by the patient and the doctor.

This book salutes all of these loyal and essential people, from the hospital administrator to the night watchman, from the doctor's wife to the patient who wonders what the doctor meant by that long word. The author hopes that this book will make your job a little more interesting. And in your battle with medical words, he promises to stay on your side.

3 Compound Terms and Combination Words

THE LARGE NUMBER of long words in both medical writings and in doctors' conversations is often confusing to persons not accustomed to medical language. Some may think that this is just an affectation on the part of doctors — an attempt to show how learned they are. This is far from the real intent. These long words, frequently combinations or compound terms, really serve a very practical purpose. Actually, they are word-savers; each of them might well be called "medical shorthand for a paragraph."

If you should happen to overhear a group of doctors discussing a medical problem informally, over their coffee, you would also inevitably hear them using these same double-barreled, long-winded compound terms. These long words are used not only because they are mutually understood shortcuts; they also automatically either pinpoint or limit the subject under discussion. They funnel the listener's attention to some precise area, or structure, or condition.

These long combination words generally assume either a definitely limiting or a widening direction. For example, the expression **cerebrovascular accident** immediately narrows and limits the discussion to a disease process — an obstructing or bursting — of a blood vessel supplying the cerebrum (the mental and motor part of the brain). It would take many words of explanation to convey the picture that these three words, linked together, immediately bring to a doctor's mind.

More comprehensive in its scope is a compound term such as **cardiovascular-renal syndrome.** This term refers to the entire symptom-complex brought on by a whole group of connected changes going on in the heart, the blood vessels, and the kidneys of a patient — changes generally related to his high blood pressure. Several long complicated phrases or even sentences would be required to describe to a lay person the picture conveyed to a doctor by these combined words, formidable as they may sound to an untrained ear.

There seem to be no hard and fast rules about the forming of these "compound derivatives," as they are sometimes called, except that they must sound right and must make good sense. Generally enough of the first word is dropped to make a euphonious combination with a definite meaning, and the words are hooked together with an -o. For instance, the joint between a rib and its connected vertebral body is called the **costovertebral joint;** the termination of the ureter in the bladder is called the **ureterovesical junction** – or the **vesicoureteral junction,** if you want to say it differently. Lots of leeway, as you see, but still precise and definite, and exclusive of everything else. Originally these words were hyphenated; lately most of the hyphens have disappeared.

This, then, is the justification for these twelve-cylinder words. The trouble is that sometimes the doctor forgets, in explaining something, that his listeners have not had the same training and background to which he was exposed. Also, the ability to simplify the explanation of something complicated without "talking down" is no small art – a real test of linguistic ability.

So, if you are working for a doctor and you have difficulty comprehending some of his medical conversation, remember that it is up to you to learn to understand the boss's language – not his responsibility to cut his terminology down to two-syllable words for your benefit. And if you are a patient and your doctor lunges off into long, complicated phrases in explaining something to you, don't automatically put him down as pompous. True, he *could* be putting up a smoke-screen to keep you from asking him "just a few simple, direct questions" to which there just aren't simple, direct answers. And, of course, he *might* be giving you a compliment by assuming that you understand. More likely, though, he is just being forgetful, and maybe just a little bit discourteous.

4 Roots and Stems — "Clues"

Dorland's Medical Dictionary, 23rd edition, in the chapter on Etymology (word origins) makes a very significant statement: "At least fifty percent of the general English vocabulary is of Greek and Latin derivation, and it is a conservative estimate that as much as seventy-five percent of the scientific element is of such origin." This is why any discussion of medical terms should emphasize the importance of these so-called *roots* and *stems* from which so many medical words originate.

Etymology — the study of word origins — is an interesting subject to anyone with a healthy amount of intellectual curiosity, and every doctor fortunate enough to have had even a little formal schooling in the classical languages continues to enjoy and appreciate the assistance he derives from some familiarity with Greek and Latin.

There seems to be considerable confusion among writers about what is a root and what makes a stem, although in nature roots and stems are most certainly not synonyms. Some authors even admit their indecision by using the term *root stems*. To simplify things, we are going to put all of them into one general word-basket and simply call them *clues*, because that is how we are going to use them.

About one-fourth of all medical words are combinations of one or more modifying syllables attached to an original *clue* element (as we said we would call it). The (*root*) clue generally establishes the "subject matter" of the word. It may not always be easy to isolate or identify because it may be surrounded by modifying *prefixes* and *suffixes*. Because these additional *prefix* and *suffix* clues are just as helpful in understanding the word as the *root* clues are, we are temporarily going to drop them into the same basket with the root clues — and explain them further in the next chapter.

The root clue usually localizes the word for you. Actually, it tells whether we are talking about the man's joints (ARTH, ARTHritis), or his heart (CARD, endoCARDitis), or whether he hurts (ALG, neur-ALGia). In analyzing a word, the root clue is generally your starting point. Here is a list of frequently used *root clues* and the hints they give you. Example words are further defined elsewhere in the text (see *INDEX*).

CLUE	HINT	EXAMPLES
ADEN	gland	adenoids, adenoma
ALG	pain	neuralgia, analgesia
ARTH	joint	arthritis, arthrodesis
BIO	life	biology, antibiotic
CALC	stone	calculus, calcification
CARD	heart	cardiac, electrocardiogram
CEPH	head	cephalic, encephalitis
CHOL	bile	cholecystitis, cholelithiasis
CHONDR	cartilage	osteochondrosis, chondrosarcoma
CIS	cut	incision, excise
CORT	bark, shell	cortex, cortisone
CORP	body	corpse, corpuscle
CUT	skin	cuticle, subcutaneous
CYST	bladder, hollow	cystocele, cholecystectomy
CYTE	cell	lymphocyte, cytology
DERM	skin	epidermis, dermatology
DORS	back	dorsal, dorsiflexion
DYS	pain, difficulty	dyspnea, dysentery
GEN	origin	pathogen, genes
GLYC	sweet	glycogen, glycosuria
GRAM, GRAPH	record, write	radiogram, urography
GYNE	woman	gynecology, gynecomastia
HEM	blood	anemia, hemoglobin
HYDR	water	hydrophobia, dehydration
LEUC, LEUK	white	leucocyte, leukemia
LITH	stone	lithotripsy, pyelolithotomy
LUMB	loin	lumbago, lumbar
MAL	bad	malnutrition, malignancy
MEG	great, large	acromegaly, megalocyte
MENS	month	menstruation, menopause
METR	measure	millimeter, optometry
MICR	small	microscope, microbe
MYO	muscle	myocardium, myositis
NEPH	kidney	nephritis, nephrogram
NEUR	nerve	neurology, neuritis
NOCT	night	nocturia, nocturnal
OPH, OP	eye	ophthalmoscope, optic
ORCH	testicle	orchitis, orchidectomy
OS	bone	ossification, periosteum
OT	ear	otitis, otosclerosis

PAR	bear or give birth	primipara, postpartum
PATH	sick, bad	psychopath, pathological
PEND	hang down	appendix, pendulous
PHLEB	vein	**phlebitis, phlebolith**
PHON	sound, voice	aphonia, phonetics
PHOT	light	photodermatitis, photosensitive
PNEUM	air	pneumonia, pneumothorax
PSYCH	mind	psychology, psychosis
PULM	lung	pulmotor, pulmonary
SALP	tube	salpingitis, salpingectomy
SCLER	hard	arteriosclerosis, sclerotic
SCOP	look at, observe	otoscope, cystoscopy
SECT	cut	resection, dissection
STOM	mouth, opening	anastomosis, stomatitis
THERM	heat	diathermy, thermometer
THROMB	clot	thrombosis, thrombophlebitis
TOME	cut	appendectomy, microtome
TOX	poison	toxemia, antitoxin
UR	urine	urology, pyuria
VAS	vessel, duct	vasectomy, vascular
VERS	turn	eversion, inverted
VIT	life	vital, vitamin

5 Prefixes, Suffixes, Combining Forms and Such — More "Clues"

IF YOU ARE going to enjoy your contact with medical words, you need to understand something about their formation.

Many medical words start out with a *prefix*. This generally consists of one or two syllables, usually of Latin or Greek origin, placed *ahead* of the *root* of the word in order to modify its meaning. The *prefix* usually indicates location, direction, time, or some other limiting condition, and so it gives you another very helpful *clue*.

If you have never studied Latin, you may find that memorizing the *prefixes* you don't already know is a little difficult, but the private satisfaction you will get from recognizing them and using them will make the effort very rewarding. Incidentally, they will also give you clues that will help you to understand many nonmedical words. Here are some of the common *prefix clues* and the hints they give.

CLUE	HINT	EXAMPLES
A, AN	no, not, without	atony, asthenic, anesthesia
AB	away from	abduct, abnormal
AD	toward, near	adduct, adrenal
ANTE	in front of (position)	antecubital, anterior
	before (time)	antefebrile, antepartum
ANTI	against	antidote, antiseptic
BI	two, double	biceps, bicornuate
CIRCUM	around	circumoral, circumcision
CO, COM, CON	with, together	coagulate, compression, consultation
CONTRA	against	contraception, contraindication
DIA	through	diapedesis, diathermy
DYS	difficult	dysfunction, dyspnea, dysmenorrhea
EC, EX	out of, out from	ectopia, exudate
END	within	endocarditis, endometrium

EPI	on, upon, over	epidermis, epiglottis, epicranium
EXTRA	outside of, beyond	extradural, extrasensory
HEMI, SEMI	half	hemiplegia, semicircular
HYPER	above normal	hyperthyroidism, hypertension
HYPO	below (position)	hypoglossal, hypodermic
	below normal	hypoglycemia, hypothyroid
INTER	between	intercostal, intervertebral
INTRA	within	intradermal, intravenous
NEO	new	neonatal, neoplasm
PARA	beside, near	parathyroid, paranasal
PER	through	perception, perforate
PERI	around	pericarditis, periosteum
POLY	many	polyarthritis, polycystic
POST	behind (position)	postnasal, postauricular
	after (time)	postmortem, postpartum
PRE	in front of (position)	prepyloric, prepatellar
	before (time)	prenatal, precancerous
RETRO	behind (position)	retrocecal, retrorectal
	backward	retrograde
SUB	below, beneath	subdural, subphrenic, sublingual
SUPER, SUPRA	above (position)	suprapubic
	beyond	supernumerary
TRANS	across, by way of	transfusion, transurethral
TRI	three	tricuspid, trimester

And then there are *suffixes*. A *suffix* is a syllable attached to the end of a word. Medical language has many words to which extra syllables have been added *after* the *root* to confer a particular meaning on that word. Suffixes perform the same function that *prefixes*, attached *ahead* of the *root*, perform: they give the root some altered meaning.

Although most of the *prefixes* are merely modifying prepositions or adverbs, many of the *suffixes* aren't that simple. They may be combinations of nouns or adjectives, added on to the root to convey some special meaning. These special combining suffixes are sometimes called *combining forms*, but they still function in the same way. Usually they attach to the root—or to each other—with the help of an -o-, although occasionally the connector is some other vowel. Enough of the preceding syllable is dropped to make the word easy to pronounce. Learn to spot suffixes as *clues*; they may indicate a condition, or a symptom, or a diagnosis, or even some sort of surgical operation. They are very informative.

Some of those *suffixes* and hints they give appear on the following page.

It is really not such a frightening list, and it certainly is a very useful and helpful one. Read it over again to give yourself some confidence: ITIS indicates inflammation; an ECTOMY removes something, by surgery; a GRAPHY records something, by some means or another; a

PEXY fixes something in position surgically; a PLASTY reshapes something; an OLOGY concentrates on some subject; and so forth.

CLUE	HINT	EXAMPLES
o-CELE	hollow protrusion	cystocele, hydrocele
EMIA	blood	hyperemia, leukemia
ECTOMY	remove (surgically) cut out	appendectomy, tonsillectomy hysterectomy
o-GENIC	origin	neurogenic, psychogenic
IASIS, ISM	condition	elephantiasis, prostatism
ITIS	inflammation, infection	arthritis, myositis, pharyngitis
OID	like, similar to	rheumatoid, dermoid
o-RRHAPHY	refashion and stabilize	herniorrhaphy, perineorrhaphy
o-SCOPY	look inside of (through a "scope")	cystoscopy, bronchoscopy endoscope
o-STOMY	cut into, leaving a "STOMA" (mouth) or opening	colostomy, tracheostomy
o-PATHY	diseased condition	adenopathy, arthropathy
o-PEXY	secure (surgically)	nephropexy, orchiopexy
o-PLASTY	reshape (surgically)	rhinoplasty, thoracoplasty
o-PTOSIS	dropping down	blepharoptosis, nephroptosis
OMA	tumor, swelling	sarcoma, osteoma
SPASM	involuntary contraction	bronchospasm, pylorospasm
OSIS	condition	lymphocytosis, nephrosis
o-LOGY	study or science of	radiology, pathology
o-GRAM	record of	urogram, electrocardiogram
o-GRAPH	the means used in making the record	radiography, electrocardiography
o-TOMY	cut into	cystotomy, craniotomy
URIA	pertaining to urine	polyuria, hematuria
THERAPY	treatment	physiotherapy, heliotherapy

II GENERAL TERMS

⑥ Nonspecific Medical and Surgical Terms

IN THIS BOOK medical terms have arbitrarily been divided into two groups which we shall call *nonspecific* and *specific*. The rationale for this unorthodox classification can be briefly explained as follows:

Under the classification *nonspecific* are grouped the terms which seem to refer to the whole general field of medicine. Some typical examples are words such as **antisepsis** (prevention of infection), **asthenia** (weakness), and **fever.** These are big, wide, inclusive words which cover a lot of medical territory.

At the other extreme are the *specific* words. These are words limited to one of the narrow fields of specialist practice. Some typical examples of *specific* words are **retina** (a part of the eye) or **pyelitis** (inflammation of a specific part of a kidney). Such words appear only in the list of terms related to the appropriate specialty.

So far, so good. But now we begin to run into exceptions to the simple *nonspecific* and *specific* classifications. Between these two obvious extremes is a group of words which seem to fit both classifications. Many terms which by definition refer to *nonspecific* medical subjects could also be included in the vocabulary of more than one of the limited medical specialties. For example, an **abscess** might be treated by a gynecologist, a proctologist, a surgeon or a urologist—to mention a few of the possibilities. It would certainly seem unnecessary to repeat *abscess* in each of these *specific* lists. Similarly, **fistula** denotes a condition we might encounter in general surgery, proctology, urology, or thoracic surgery. So there is obviously a problem. The purpose and limited scope of this book would seem to be best served by including these words in the *nonspecific* list. This seems to be the least confusing way of handling them, and accordingly the following list includes also these "related" terms.

We have casually disposed of one trouble maker but there are still two situations in which repetition is unavoidable. Certain *nonspecific* terms are so inextricably connected with a specific field of practice that it seems illogical to omit them from that specific list. For instance, one can hardly think of *orthopedic surgery* without including **fracture,** no matter how nonspecific the term *fracture* may have become. Words of this type will necessarily appear more than once.

A multiple listing of a term is also required when the same term has acquired a different meaning or connotation in different branches of medicine. For instance, **auricle** may refer to the external ear or to a part of the heart; **myelitis** implies inflammation of the spinal cord to neurologists, and a disorder of the bone marrow to orthopedists; **fundus** may indicate to different specialists the body of the uterus, the top of the bladder, a portion of the stomach, or a part of the eye!

CONSULTANTS

Frank W. Norman, M.D.
Former President, California Academy of General Practice
Santa Rosa, California

Harding Clegg, M. D.
Santa Rosa, California

abrasion (a-brā′zhun). A scraping off of tissue; also, the scraped skin surface.

abscess (ab′ses). A localized collection of pus.

abuse. *See* **addiction.**

acetanilid (as-e-tan′il-id). A commonly-used drug similar to aspirin. It relieves pain and lowers temperature.

acidosis (as-id-ō′sis). An acid-base imbalance in the body (acids predominating over bases). *See* **alkalosis.**

acute (a-kyūt′). *adj.* The term generally refers to disease or pain which is characterized by sudden onset, and a relatively short, severe course. (Opposite of **chronic.**)

addict (ad′dikt). A person who is under the control of an **addiction.**

addiction (ad-dik′shun). An uncontrollable habit, or a dependence on the use of certain substances. "Habituation" is sometimes used as a synonym for "addiction."

adenitis (ad-en-ī′tis). ADEN=gland; ITIS=inflammation. Inflammation of, or in, a **lymphatic** gland.

adenopathy (ad-en-op′a-thē). A general term indicating any disease of the **lymphatic** glands; however, gland enlargement is generally implied.

adhesion (ad-hē′zhun). An abnormal sticking together of tissues; also, the result of their sticking together.

adiposity (ad-i-pos′i-tē.) ADIP=fat. An abnormal, general deposition of fat throughout the body tissues (**obesity**).

adventitious (ad-ven-tish′us). *adj.* Growing unnaturally, or situated in an abnormal position.

Aesculapius (es-kūl-ā′pē-us). The mythical Roman god of healing. (*adj.* – aescula′pian.)

agglutination (ag-glū′tin-ā-shun). A clumping or sticking together, generally referring to blood cells or bacteria.

alcoholism (al′kō-hall-izm). A physiologic state or a chronic behavioral disorder referring to an abnormal craving for, or an inability to tolerate, alcohol.

alkaline (al′ka-lin). *adj.* Referring to a chemical substance, or condition, which is basic in type. (Opposite of acid.)

alkaloid (al′ka-loyd). One of a large group of basic substances found in plants. Is the case of plants used medicinally, the alkaloid generally forms the active principle of the drug. Alkaloids are generally bitter, and their names frequently end in – ine, as atropine, caffeine, and strychnine.

allergy (al′er-jē). The condition of being hypersensitive to something. (*adj.* – aller′gic.)

ameba — amoeba (a-mē′ba). A one-celled animal that can cause disease. (*adj.*, – ame′bic.)

amnesia (am-nēz′ē-a *or* –zha). The temporary or permanent loss of memory. (*adj.* – amnes′ic.)

amorphous (ā-morf′us). *adj.* Having no consistent shape or form.

ampule (am′pyūl). A small glass container generally containing sterile solutions.

analgesia (an-al-jēz′ē-a *or* –zha). AIG= pain. The absence or loss of the normal sense of pain.

analgesic (an-al-jēz′ik). A drug given to alleviate or control pain. The term is also used as an adjective.

analogue (an′a-log). An organ similar to another in function but differing in structure and evolutionary origin; for example, the lungs of man and the gills of fish. (*adj.* – anal′ogous.)

anaphylaxis (an-a-fil-aks′is). An exaggerated or unusual reaction to a drug or agent, generally related to pre-vious contact with it.

anemia (a-nēm'ē-a). A deficiency in the quality or quantity of blood. (*adj.* — anem'ic).

anesthesia (an-es-thēz'ē-a *or* — zha). ESTHE=feeling. The absence or loss of sensation or feeling. (*adj.* — anesthet'ic.)

angina (an-jīn'a *or* an'ji-na). A severe chest pain, generally referring to that caused by cardiovascular spasm or occlusion.

annular — **anular** (an'yūl-ar). *adj.* Ring-shaped, referring particularly to a skin lesion.

anodyne (an'ō-dīn). An old name for a drug or medicine which relieves pain. The term is also used as an adjective.

anomaly (a-nom'a-lē). An abnormal structure or condition, generally congenital. (*adj.* — anom'alous.)

anorexia (an-or-reks'ē-a). A lack or loss of appetite for food.

antefebrile (an-tē-fēb'rīl). *adj.* Referring to the interval of time between the first symptoms of a disease and the beginning of the febrile (**fever**) stage.

antemortem (ant-ē-mort'em). *adj.* Be-fore death.

antibiotic (an-te-bī-ot'ik). BIO=life. A chemical substance produced by molds or bacteria, which destroys or suppresses the growth of other **bacteria**. Antibiotics are used largely in the treatment of infectious diseases. (Also used as an adjective.)

antidote (an'ti-dōt). A remedy for coun-teracting a particular poison or a group of poisons.

antigen (an'ti-jen). A substance which stimulates a specific resistance re-sponse and promotes antibody for-mation. (*adj.* — antigen'ic.)

antisepsis (an-ti-sep'sis). SEP=decay. The prevention of infection. (*adj.* — antisep'tic.)

antiseptic (an-ti-sep'tik). An agent used in the prevention or treatment of infection. (Also used as an adjective.)

antispasmodic (an-tē-spaz-mod'ik). An agent which relieves spasm. (Also used as an adjective.)

antitoxin (an-ti-toks'in). A counteract-ing substance produced in the blood stream of animals that have been in-jected with the **toxins** (poisons) of certain bacteria. Injection of this antitoxin into a person suffering from the same infection gives him in-creased resistance.

antivivisection (an-tē-viv-i-sek'shun). Opposition to animal experimenta-tion, particularly operating on live animals.

aphrodisiac (af-rō-diz'ē-ak). Any drug that arouses sexual impulses.

aplasia (a-plāz'ē-a *or* a-plā'zha). The congenital absence or underdevelop-ment of a part or organ of the body. (*adj.* — aplas'tic.)

apoplexy (ap'ō-pleks-ē). A condition caused by the bursting or blocking of a blood vessel leading to the brain (a "stroke" or a "C.V.A.").

aqua (ak'wa). Latin for water. (*See aq. dest.* in Medical Abbreviations.)

aqueous (ā'kwē-us). *adj.* Pertaining to or consisting of water; watery.

arteriosclerosis (ar-tē-rē-ō-skler-ō'sis). SCLER=hard. The hardening, thick-ening, or loss of elasticity of the wall of an artery. (*adj.* — arteriosclerot'ic.)

arthritis (arth-rīt'is). ARTH=joint. Inflammation of or in a joint. (*adj.* — arthrit'ic.)

asepsis (ā-sep'sis). The absence of infection. (*adj.* — asep'tic.)

asphyxia (as-fiks'ē-a). Suffocation; death from lack of oxygen.

asthenia (as-sthēn'ē-a). STHEN= strength. A lack of strength; weak-ness.

atopic (ā-top'ik). *adj.* Out of its normal or ordinary position.

atrophy (at'rō-fē). The wasting away of a previously normal part or entire organ. (*adj.* — atroph'ic.)

attenuate (at-ten'yū-āt). To weaken or to thin, particularly to make less virulent as in the case of disease-causing bacteria.

atypical (ā-tip′ē-kl). *adj.* Different from its usual character or form.

autoclave (aw′-tō-klāv). A piece of equipment for sterilizing surgical supplies or instruments; also a verb, to sterilize by means of steam under pressure.

autogenous (au-toj′jen-us). *adj.* Produced or originating within the patient's own body.

azygous (az′i-gus). *adj.* Unpaired; having no corresponding part on the opposite side of the body.

bacteria (bak-tēr′ē-a). *plural.* In common usage, a general term which includes the organisms causing disease, exclusive of **viruses.**

benign (bē-nīn′). *adj.* A general term referring to some tumors, indicating their nonmalignant and essentially harmless nature. (Opposite of **malignant.)**

bilateral (bī-lat′er-al). BI=two; LAT= side. *adj.* Two-sided, or relating to both sides of the body.

bilocular (bī-lok′yūl-ar). *adj.* Having two compartments, as a bilocular **cyst.**

biopsy (bī′ op-sē). The surgical removal of a small portion of tissue for examination and diagnosis. (Also used as a verb; and as a noun, meaning the tissue removed.)

boric acid (bōr′ik). An antiseptic powder generally used in solution.

Bright's disease. A common name for noninflammatory, degenerative **nephritis.**

"B.U.N." Abbreviation for the blood urea-nitrogen level (a measure of the amount of nitrogenous waste material in the blood stream).

bursitis (burs-īt′is). An inflamed condition of a **bursa.**

"C.A." (sē-ā). Medical lingo for **cancer.**

cachexia (ka-kek′sē-a). The condition of wasting away, generally associated with malnutrition.

cadaver (ka-dav′er). A dead human body, particularly one prepared for dissection purposes.

caduceus (ka-dūs′ē-us). The emblem of the medical profession (two serpents coiled around a staff).

calorie — calory (kal′o-rē). Although technically meaning the amount of heat required to produce a specific chemical result, in common usage the term refers to a measurement of the heat energy generated by a stated amount of food when digested and **oxidized** in the body.

cancer (kan′ser). A general term covering any **malignant** cellular tumor.

canula — cannula (kan′yūl-a). A small hollow tube which is introduced into a body cavity for carrying out certain treatments or to accomplish a specific result such as introducing medicine or withdrawing fluid.

capsule (kap′sul). A gelatin covering for a dose of medicine; also the **fibrous** covering of a joint, or of certain organs or structures.

carbon dioxide (dī-oks′īd). A gaseous waste produced in the tissues by normal life processes. It is expelled into the blood by the capillaries and carried to the lungs where it is eliminated from the body by means of expired air.

carcinogenic (kar-sin-ō-jen′ik). *adj.* GEN=origin. Capable of, or conducive to, the production of **cancer.**

case. A medical term referring to a specific incidence of disease, as a case of pneumonia. It does **not** refer to the patient, but to the disease with which he is afflicted.

casein (kā′sēn). A protein found in milk.

catgut. Absorbable cord used for **ligating** (tying) blood vessels or suturing tissues. (It is actually produced from sheep intestines, not from cats.)

catheter (kath′e-ter). A flexible hollow surgical instrument used for withdrawing liquids from, or introducing liquids into, a hollow space in the body.

catheterization (kath-e-ter-i-zā′shun). The inserting of a **catheter.**

cautery (kaw′ter-ē). An agent used for searing or burning tissue by means of heat, electric current, or corrosive chemicals.

cavity (kav′i-tē). A hollow or a space, especially one within an organ or within the body. Most body cavities are in reality only *potential* open spaces.

"CBC" Medical jargon for a "complete blood count." A complete blood count consists of a hemoglobin and hematocrit determination, a red cell count, a white cell count, and a differential count of the white cells.

centigrade scale (sent′i-grād). One of the scales used for the measuring temperature.

chemotherapy (kēm-ō-ther′a-pē). A general term for the treatment or prevention of disease by the use of chemical compounds.

chiropractic (kīr-ō-prak′tik). A non-medical system of treatment based on the theory that disease is caused by abnormal functioning of the nervous system, particularly centered in those nerves emanating from the spinal column. The theory states that this abnormal functioning is, for the most part, due to pressures exerted on the spinal nerves by derangements of the spinal column. Treatment is, therefore, manipulative, concentrating on the spinal column and the spinal ligaments, and is aimed at relieving these pressures and thus reestablishing normal conditions and normal function. Chiropractors are generally prohibited from prescribing drugs.

chronic (kron′ik). *adj.* Referring to a disease condition of slow onset and of long duration. (Opposite of **acute.**)

cicatrix (sik′a′triks). An erudite name for a scar. (*plural* – cicat′rices.)

clinic (klin′ik). An institution or establishment in which patients, generally ambulatory, are studied by medical students under supervision, or by a group of physicians practicing together.

clinical (klin′i-kl). *adj.* Referring to the actual bedside symptoms, the observed findings, or the course of a disease, as opposed to conditions theoretically accompanying it.

clinician (klin-ish′un). A practicing physician, as distinguished from one whose work does not include the actual care of patients.

clysis (klī′sis). The giving of fluids by other routes than by mouth. Generally the fluid is given for therapeutic purposes. The term is also used to indicate the solution administered

colic (kol′ik). Pain occurring in spasms.

coma (kōm′a). A state of insensibility or deep stupor. (*adj.* – com′atose.)

compensatory (kom-pens′a′tō-re). *adj.* Referring to the making up for the lack of function of another part, particularly a fellow part or an opposite part.

congenital (kon-jen′i-tal). *adj.* Referring to conditions or states existing at birth, particularly those which are abnormal.

congestion (kon-jest′chun). Local excessive accumulation of blood or body fluid in tissues.

contagious (kon-tāj′us). *adj.* A term referring to an infectious disease which can be communicated from one person to another.

contraceptive (kon-tra-sep′tiv). CONTRA=against. A means used to prevent conception or to accomplish "birth control." (Also used as an adjective.)

contraindication (kon-tra-in-di-kā′-shun). A (subjective) symptom, an (objective) sign or finding, or a circumstance which makes a contemplated patient-procedure inadvisable.

contralateral (kon-tra-lat′er-al). *adj.* On the opposite side, generally referring to a similar structure on the opposite side of the body.

contusion (kon-tūzh′un). A bruise.

convalescence (kon-val-es′sens). The period of recovery from an illness or an accident. (*adj.* — convales′cent.)

convalescent (kon-val-es′sent). A patient in the recovery stage.

convulsion (kon-vul′shun). A series of violent, uncontrollable, muscle contractions.

"coronary" (kor′ō-nair-ē). COR=heart. A common name for a "heart attack," generally referring to the partial or complete blocking of a coronary artery.

corpse (korps). A dead human body.

corpus (kor′pus). The main part of any organ. (*plural* — cor′pora.)

cryptogenic   (krip-to-jen′ik) — *adj.* CRYPT=hidden. GEN=origin. Of obscure or doubtful origin.

curettage (kyūr-et-tazh′). The surgical scraping of the lining of a cavity with a **curet.**

"C.V.A." Medical lingo for a **cerebrovascular accident** (a "stroke").

cyanosis (sī-an-ō′sis). Bluish discoloration of the skin or of the **mucous membranes** due to a lack of oxygen in the blood.

cyst (sist). A hollow, sac-like tumor, generally containing fluid of some sort. Cysts are usually **benign.**

cytology (sī-tol′ō-jē). The study of cells, particularly for the purpose of detecting cancer cells.

debility (dē-bil′i-tē). Weakness or loss of strength.

decongestant   (dē-kon-jes′tant).   An agent that reduces congestion.

degeneration (dē-jen-er-ā′shun). Deterioration or retrogressive change in cells or tissue, generally resulting in progressive loss of function. (*adj.* — degen′erative.)

dehydration (dē-hī-drā′shun). HYDR= water. The loss or elimination of water from body tissues.

Demerol (Dem′er-ol). A proprietary brand of meperidine hydrochloride commonly used for its analgesic, antispasmodic, and hypnotic effects. It may be habit-forming.

dentition (den-tish′un). A term referring to the natural teeth, particularly to their eruption and development.

depilatory (dē-pil′a-to-rē). PIL=hair. An agent used for the removal of hairs. (Also used as an adjective.)

dextrose (deks′trōs). A name given to d-glucose, the most important of the sugars found in the body. It is used extensively as a nutrient because of its easy assimilation. Abnormally high concentrations in the urine and in the blood indicate diabetes.

diabetic (dī-a-bet′ik). A person afflicted with diabetes. (Also used as an adjective.)

diagnosis (dī-ag-nō′sis). GNOS=know. The identification of the nature of a disease ("What's the matter with me, Doc?"). (*adj.* — diagnos′tic; *verb* — diagnose.)

diagnostician   (dī-ag-nos-tish′un).   A term frequently applied to a specialist in internal medicine who is an expert in diagnosing diseases.

diaphoresis (dī-a-for-ē′sis). Perspiration, especially profuse perspiration.

diarrhea (dī-ar-rē′a). Frequent (generally watery) fecal discharges.

diastolic blood pressure (dī-a-stol′ik). The pressure maintained in the arteries even while the heart is at rest (two-thirds of the total time occupied by a **cardiac cycle**).

dietetics (dī-et-tet′iks). The science and study of proper diet.

dilatation (dil-a-tā′shun). A stretched (or **dilated**) state of an organ.

dilation (dīl-ā′shun). The stretching or opening of a narrowed tube, channel, or hollow organ. (*verb* — dilate.)

diluent (dil′yū-ent). An agent used for thinning or diluting medication.

diphtheria (dif-thēr′ē-a). An acute, communicable, infectious disease, generally affecting the throat (now rarely seen).

discrete (dis-krēt′). *adj.* Well separated, distinct, not running together.

disease (diz-ēz′). An illness or an abnormal state having a definite pattern of symptoms.

disinfectant (dis-in-fek'tant). An agent used to destroy disease-causing bacteria. (Also used as an adjective.)

dissection (dis-sek'shun). The process of separating tissues along their natural lines of separation from each other.

diuresis (di-yūr-ē'sis). Increased output of urine, particularly caused by the use of medication. (*adj.,* – diuret'ic).

diuretic (dī-yūr-et'ik). A drug used to induce **diuresis.**

diurnal (dī-urn'al). *adj.* Relating to something which occurs during the daytime.

donor. One who donates his blood for transfusion.

dormant (dor'mant). *adj.* Inactive; in medicine it usually refers to the course of a disease.

dose (dōs). The proper amount of medication to be taken in a single administration.

Dramamine (Dram'a-mēn). A proprietary drug used to combat nausea and various forms of motion sickness.

dropsy. An old name for the accumulation of serous fluid in tissues and body cavities. (*adj.,* – drop'sical) *See* **ascites, edema, effusion.**

dysentery (dis'en-tair-ē). An acute **diarrhea** in which blood or **mucus,** or both, appear in the fecal discharge.

dysfunction (dis-funk'shun). Impaired or improper function of an organ.

dyspnea (disp'nē-a *or* disp-nē'a). Difficulty in breathing.

ecchymosis (ek-i-mō'sis). A **hemorrhagic** discoloration in or beneath the skin, generally caused by bruising ("black and blue"). (*adj.,* – ecchymot'ic; *plural* – ecchymo'ses.)

ectopia (ek-tōp'ē-a). The condition of being out of, or away from, the normal location. (*adj.,* – ectop'ic.)

eczema (eks'e-ma). A skin disease frequently due to an **allergy** or to hypersensitivity.

edema (e-dēm'a). Excessive accumulation of **serous** fluid in the body tissues. (*adj.* – edem'atous.) *See* **dropsy.**

effusion (ef-fyū'zhun). An abnormal escape or excretion of fluid; also, free fluid within a joint or a cavity.

electrolyte (ē-lek'trō-līt). Any compound which, in solution in the body, is capable of conducting an electric current.

electrolyte balance. The relative proportion in which various vital body electrolytes are present in the blood.

emaciation (ē-mās-ē-ā'shun). A wasting away of body tissues.

emesis (em'e-sis). The act of vomiting.

emetic (e-met'ik). Something given or taken to induce vomiting.

enema (en'e-ma). Liquid introduced into the rectum for laxative or medicinal purposes.

epidemic (ep-i-dem'ik). The presence of an infectious disease which simultaneously attacks large numbers of people in the same geographic area.

etiology (ē-ti-ol'ō-jē). The study of the causes of a disease, or of an abnormal condition. (*adj.* – etiolog'ic.)

expectorant (eks-pek'tor-ant). A drug which aids in thinning bronchial secretions.

expiration (eks-spir-ā'shun). The breathing out of air from the lungs; also, the act of dying.

exudate (eks'yū-dāt). Fluid thrown out by body tissues in the presence of irritation, damage, or inflammation.

familial (fam-il'ē-al). *adj.* Involving or common to other members of the same family.

fertile (fer'til). *adj.* Capable of producing offspring.

fever. Body temperature above the normal level. (*adj.* – feb'rile *or* fev'erish.)

findings. The objective, discernible features present at a stated time in the course of a disease, such as a dry, coated tongue, or a fast, bounding pulse. *See* **symptom.**

flaccid (flak'sid). *adj.* Relaxed, opposed to contracted or tense.

flatulence (flat'yūl-ens). A distending collection of air or gas in the gastrointestinal tract. (*adj.* – flat'ulent.)

flatus (flāt'us). Gas or air in the stomach or intestines.

fracture (frak'tchur). A sudden breaking, particularly of a bone. (Also used as a verb.) (Fig. 15, p. 138)

functional. *adj.* In medicine, this term generally refers to some unusual finding associated with the function of an organ rather than with an anatomical or structural defect. For this reason, the word has acquired a connotation of relative insignificance.

fungus (fung'gus). A primitive form of plant life which may cause infection in humans.

gangrene (gang-grēn'). Death of tissue, particularly from lack of blood supply, with or without infection. (*adj.* — gang'renous.)

generic (jen-er'ik). *adj.* In medicine, a term applied to pharmaceutical names which (generally) describe or indicate the composition of the medicine or drug. Generic names are not capitalized. *See* **proprietary.**

genus (jēn'us). Biologically, a division ranking below the family and next above the species. In descending rank are family, genus, species, and class.

geriatrics (jer-ē-at'riks). The study and treatment of problems related to old age.

germicide (jerm'i-sīd). A general term for an externally-applied agent which kills bacteria.

germs. *plural.* An old name for **bacteria.**

giantism (jī'ant-izm) — gigantism (jī-gant'izm). Excessive size of the body or of any of its parts.

granulation tissue (gran-yūl-ā'shun). The new, soft, whitish tissue generally seen in the healing of an open wound ("proud flesh").

gurney (gur'nē). The clumsy, four-wheeled, undignified, hospital conveyance on which patients or linen and other gear are transported up and down the corridors.

habitus (hab'i-tus). Appearance or physique suggesting a predisposition toward a particular condition or disease.

halitosis (hal-i-tō'sis). Bad breath.

hemiplegia (hem-i-plēj'ē-a *or* –plē'ja). HEMI=half; PLEG=paralysis. Paralysis of one side of the body. (*adj.* — hemipleg'ic.)

hemiplegic (hem-i-plēj'ik). A person afflicted with **hemiplegia.**

hemorrhage (hem'or-rāj). Extensive bleeding from a blood vessel. (Also used as a verb.)

hernia (her'nē-a). The abnormal protrusion of part of an organ through a weakened muscle or through a dilated opening.

heroin (hair'ō-in). A habit-forming analgesic and sedative drug related to morphine.

Hippocrates (Hip-pok'ra-tēz). A Greek physician who is called the father of medicine. (*adj.* — hippocrat'ic.)

hirsutism (hir'sūt-izm). Abnormal hairiness. (*adj.* — hir'sute.)

homogeneous (hōm-ō-jēn'ēus). *adj.* HOM=common, same. Of uniform composition throughout.

homologue (hom'ō-log). A part or a structure having the same location, structure, and evolutionary origin as a corresponding part; for example, a bird's wing and a man's arm. (*adj.* — homol'ogous.) *See* **analogue.**

hydrophobia (hī-drō-fōb'ē-a). **Rabies.**

hygiene (hī'jēn). The science and study of health and of its standards.

hyperpyrexia (hī-per-pī-reks'ē-a). PYR= fire. Excessively high body temperature, especially one artificially produced.

hypertension (hī-per-ten'shun). Abnormally high blood pressure. (*adj.* — hyperten'sive.)

"hypo". Medical jargon for a syringe used for injecting fluid medication beneath the skin; also, the material injected.

hypochondriac (hī-pō-kond'rē-ak). A person who shows undue anxiety about his health, and who is constantly worried by unusual body sensations.

hypodermic (hī-pō-derm'ik). *adj.* Referring to a position beneath the skin. *See* "hypo".

intensive care unit. A section of the hospital where acutely ill, medical or post-surgical patients are concentrated and given intensive treatment. (*Abbr.* – I.C.U.)

idiopathic (id-ē-ō-path'ik). *adj.* Without known cause.

idiosyncrasy (id-ē-ō-sin'kra-sē). A state or condition peculiar to an individual, which causes him to react to a stimulus in other than the usual manner.

impaction (im-pak'shun). A solidly packed mass, generally referring to feces in the rectum, or to a **fracture** in which the broken bone ends are driven into each other.

imperforate (im-per'for-āt). *adj.* Lacking a normally-present opening, usually referring to a congenital anal condition.

incarcerated (in-kar'ser-āt-ed). *adj.* Unnaturally retained or confined in one position, generally referring to a **hernia.**

incision (in-sizh'un). CIS=cut. A cut, particularly one made for surgical purposes.

incontinence (in-kont'i-nens). Inability to control involuntary evacuation of urine or feces. (*adj.* – incont'inent.)

indication (ind-i-kā'shun). A subjective symptom, objective sign or finding, or a circumstance which makes a contemplated patient-procedure advisable.

indigestion. An undefinite, unscientific term referring to the lack or failure of one or more of the early digestive processes. It may indicate serious disease or be due to emotional factors.

indurated (in'dūr-āt-ed). *adj.* DUR= hard. Hardened, in a specific way, such as soft tissues becoming firm, but not as hard as bone.

induration (in-dūr-ā'shun). The condition or process of abnormal hardening of tissue.

infection. The invasion of the body by bacteria; also, the condition resulting from it. (*adj.* – infec'tious.)

infiltration (in-fil-trā'shun). A firmness sometimes produced in tissue by trauma, or by the presence of a foreign substance or growth; also the process of filling tissue with fluid introduced under pressure.

inflammation. Redness and swelling of a body part generally related to or resulting from **infection.**

influenza (in-flū-en'za). A common, vaguely-defined, infection or illness, formerly called *"grippe"* and now commonly referred to as *"flu."*

infusion (in-fyū'zhun). The therapeutic introduction of fluid into the body by gravity flow; also, the material introduced.

inhalation (in-hal-ā'shun). The act of drawing gaseous or other materials into the lungs by sucking. It differs slightly from **inspiration** which is automatic inhalation.

injection. The forcible introduction of a solution into the body with a syringe; also the material injected. *See also* "Ophthalmology" chapter.

"in situ" (in sī'tū). A phrase meaning "in its present location" or "in its original location."

insomnia (in-som'nē-a). The habitual inability to sleep.

instillation (in-stil-lā'shun). The introduction of a liquid into a cavity, usually by drops. *See also* "Ophthalmology" chapter.

insufflation (in-suf-flā'shun). The introduction of powder or gas into a cavity by blowing.

interaction. In medicine, the enhanced or diminished drug effect produced by the simultaneous administration of two or more drugs.

intercurrent disease (in-ter-kur'rent). One that breaks into and modifies the course of an already-present disease.

intradermal (in-tra-derm′al). *adj*. IN-TRA=into, within. Within or into the skin.

intraluminal (in-tra-lūm′in-al). *adj*. Within or into the cavity or interior of any tubular body structure.

intramedullary (in-tra-med′yūl-air-ē). *adj*. Within or into the marrow of a bone.

intramuscular (in-tra-mus′kyūl-ar). *adj*. Within or into a muscle. (*Abbr.*—I.M.)

intravenous (in-tra-vēn′us). *adj*. Within or into a vein. (*Abbr.*—I.V.)

invagination (in-vaj-in-ā′shun). The infolding of one part within another, e.g., to form a double-layered cup; also, the result of the infolding.

irrigation. The washing or cleansing of a cavity or a passage by means of a stream of liquid.

ischemia (is-kēm′ē-a). A condition of localized diminished blood supply.

labile (lā′bīl). *adj*. Unstable, not fixed (particularly in reference to its physical state).

laceration (las-er-ā′shun). An accidental wound made by tearing or cutting.

laparotomy (lap-a-rot′ō-mē). A broad term covering any intra-abdominal surgical procedure.

latent (lā′tent). *adj*. Concealed or hidden, generally referring to a disease process.

lavage (la-vahzh′). The cleansing irrigation of an organ or a cavity. (Also used as a verb.)

lesion (lēzh′un). The change in a part caused by a disease or an injury.

leukocytosis (lūk-ō-sīt-ō′sis). Increase in the number of white corpuscles in the blood, generally caused by an infection.

ligation (lī-gā′shun). The surgical placing of a constricting tie, generally done to control bleeding.

ligature (lig′a-tchūr). Thread, catgut, or wire used to constrict or close the end of a blood vessel or tube. (*verb.*—li′gate.)

lues (lū′ēz). An old name for **syphilis.**

lumbago (lum-bāg′ō). A vague term sometimes used to describe a vague pain in the lower back.

lumen (lūm′en). A cavity or channel within an organ or a tubular structure.

malaise (mā-lāz′). MAL=abnormal. Indistinct, vague body fatigue or discomfort ("Doc, I just don't feel well.").

malformation (mal-form-ā′shun). Imperfect development of a part, usually congenital.

malignancy (mal-ig′nan-sē). A general term describing the malignant nature of a tumor; also, the tumor itself.

malignant (mal-ig′nant). *adj*. A term generally referring to certain **tumors,** indicating their tendency to spread to and invade neighboring or distant parts of the body. (Opposite of **benign.**) The term may also indicate an unusually severe, almost uncontrollable disease condition, such as malignant **hypertension.**

malingerer (mal-ing′ger-er *or* mal-inj′jer-er). One who feigns conditions or symptoms for purposes of gain.

malnutrition (mal-nū-trish′un). MAL=sick. Faulty or imperfect assimilation of the end products of digestion; also lack of available food. Either or both generally result in loss of weight.

manipulation (man-ip-yūl-ā′shun). MAN=hand. A procedure or treatment given with the hands.

manometer (man-om′e-ter). METR, MET=measure. An instrument for measuring pressure of gases or liquids.

metastasis (mē-tas′ta-sis). The appearance of a disease or of a malignant tumor in a region not adjacent to the primary site of the process.

microbe (mīk′rōb). *See* **microorganism.**

microorganism (mīk-rō-or′gan-izm). A general term referring to one-celled organisms capable of causing disease. They include **bacteria, fungi, protozoa,** and **viruses.**

microscope (mīk′-rō-skōp). An instrument which magnifies minute objects.

Types of microscopes are simple, compound, monocular, binoculai, electron, and otomicroscope microscopes.

migraine (mī'grān). "Sick headache," sometimes due to an allergic factor.

morbid. *adj.* MOR=sick. Diseased.

moribund (mor'i-bund). *adj.* In a dying state.

mortality rate. The ratio between the number of deaths and the total number of cases of a particular disease or surgical procedure.

mumps. A contagious disease involving the salivary glands; also called **paroti'tis.**

myositis (mī-ō-sīt'is). MYO=muscle. Inflammation in or of a muscle, particularly a voluntary muscle.

narcosis (nark-ō'sis). NARC=sleep. A state of deep stupor or unconsciousness, particularly one produced by the action of a drug.

nausea (nawz'ē-a). An abdominal uneasiness generally including a tendency toward vomiting. It may be gastric in origin, or be brought on by sensory or emotional factors.

Nembutal (Nem'byū-tawl). A proprietary barbiturate sedative.

neoplasm (ne-ō-plasm). An abnormal growth of benign or malignant nature.

neurosis (nūr-ō'sis). A type of mental disorder, generally with no obvious physical causes. (*Plural*—neuro'ses.) *See* **psychoneurosis.**

nocturnal (nok-tern'al). *adj.* During the night.

nodule (nod'yūl). A small swelling.

nonviable (non-vī'a-bl). Unable to sustain life.

obese (ō-bēs'). *adj.* Excessively fat or corpulent.

obesity (ō-bēs'i-tē). Excessive increase of body fat.

occlusion (ok-klū'zhun). The process of closing or being closed, particularly referring to an artery; also the relation of opposing teeth when the jaws are closed.

oliguria (ol-i-gūr'ē-a). Diminished output of urine.

optimum (op'ti-mum). The condition of maximum favorability. (*adj.*—optimal.)

organism. Any living thing, plant or animal. Unicellular organisms include **bacteria** and plant cells; multicellular organisms may include man and animals.

organotherapy (or-gan-ō-ther'a-pē). A broad term covering the treatment of disease by the administration of dehydrated animal organs or of their extracts.

orthopnea (or-thop'nē-a). The ability to breathe comfortably only with the chest in a vertical or propped-up position. (*adj.*—orthopne'ic.)

orthostatic (or-thō-stat'ik). *adj.* Produced as the result of standing erect.

osmotic pressure (oz-mot'ik). The force exerted when solutions of different concentrations are diffused through a membrane. The process is vitally concerned with diffusion through the walls of capillaries.

osteoarthritis (os-te-ō-arth-rī'tis). OS= bone; ARTH=joint. A chronic disease of the joints, usually of older people (**"wear and tear" arthritis** *or* **"degenerative" arthritis**).

osteopathy (os-tē-op'path-ē). A system of medical treatment based on the broad theory that when the body is in "correct structural relationship" it is able to overcome most of its problems. The manipulative and mechanical means of therapy are gradually being given less prominence and most osteopaths rely on, and are licensed to carry out, the usual medical and surgical measures.

osteoporosis (os-tē-ō-por-ō'sis). An abnormal, increased porousness (**decalcification**) of one or more bones. (*adj.*—osteoporot'ic.)

outpatient. Someone who goes to a clinic or a hospital for diagnosis or treatment, but who is not a "bedpatient." (Also used as an adjective.)

oxygen (oks'i-jen). An essential part of the air which, when breathed into the lungs, is diffused into the blood stream and is transported to the body cells, where it is essential to **metabolism.**

pallor (pal'lor). Unnatural paleness of the skin.

palpation (pal-pā'shun). PALP=to touch softly. A diagnostic examining maneuver carried out with the hands (or fingers) placed against the external surface of the body.

paralysis (pa-ral'i-sis). Partial or complete loss of motor function of a part resulting from a lesion of nervous or muscular origin. (*adj.* — paralyt'ic.)

parasite (pair'a-sīt). An organism that is dependent on another in order to live. (*adj.* — parasit'ic.)

parenteral (par-ent'er-al). *adj.* Referring to the introduction of substances into the body by some way other than by mouth or by rectum. (*adv.* — parenterally.)

paroxysm (pair'oks-izm). An uncontrollable seizure generally spastic in nature. (*adj.* — paroxys'mal.)

patent (pāt'ent). *adj.* In medicine, open or patulent, particularly referring to a tube or **duct.**

pathogen (path'ō-jen). PATH=sickness. A broad term covering any microorganism or material that produces disease (*adj.* — pathogen' ic.)

pathogenesis (path-ō-jen'e-sis). The origin or mode of development of a disease.

pathognomonic (path-ō-nō-mon'ik). *adj.* Referring to a symptom or a physical condition which is definitely indicative of the existence of a particular disease.

pathology (path-ol'ō-jē). The study of the structural and functional changes in body tissues and organs caused by a disease. (*adj.* — patholog'ical *or* patholog'ic.)

pendulous (pend'yūl-us). *adj.* Hanging freely or loosely.

penicillin (pen-i-sil'lin). An **antibiotic** derived from a genus of molds, which is used to combat numerous bacteria and other microorganisms.

petechia (pē-tēk'ē-a). A pinpoint **hemorrhage** in the skin or mucous membrane. (*Plural* — petech'iae.)

pharmacist (farm'a-sist). An individual holding a license to dispense drugs and prepare prescriptions. (Also called an **apothecary** or a **druggist.**)

pharmacology (farm-a-kol'ō-jē). The science which deals with drugs and their action. It is a required course in medical schools.

pharmacopeia (farm-a-kō-pē'a). An authoritative listing of drugs and their preparation. It also lists average dosages of drugs.

phenacetin (fen-as'e-tin). A drug similar to aspirin in uses and effects.

phlegm (flem). Thick, heavy mucus, generally copious, particularly referring to that ejected from the mouth.

phonetics (fōn-et'iks). The science of vocal sounds.

phthisis (tī'sis, tis'is, thī'sis, *or* thē'sis). An old word meaning **tuberculosis,** or a wasting away. (Choose your own pronunciation.)

physiology (fiz-ē-ol'ō-jē). The scientific study that deals with living things and their normal vital processes.

placebo (pla-sēb'o). Inactive, harmless material sometimes temporarily substituted for other prescribed medication. Although mainly used in drug evaluation studies, a physician may administer a placebo ("sugar pill") to determine the actual need or effectiveness of some medication.

podiatry (pō-dī'a-trē). A system of manipulative treatment for minor disorders of the feet. A **podiatrist** (formerly called a **chiropodist**) practices under a license issued by a special state board.

poliomyelitis (pō-lē-ō-mī-el-ī'tis). The formal name of the disease previously called *infantile paralysis.*

polydipsia (pol-ē-dip'sē-a). Excessive thirst.

polyethylene (pol-ē-eth'e-lēn). A type of plastic used in the manufacture of most surgical tubing.

polyp (pol'ip). A type of tumor generally protruding into a body cavity from a narrow base. Polyps are usually **benign** (*plural* — polyps *or* pol'ypi.)

prognosis (prog-nō'sis). A prediction regarding the course of a disease and its probable outcome. (*adj.* — prognos'tic; *verb* — prognos'ticate.)

prolapse (prō'laps). The abnormal dropping down of an organ from its usual position, particularly the uterus, kidney or stomach.

prophylaxis (prō-fil-aks'is). Treatment designed to prevent a disease before its onset. This may consist of **vaccination, immunization,** or measures recommended for use before or after contact with potentially infectious persons or situations.

proprietary (prō-prī'e-ter-ē). *adj.* A classification applied to drugs or medications which are marketed only under a patented or copyrighted name. A proprietary name is capitalized. *See* **gener'ic.**

prosthesis (pros-thē'sis). An artificial part substituting for or replacing one that has been lost.

prostration (pros-trā'shun). The condition of extreme body exhaustion from any cause.

pruritus (prūr-ī'tus). Itching, particularly intense itching.

psittacosis (sit-a-kō'sis). Parrot fever, sometimes transmitted to man.

psychogenic (sīk-ō-jen'ik). *adj.* Referring to a symptom which has an emotional origin rather than an organic basis.

psychoneurosis (sīk-ō-nūr-ō'sis). One of the two major classes of emotional illnesses. The other category is **psychosis.** *See also* "Psychiatry" chapter.

psychosomatic (sīk-ō-sō-mat'ik). *adj.* Referring to body symptoms which are partially or completely due to emotional factors.

psychosis (sīk-ō'sis). A severe mental disorder in which the patient at least temporarily loses touch with reality.

"ptomaine" (tō'mān). An indefinite term applied to any one of a group of food poisonings. Although a ptomaine is a definite chemical entity, "ptomaine poisoning" is an inaccurate name given by lay persons to indicate almost any food poisoning.

ptosis (tō'sis). Prolapse of an organ such as an eyelid, kidney or stomach.

puberty (pyūb'er-tē). The age at which the secondary sex characteristics appear and the genital organs become functionally operative.

pulmotor (pul'mō-tor). An apparatus for providing artificial respiration.

pulsation (pul-sā'shun). A rhythmical beat or impulse.

pulse. The palpable, generally rhythmic, **dilating** of an artery as it receives the increased volume of blood caused by a heart **contraction.**

pulse deficit. A pulse beat that is not palpable at the wrist in spite of a heart beat.

purulent (pyur'yūl-ent). *adj.* Consisting of or containing pus.

putrefaction (pyū-tre-fak'shun). Foul-smelling decomposition, particularly of body tissue. The odor is caused by the interaction of **enzymes** and protein substances.

pyrexia (pī-reks'e-a). A body temperature above the normal level (another name for a **fever**). It is usually spoken of as **hyperpyrexia.**

rabies (rāb'ēz). A specific disease, generally transmitted to man through the bite of an infected animal. (*adj.* — rabid.) *See* **hydrophobia.**

radiolucent (rād-ē-ō-lūs'ent). *adj.* Transparent or nearly transparent to x-rays; therefore casting no shadow, or practically no shadow, on a film or radiographic screen; nonopaque.

radiopaque (rād-ē-ō-pāk'). *adj.* Opaque to x-rays. Radiolucent areas appear dark on an exposed x-ray film while radiopaque areas appear light. (Opposite of **radiolucent.**)

rash. A skin eruption originating from causes within the body. Rashes are generally temporary, often wide spread, and are frequently associated with childhood contagious diseases, allergies or drug reactions.

regurgitation (rē-gurj-i-tā'shun). A backward flowing, generally referring to undigested food coming back up into the throat.

rehabilitation (rē-hab-il-i-tā'shun). The restoration of a patient to normal activities.

relapse. The return of a disease after its apparent cessation.

resect (rē-sekt'). *verb.* To excise or remove all, or a large portion, of an organ.

resonance (rez'ō-nens). A hollow sound produced by percussion over air-containing organs or regions of the body.

respirator (res'spir-ā-tor). Equipment which can perform respiration artificially.

resuscitation (rē-sus-si-tā'shun). The act of restoring an apparently dead person to life or consciousness.

rheumatism (rūm'a-tizm). A word commonly used to designate many diseases assciated with joints, tendons, muscles or bones.

rupture (rup'tchur). A tearing or breaking apart of nonbony tissue; also a common name for a **hernia.**

sanitation. The establishment of conditions conducive to cleanliness and better health.

sciatica (sī-at'i-ka). Pain along the course of the great sciatic nerve (hip, thigh, leg, foot).

sclerosis (skler-ō'sis). SCLER=hard. A general term indicating the abnormal hardening of tissue, particularly of the arteries (**arteriosclerosis**).

sedation (sēd-ā'shun). The administration of a quieting drug, or the actual state of calmness produced.

sedative (sed'a-tiv). The common name for medication given to achieve or produce a state of calmness. (Also used as an adjective.)

seizure (sē'zhur). The sudden onset of severe pain or of the symptoms of a disease. More commonly it refers to **convulsions.**

senility (sen-il'i-tē). The degenerative changes associated with old age, particularly mental changes. (*adj.*—senile.)

sepsis (sep'sis). Poisoning resulting from putrefaction and/or from bacterial decomposition. (*adj.*—sep'tic.)

septicemia (sep-ti-sēm'ē-a). The presence of bacteria or bacterial poisons in the blood stream.

serum (sēr'um). 1. The clear fluid exuded from injured or inflamed portions of the body. (*adj.*—ser'ous.) 2. The clear portion of the blood, exclusive of its formed structures, which separates in the clotting of blood. (*adj.*—ser'ous.) 3. Blood serum obtained from animals inoculated with **bacteria** or their toxins. It is given to patients to produce an **immunity.**

sibling (sib'ling). A full brother or sister.

sign (sīn). A change or manifestation indicating a disease process which can be perceived objectively. (*See* **symptom.**)

Silastic (Sī-las'tik). The proprietary name of a semi-rigid plastic material sometimes implanted into the body.

slough (sluff). Devitalized tissue cast-off or separated from living tissue; also, used as a verb meaning to cast off.

soporific (sōp-or-if'ik). SOPOR=sleep. A drug causing profound sleep. (Also used as an adjective.)

spastic. *adj.* Referring to a condition characterized by muscular spasms; also, a name commonly used to designate a person suffering from spastic paralysis ("a spastic").

specimen. A sample.

speculum (spek'yū-lum). A tubular instrument through which the interior of a hollow organ or part can be examined visually or treated.

splint. A rigid appliance used to support or immobilize a part of the body.

sputum (spyū'tum). Material ejected from the mouth, especially that coughed up from the lungs or bronchial tubes.

stenosis (sten-ō'sis). Narrowing of a **duct** or canal, sometimes to the point of closure. Generally, it is a congenital failure.

stethoscope (steth'ō-skōp). An instrument placed over the examined area and connected to ear pieces for the purpose of listening to various sounds in the detection and diagnosis of disease.

stool. A term applied to all fecal matter discharged from the bowel: **feces.**

strangulation (strang'gyū-lā'shun). The active shutting off of air by compression of the air passages; also, the shutting off of blood from tissues by constriction of their blood supply, as in a strangulated **hernia.**

streptomycin (strep-tō-mī'sin). An antibiotic derived from the soil. It is one of the few antibiotics effective against the tubercle bacillus which causes **tuberculosis.**

stricture (strik'tchur). Scarring causing a diminution in the size of the channel of a tube or **duct.**

stupor (stūp'or). A state of deadened or dazed sensibility with little or no awareness of surroundings.

subacute (sub-a-kyūt'). *adj.* Referring to a stage or degree (between **acute** and **chronic**) of the onset or course of an illness.

subcutaneous (sub-kyūt-ān'ē-us). *adj.* CUT=skin. Beneath the skin.

suppuration (sup-pyūr-ā'shun). The formation of pus. The term also generally infers its subsequent discharge from the body.

suture (sū'cher). The material used for stitching together surgically, as in closing a wound; also, used as a verb, to close by sewing.

symptom (simp'tom). Any subjective change from the normal of which the patient complains ("What bothers you, Mr. Smith?"). (*adj.* — symptomat'ic.) *See* **findings.**

symptomatology (simp-tom-a-tol'ō-jē). The study and consideration of all of the symptoms of a disease, particularly for purposes of review, teaching or discussion.

syncope (sin'kō-pē). A fainting spell.

synthesis (sin'the-sis). The process of building up therapeutic compounds by artificially combining their elements.

syphilis (sif'i-lis). A **venereal disease** often characterized by three stages if its course is not interrupted by treatment. (*adj.* — syphilit'ic.)

syringe (sir'inj). An instrument used for injecting liquid into or withdrawing liquid out of, the body.

systemic (sis-tem'ik). *adj.* Pertaining to the body as a whole.

systolic pressure (sis-tol'ik). The temporary peak of the blood pressure level present at the time of maximum heart contraction.

tactile (tak'til). *adj.* Relating to the act of touching, particularly recognition by touching.

therapy (ther'-a-pē). The treatment of disease. (*adj.* — therapeu'tic.)

thermometer (ther-mom'e-ter). THERM=heat; MET=measure. An instrument for recording body temperature. The present tendency is for the Centigrade scale to replace the Fahrenheit system.

thrombosis (throm-bō'sis). The formation or the presence of a **thrombus** on the inner surface of the wall of a blood vessel.

thrombus (throm'bus). A blood clot which remains at the site of its formation in the circulatory system. (When it breaks loose, it becomes an **embolus.**) (*adj.* — thrombot'ic.)

torsion (tor'shun). TORS=twist. A twisting, as of the mesentery of the bowel, or of an ovary, or of the stem of a polyp, or of the spermatic cord.

tourniquet (turn'i-ket). A constricting band which is applied tightly to interrupt normal blood flow to or from an extremity.

toxemia (toks-em'ē-a). TOX=poison. A generalized state of poisoning; actually, poison in the blood stream.

toxic (toks'ik). *adj.* TOX=poison. Poisonous, or capable of producing a state of poisoning.

toxicity (toks-is'i-tē). The potential or strength of a poison. The term may also refer to the adverse effect of drugs.

toxicology (toks-i-kol'ō-jē). The study of poisons, their actions, their detection, and the treatment of conditions produced by them.

transfusion (trans-fūzh'un). The addition of fluid to the circulating blood, generally referring to the addition of blood or blood derivatives.

trauma (trawm'a). A wound or injury caused by force. The term may also refer to the force causing the injury. (*adj.* — traumat'ic.)

tumor. Actually any swelling or enlargement, but generally referring to an independent, useless new growth.

ulcer (ul'ser). Any open sore on a **mucous membrane** or a skin surface which shows little or no tendency to heal. (*adj.* — ul'cerous.)

unconscious. *adj.* Insensible to the reception of any stimuli and incapable of performing or experiencing any controlled functions.

unilateral. *adj.* In medicine, one-sided, or referring to only one side of the body.

uremia (yūr-ēm'ē-a). The toxic condition resulting from the presence in the blood of excessive amounts of nitrogenous waste material normally excreted by the kidneys.

urinal (yūr'i-nal). A receptacle for receiving urine.

venereal disease (ven-ēr'ē-al). A disease related to, or contracted by, sexual intercourse (**gonorrhea, syphilis, chancroid,** etc.).

vermiform (verm'i-form). *adj.* Worm-shaped, generally referring to the **vermiform appendix.**

vestigial (ves-tij'ē-al). *adj.* Referring to persisting rudimentary parts (generally embryonic) which have no use or function following birth.

viability (vī-a-bil'i-tē). The ability to remain alive, or to sustain life.

virilism (vir'il-izm). The development or presence of male characteristics or tendencies in a female.

virility (vir-il'i-tē). The possession of normal powers of reproduction in the male.

virulent (vir'yūl-ent). *adj.* Referring to the disease-producing power of a microorganism. (*noun* — virulence.)

virus (vīr'us). A term referring to a number of infectious agents which are too small to be seen through the usual light microscope. (*plural* — viruses.)

viscous (vis'kus). *adj.* Sticky or gummy. *See* **viscus.**

vitamin (vīt'a-min). A general term referring to various compounds vital to the metabolic processes. Most of the vitamins are present naturally in various foods. Vitamins do not supply energy as foods do; neither do they supply substances from which tissue is built. Vitamins are best studied by noting the abnormalities that result when they are *absent* from the body.

void (voyd). *verb.* To pass wastes from the body, particularly urine. The term also is applied to defecation.

vomitus (vom'i-tus). Vomited or regurgitated material.

7 The Parts and Normal Functions of the Body

ATTEMPTING TO CLASSIFY medical terms according to special fields of practice runs into another problem of repetition because of the overlapping and intermeshing of these various specialties. The various parts and normal functions of the body will naturally have to be repeated many times throughout the book. For instance, the many structures of the neck region, by their very nature, automatically suggest several specialized medical fields. Thyroid gland secretion, which occurs in the neck region, specifically affects several separate parts of the body and many divergent functions, in addition to affecting the entire body. The overlapping of the specialties also applies to other neck region involvements such as swallowing (**deglutition**), and the transmission of blood to and from the brain.

Since our purpose is to explain medical terms rather than to teach anatomy or physiology, a general list of the parts and various normal functions of the body precedes the lists of words which apply to the various specialties. Naturally, the names of some of the body parts will reappear, and the various body functions will be elaborated on in the subsequent specialty lists.

CONSULTANTS

Harding Clegg, M.D.
Santa Rosa, California

Frank W. Norman, M.D.
*Former President, California Academy
of General Practice
Santa Rosa, California*

abdomen (ab-dō'men *or* ab'dō-men). That portion of the body between the chest and the pelvis. (*adj.*—abdominal.) (Fig. 22, p. 218; Fig. 2, p. 8)

Achilles tendon (A-kil'ēz ten'don). The large heel tendon.

adenoids (ad'e-noydz). *plural*. ADEN= gland. Glandular tissue normally found in the **nasopharynx** of a child.

adrenal cortex (ad-rēn'al kor'teks'). The outer portion of the **adrenal gland** which secretes the hormone **epinephrine.**

adrenal glands (glandz). *plural*. REN= kidney. Paired, vital, hormone-producing glands located above the kidneys. *See* **suprarenal glands.** (Fig. 25, p. 241)

alveolus (al-vē'ō-lus). One of the many small air sacs making up the bulk of the lungs. (*adj.*—alve'olar; *plural*— alve'oli.)

amino acid (am'ē-nō). The basic component of most proteins.

ampulla (am-pul'la). A dilated portion of a tubular structure of the body which accomplishes a particular function; for example, ampulla of the rectum.

amylase (am'il-as). A digestive enzyme which helps to convert starch into sugar.

antibody (an'tē-bod-ē). A protective body substance produced as a result of exposure to an **antigen.**

anus (ān'us). The exterior outlet of the intestinal canal. (*adj.*—an'al.) (Fig. 19, p. 186; Fig. 20, p. 190)

aorta (ā-or'ta). The main arterial vessel, receiving the blood from the left side of the heart. The two coronary arter-

ies are its first branches. (*adj.*—āor'tic.) (Fig. 8, p. 85; Fig. 9, p. 88)

appendage (ap-pend'aj). PEND=hang. A general term designating a subordinate part attached to a main structure.

appendix (ap-pend'iks). The common name for the **vermiform appendix.** (Fig. 20, p. 190; Fig. 21, p. 212)

areola (a-rē'ō-la). The central pigmented area surrounding the nipple of a breast. (*plural*—are'olae.)

areolar tissue (a-rē'ō-lar). One of the component parts of connective tissue.

arteriole (ar-tēr'ē-ōl). A terminal branch of an **artery.**

artery (ar'ter-ē). A blood vessel carrying blood in the direction away from the heart. (*adj.*—arter'ial.) *See* the list of arteries at the end of the chapter.

articulation (ar-tik-yūl-ā'shun). The more-or-less-movable fitting together of two or more adjacent bones, as in a joint. (*adj.*—artic'ular.)

assimilation (as-sim-i-lā'shun). The intestinal absorption and the body use of the end products of digestion.

atlas (at'las). A name given to the first cervical **vertebra,** upon which the skull rests. (Named for Atlas, who carried the world on his shoulders.)

atrium (āt'rē-um). One of the two paired upper chambers of the heart into which the veins discharge blood. (*plural*—a'tria) Also called an **auricle.** (Fig. 8, p. 85; Fig. 9, p. 88)

auricle (awr'i-kl). An older term for one of the two upper chambers of the heart; also, the projecting portion of the ear. (Fig. 17, p. 146)

axilla (aks-il'a). The armpit. (*adj.*—ax'illary.)

biceps (bī'seps). The large muscle on the front side of the upper arm; its main function is to bend the elbow.

bile (bīl). The digestive secretion produced by the liver; the excess is temporarily stored in the gallbladder (bile was formerly called "gall"). (*adj.*—bil'iary.) *See* **gallbladder.**

bladder (blad'er). The reservoir for the temporary storing of the urine. (*adj.*—ves'ical.) (Fig. 12, p. 119; Fig. 25, p. 241; Fig. 26, p. 245)

bone. The hard substance comprising most of the skeleton. *See* the list of bones at the end of the chapter. (Fig. 15, p. 138)

bronchiole (brong'kē-ōl). A small division of a bronchus. *See* **bronchus.**

bronchus (brong'kus). One of the two terminal divisions of the trachea, each carrying air to one lung. (*adj.*—bron'chial; *plural*—bron'chi.) (Fig. 24, p. 232)

bursa (burs'a). A friction-reducing sac or pocket frequently found near a joint, generally between the bone and an overlying tendon, or in the subcutaneous tissues. (*adj.*—burs'al; *plural*—burs'ae.)

capillaries (kap'il-lair-ēz). *plural.* The fine network of small blood vessels connecting the terminal arteries with the veins. The thin walls of the capillaries allow the vital exchange of nu-

triments and waste products between the tissues and the blood.

carpals (kar'plz). *plural.* A composite term referring to the eight bones making up the wrist joint. (Fig. 3, below)

cartilage (kar'ti-lej). The dense connective tissue termination of most bones, particularly the smooth substance covering the joint surfaces of the bones.

cecum (sē'kum). The first part of the **colon,** located in the right lower abdomen; the **ileum** discharges its contents into it at the **ileocecal valve.** (Fig. 20, p. 190; Fig. 21, p. 212)

celiac (sēl'ē-ak). *adj.* Pertaining to the abdomen.

cerebellum (ser-ē-bel'um). The portion of the brain, located near its base, that controls coordination and equilibrium. (*adj.*—cerebel'lar.)

cerebrum (ser'ē-brum *or* ser-ē'brum). The large upper portion of the brain which is the main seat of conscious thought, action and sensation. (*adj.*—cere'bral.)

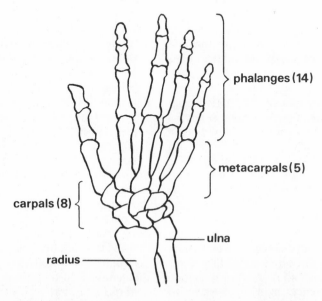

phalanges (14)

metacarpals (5)

carpals (8)

ulna

radius

FIG. 3. Bones of the Fingers, Hand, and Wrist

cervix uteri (ser'viks yūt'er-ī). The mouth of the uterus, which projects into the upper part of the vagina. **Pap smears** are usually made from the cervix uteri. (Fig. 12, p. 119)

cilium (sil'ē-um). An eyelash. (*plural*— cil'ia.)

circulation (ser-kyū-lā'shun). The round-and-round movement of the blood through the body; each circuit normally takes 17 seconds.

clitoris (klit'ō-ris). A female sexual organ which is the homologue of the male **penis.**

coagulation (kō-ag-yūl-ā'shun). The formation or production of a blood clot (a **coagulum**).

colon (kō'ln). The large intestine, exclusive of the **rectum.** (*adj.*—colon'ic.) (Fig. 20, p. 190)

conception (kon-sep'shun). The fertilization of the ovum by the male sperm.

connective tissue. The tissue that supports and binds together the various structures of the body.

copulation (kop-yūl-ā'shun). Sexual intercourse.

coronary arteries (kor'ō-nair-ē). COR= heart. The paired arterial blood vessels which supply the heart muscle with blood; they arise from the first portion of the **aorta,** behind the cusps of the aortic valve. (Fig. 8, p. 85; Fig. 9, p. 88)

corpuscle (kor'pus-sel). CORP=body. In medicine, a general term referring to any of the various kinds of cells in the blood.

cortex (kor'teks). CORT=shell. The outer layer of an organ or of the hard bones. (*adj.*—cor'tical; *plural*—cor' tices.)

corticosterone (kor-ti-kō-stēr-ōn' *or* kort-i-kost'er-ōn). A vital hormone secreted by the **adrenal cortex** which influences carbohydrate **metabolism.**

cortisone (kort'i-sōn). A vital hormone which influences many processes and is produced principally by the **adrenal cortex.**

cranium (krān'ē-um). CRAN=skull. The portion of the skull which supports and encloses the brain. (*adj.*— cranial.)

cuticle (kyūt'i-kl). CUT=skin. The outer layer of the skin; in common usage, generally refers to the hard **epidermis** at the junction of the skin and the upper surface of the nails.

cytoplasm (sīt'ō-plasm). CYTO=cell. The **protoplasm** making up a cell, exclusive of the cell nucleus. Also called protoplasmic cytoplasm.

defecation (def-ē-kā'shun). The act of eliminating fecal material from the body.

deglutition (deg-lū-tish'un). The act of swallowing.

dermis (derm'is). DERM=skin. The "true skin," beneath the **epidermis.**

diapedesis (dī-a-ped-ē'sis). The continuous outward oozing of the blood, particularly its **corpuscles,** through the intact walls of the blood conveying system, especially the **capillaries.**

diaphragm (dī'a-fram). The muscular partition separating the thoracic and abdominal cavities. (*adj.*—diaphragmat'ic.) (Fig. 22, p. 217; Fig. 23, p. 230)

diastolic pressure (dī-as-tol'ik). The blood pressure constantly maintained within the **arteries,** even during the phase of greatest cardiac relaxation.

digestion (di-jes'tchun). The natural process of reducing food to its simplest forms for the purpose of absorption from the gastrointestinal tract.

digit (dij'it). Any one of the fingers or toes.

dorsum (dors'um). The back surface of a part of the body. (*adj.*—dors'al.)

duct (dukt). A channel with definite walls for the conveying of fluids, particularly secretions.

duodenum (dū-ō-dēn'um *or* dū-od'e- num.) The first twelve inches of the small intestine, beginning at the pylorus. (*adj.*—duoden'al or duod'enal)

(Fig. 5, p. 51; Fig. 22, p. 217; Fig. 23, p. 230)

ear drum A common name for the tympanic membrane which transmits sound vibrations to the ossicles and eventually to the cochlea and the auditory nerve. (Fig. 17, p. 146)

ejaculation (ē-jak-yūl-ā'shun). The emission of **seminal fluid** — the climax of sexual intercourse in the male. (*adj.* — ejac'ulatory.)

endocardium (end-ō-kard'ē-um). CARD=heart. The inner lining of the heart.

endocrine gland (en'dō-krēn). One of the group of ductless glands which secrete directly into the bloodstream a substance which affects other organs or parts.

endothelium (end-ō-thēl'ē-um). The layer of flat (**epithelial**) cells which lines the inner surface of the entire circulatory system. (*adj.* — endothel' ial.)

enzyme (en'zīm). A substance or compound capable of initiating chemical changes in the body.

epidermis (ep-i-derm'is). DERM=skin. The outermost layer of the skin.

epigastrium (ep-i-gast'rē-um). GAST= stomach. The upper middle portion of the abdomen, sometimes called the "pit of the stomach."

epiglottis (ep-i-glot'tis). The cartilaginous covering, or lid, of the **larynx**; it prevents food and liquid from entering the larynx as they pass over it while moving from the mouth to the esophagus. (Fig. 18, p. 148)

epiphysis (ē-pif'i-sis). The region near the ends of long bones where most of the growth in their length occurs.

epithelium (ep-i-thēl'ē-um). The outer layer of cells covering the internal and external surfaces of the body, including its cavities and vessels. (*adj.* — epithel'ial.)

erythrocyte (ē-rith'rō-sīt). ERYTHR= red. One of the millions of red blood corpuscles which carry most of the **hemoglobin** and **oxygen.**

esophagus (ē-sof'a-gus). PHAG=swallow. The muscular tube conveying food from the throat (**pharynx**) to the stomach. (Fig. 5, p. 51; Fig. 18, p. 148; Fig. 23, p. 230)

estrogen (est'rō-jen). ESTR=woman; GEN=origin. An ovarian hormone, commonly called "the female hormone."

eustachian tube (yūs-tāk'ē-an). The paired tube connecting the **nasopharynx** with the middle ear. (Fig. 17, p. 146)

evacuation (ē-vak-yū-ā'shun). The emptying out of the bladder or the rectum; also, the surgical procedure of emptying out the contents of one of the hollow body structures.

expiration (eks-pir-ā'shun). The breathing out of air from the lungs. (*adj.* — expir'atory.) *See* **inspiration.**

extension (eks-ten'shun). The straightening of a part of the body, or the moving of it toward a straightened position. (Opposite of **flexion.**)

extensor (eks-ten'sor). A general term applying to any one of the muscles which accomplish extension.

fallopian tube (fal-ō'pē-an). One of the paired tubes conveying the ovum from an ovary to the uterus. (Fig. 12, p. 119)

fascia (fash'ya). The sheet of fibrous tissue enveloping and sometimes joining together many of the muscles and organs of the body.

femur (fēm'ur). The thigh bone. (*adj.* — fem'oral.) (Fig. 4, p. 50; Fig. 16, p. 143)

fertility (fer-til'i-tē). The ability to conceive or to cause conception.

fibula (fib'yūl-a). The outer and smaller of the two bones of the leg, located below the knee. (Fig. 4, p. 50)

flexion (fleks'shun). FLEX=bend. The bending of a part of the body or the moving of it toward a more angulated position. (Opposite of **extension.**)

flexor (fleks'or). Any muscle which produces **flexion.**

follicle (fol'i-kl). A small gland or sac which produces either a growing part or some secretion.

fontanel — fontanelle (fon-ta-nel'). The "soft spot" in the top of a baby's skull.

foramen (fōr-ām'en). A natural aperture, hole or perforation, particularly in a bone, forming the passageway for a nerve or blood vessel.

forearm (fōr'arm). The part of the arm between the elbow and the wrist.

fossa (fos'a). A pit, excavation, or depression. (*pl.* — fos'sae.)

frenum (frēn'um) — **frenulum** (fren'yūl-um). A small fold originating from either skin or **mucous membrane** which limits the movement of the organ or part.

fundus (fund'us). The dome or top of any hollow or sacular organ, particularly the uterus or the bladder. (Fig. 5, p. 51; Fig. 12, p. 119)

gallbladder (gawlblad'er). The sac-like organ located just beneath the liver which stores some of the **bile** until it is used. (Fig. 10, p. 93; Fig. 22, p. 217)

ganglion (gang'glē-on). A collection of nerve cells for transmitting or sending nervous impulses. (*pl.* — gang'lia.)

gingiva (jin'jiv-a). The gum tissue surrounding the teeth. (*pl.* — gingivae)

glottis (glot'tis). The sound-producing portion of the **larynx.**

gluteus (glūt-ē'us *or* glūt'ē-us). A composite name for a group of three muscles forming each buttock. (*pl.* — glut'ei.)

gonad (gōn'ad). A general name referring to the primary sex gland (male or female).

groin (groyn). The junction of the lower abdomen and the thigh. (*adj.* — in'guinal.)

"hamstrings" (ham'strings). The tendons of the posterior thigh muscles which flex the leg at the knee.

hematopoiesis (hēm-a-tō-poy-ē'sis). HEM=blood. The process of blood cell formation.

hemoglobin (hēm'ō-glōb-in). The pigment of the red blood cells; it carries and delivers oxygen. (*Abbr.* — hb.)

heparin (hep'ar-in). HEPAR=liver. A secretion of the liver which makes the blood less susceptible to clotting.

hepatic (hep-at'ik). *adj.* Referring to the liver.

hiatus (hī-ā'tus). A cleft or gap in the normal body architecture.

histamine (hist'a-mēn). A substance produced by the body when exposed to allergic or inflammatory stimuli.

hormone (hor'mōn). One of the many secretions of the ductless glands which is absorbed by the body and which controls some of the body processes. (*adj.* — hormon'al.)

humerus (hyūm'er-us). The large bone of the upper arm. (Fig. 4, p. 50)

hydrolysis (hī-drol'i-sis). HYDR=water; LYS=destroy. The chemical breaking down of compounds by the addition of water.

hymen (hī'men). The membrane which partially covers the external orifice of the vagina.

hypochondrium (hī-pō-kond'rē-um). The paired upper, lateral region of the abdomen. (*adj.* — hypochond'riac.)

hypogastrium (hī-pō-gast'rē-um). The lower middle portion of the abdomen. (*adj.* — hypogast'ric.)

hypophysis (hī-pof'i-sis). A name referring to the pituitary body — a gland located beneath, and attached to, the brain. Its two parts supply distinct, separate internal secretions important to body processes, notably those of growth and development.

hypothalamus (hī-pō-thal'a-mus). A portion of the brain which regulates body temperature, among other functions.

hypothenar eminence (hī-pō-thēn'ar em'i-nens). The medial fleshy border of the palm beneath the little finger.

ileum (il'ē-um). The long terminal portion of the small intestine which ends at the **cecum.**

ilium (il'ē-um). The uppermost, flared portion of the three fused bones forming the bony pelvis. (Fig. 4, p. 50; Fig. 16, p. 143)

immune (im-myūn'). *adj.* Referring to the body's ability to resist certain illnesses or toxins.

immunity (im-myūn'i-tē). Natural or acquired security against a disease or against the effects of a poison.

ingestion (in-jest'chun). The act of taking a substance into the body by swallowing it.

inguinal (ing'gwin-al). *adj.* Pertaining to the region of the groin.

insertion (in-ser'shun). The place of attachment of a muscle or its tendon to the part of the skeleton which it moves when the muscle contracts and shortens.

inspiration (in-spir-ā'shun). The drawing-in phase of **respiration.**

insulin (in'sul-in). A natural pancreatic hormone involved in the **metabolism** of sugar in the body, and therefore with the presence and treatment of diabetes. It is also produced commercially.

integument (in-teg'yū-ment). A general term referring to the entire body skin.

interstices (in-ter'sti-sēz). *plural.* The small spaces between the cells of tissue. (*adj.* – intersti'tial.)

intervertebral disk (in-ter-ver-tē'bral). One of the fibrous, flat, cushion-like structures separating each two adjacent vertebral bodies which are not normally fused together.

intestine (in-tes'tin). A composite term for the entire digestive tract beyond the stomach.

introitus (in-trō'i-tus). The natural entrance to any body cavity, generally referring to the vagina.

involution (in-vol-lū'shun). The return of a part of the body to normal size, as of the uterus following childbirth.

jejunum (je-jūn'um). The middle portion of the small intestine; the segment located between the **duodenum** and the **ileum.**

jugular veins (jug'yūl-ar). *plural.* The large superficial veins of the neck by which much of the blood returns from the head.

kidney (kid'nē). One of the two paired organs which form and excrete the urine. (*adj.* – ren'al.) (Fig. 25, p. 241)

labium (lāb'ē-um). LAB=lip. A lip or lip-shaped structure, but usually referring to the "lips" of the vagina. (*pl.* – lab'ia.)

lacrimal glands (lak'rim-al). LACR= tears. The paired glands which secrete tears. (Fig. 14, p. 129)

lacrimation (lak-rim-ā'shun). The secretion of tears by the **lacrimal glands.**

lactation (lak-tā'shun). LAC=milk. The secretion of milk by the breasts.

larynx (lair'inks). The "voice box" situated at the upper end of the trachea. (*adj.* – laryn'geal.)

leukocyte (lūk'ō-sīt). LEUK=white. Any one of the several kinds of *white* blood cells.

ligament (lig'a-ment). Any one of the fibrous bands or folds which support organs, hold bones together, or attach some muscles to the bones they act upon. *See* the list of ligaments at the end of the chapter.

linea alba (lin'ē-a alb'a). The vertical line running down the middle of the *anterior* abdominal wall.

lingua (ling'gwa). The tongue; the term is used in naming several conditions affecting the tongue. (Fig. 18, p. 148)

liver (liv'er). The body's largest internal organ; it has many functions. *See* **hepatic.** (Fig. 10, p. 93; Fig. 22, p. 217)

locomotion (lō-kō-mō'shun). The voluntary, active movement of the body from one place to another. (*adj.* – locomotor.)

loin (loyn). The *paired* part of the back between the **thorax** and the pelvis. (*adj.* – lum'bar.)

lumbar (lum'bar). *adj.* Relating to the loins or to the lower back.

lung. One of the two paired main organs of respiration. (*adj.*—pul'monary.) (Fig. 24, p. 232)

lymph (limf). A transparent, slightly yellow body fluid present in the lymph spaces and in the lymph vessels. (*adj.*—lymph *or* lymphoid.)

lymphatic system (lim-fat'ik). The system of channels and other structures through which **lymph** circulates in the body.

lymphocyte (limf'ō-sīt). A class of **leukocytes** having clear **cytoplasm.**

mammary gland (mam'er-ē). MAMM= breast. The *paired* breast, generally referring to the female milk-secreting gland.

marrow (mair'ō). The soft material which fills the hollow bones. It is also involved in the production of the blood cells.

mastication (mas-ti-kā'shun). The act of chewing.

mastoid (mas'toyd). *adj.* Referring to the bony, pointed projection from each temporal bone. It contains the mastoid cells and is located behind the ear. The term is also frequently used as a noun.

meatus (mē-ā'tus). An opening, particularly the "downstream" end of a body channel. (*plural*—meat'uses.)

mediastinum (mē-dē-as-tīn'um). The mass of tissue in the middle of the chest which separates the two lungs and contains the heart, esophagus, and many other vital structures. (*adj.*—mediastin'al.)

medulla (med-dul'la). The central portion (not the **cortex**) of an organ.

medulla oblongata (ob-long-ga'ta). The downward continuation of the brain proper, terminating in the spinal cord.

membrane (mem'brān). A thin sheet of tissue, generally a divider or a lining.

menopause (men'ō-paws). MEN= month. The cessation of **menstruation** ("change of life").

menses (men'sēz). Another name for **menstruation;** the cyclic bleeding from the lining of the uterus which occurs approximately monthly from the onset of menstruation until the **menopause.**

menstruation (men-strā'shun). *See* **menses.**

mesentery (mes'en-ter-ē). An extension or fold originating from the posterior wall of the **peritoneal** cavity; it suspends the intestines within the abdomen. (*adj.*—mesenter'ic.)

metabolism (mē-tab'ō-lizm). The sum of the energy expended in carrying on the normal body processes.

mucocutaneous (myū-kō-kyūt-ān'ē-us). *adj.* MUC=mucus; CUT=skin. An adjective referring to the meeting place of the **mucous** lining of body cavities with the skin.

mucosa (myū-kō'sa). A general term referring to any one of the **mucous membranes.**

mucous membrane (myū'kus mem'brān). The smooth lining of those body cavities which communicate with the exterior, notably the alimentary, the respiratory, and the urinary tracts. Unlike the serous membranes, mucous membranes secrete **mucus.**

mucus (myū'kus). A complex sticky substance produced by the lining of certain body cavities. (*adj.*—mu'cous.) *See* **mucous membrane.**

muscle (mus'el). Body tissues which, by their ability to shorten, can cause voluntary or involuntary movement within the body. *See* the list of muscles at the end of the chapter.

myocardium (mī-ō-kard'ē-um). MYO= muscle; CARD=heart. The muscular substance making up most of the bulk of the heart.

nape (nāp). Another name for the back or scruff of the neck. (*adj.*—nuch'al.)

nares (nair'ēz). *plural.* The two external nasal openings. (*Singular*—nar'is.)

nasopharynx (nā-zō-fair'inks). NASO= nose. The space above the roof of the mouth, connecting the nose and the throat. (Fig. 18, p. 149)

navel (nāv'al). The **umbilicus.**

nerve. One of the cord-like structures which form a portion of the nervous system and convey impulses throughout the body. (*adj.* — neural.) *See* the list of nerves at the end of the chapter.

nostril (nos'tril). One of the paired openings of the nose. *See* **nares.**

nutrition (nū-trish'un). The assimilation and use of digested food.

occiput (ok'si-put). The back of the head. (*adj.* — occip'ital.)

olfactory (ol-fak'tō-rē). *adj.* An adjective referring to the sense of smell.

omentum (ō-men'tum). The "apron" of fatty tissue suspended principally from the stomach, in the anterior part of the abdominal cavity.

oral (or'al). *adj.* Referring to or by way of the mouth.

orbit (orb'it). The bony eye socket.

orgasm (or'gazm). The climax of sexual excitement.

orifice (or'if-is). An opening — either an entrance or an outlet — to any body cavity.

ossicle (os'i-kl). OS=bone. Any small bone, but generally referring to one of the three small bones of the middle ear. (Fig. 17, p. 146)

ossification (os-sif-i-kā'shun). The normal process of the hardening or forming of bone through the deposition of calcium.

ovary (ōv'er-ē). OVA=egg. The paired female reproductive gland. (Fig. 12, p. 119)

ovulation (ov-yūl-ā'shun). The cyclic freeing of an **ovum** from the ovary.

ovum (ōv'um). The female reproductive cell (or egg). (*plural* — ov'a.)

oxidation (oks-i-dā'shun). A vital **metabolic** process involving the combination of oxygen with body tissues.

palate (pal'et). The roof of the mouth. *See* **soft palate.**

palpebra (pal-pē'bra). PALPEB=eyelid. Another name for any one of the four eyelids. (*adj.* — palpe'bral; *plural* — palpe'brae.)

pancreas (pan'krē-as). An abdominal gland which produces both an internal secretion (**insulin**) and a digestive juice; the latter is passed into the small intestine by way of the pancreatic duct and aids in the digestion of fats. (*adj.* — pancreat'ic.) (Fig. 10, p. 93; Fig. 22, p. 217)

parathyroid (pair-a-thī'royd). One of a group of small glands located in the neck; their secretion is vital to the **calcium metabolism** of the body. Their proximity to the thyroid makes their location important to surgeons doing **thyroidectomies.**

parenchyma (par-eng'ki-ma). The vital functioning part of an organ as distinguished from the total bulk. (*adj.* — paren'chymal.)

parotid gland (par-ot'id). One of the paired sets of saliva-producing glands.

parturition (par-tyūr-ish'un *or* par-tūr-ish'un). A fancy medical name for the universal process of "having a baby."

patella (pa-tel'la). The knee cap.

pelvis (pel'vis). The bony framework at the lower end of the trunk to which the lower extremities are attached. (*Plural* — pel'ves.)

penis (pēn'is). The male sexual organ (**phallus**). (*adj.* — pen'ile.) (Fig. 26, p. 245)

pepsin (pep'sin). One of the **enzymes** of the digestive juice secreted in the stomach; it assists in the digestion of proteins.

pericardium (per-i-kard'ē-um). CARD =heart. The fibrous sac which surrounds the heart, helping to hold it in position and isolating it from the other contents of the thoracic cavity and of the **mediastinum.** (Fig. 8, p. 85)

perineum (per-i-nē'um). The region between the external genitalia and the anus. (*adj.* — perine'al.)

periosteum (per-ē-os'tē-um). The tightly adherent membrane covering the bones.

peristalsis (per-i-stal'sis). A muscular contraction wave passing along the wall of a hollow tube or organ and propelling the contents forward, particularly noticeable in the esophagus, intestines, and ureters.

peritoneum (per-i-tōn-ē'um). The thin membrane which lines the abdominal cavity; it also envelopes the abdominal organs and helps to keep them in position by forming their **mesenteries.**

phalanx (fā'lanks). Any one of the 56 bones of the fingers and toes. (*plural* – phalan'ges.) (Fig. 3, p. 41)

phallus (fal'lus). The penis. (*adj.* – pen' ile.)

pharynx (fair'inks). The throat.

pituitary gland (pit-ū-i-tair'ē). *See* **hypophysis.**

plantar (plan'tar). *adj.* An adjective referring to the sole or the underside of the foot.

plasma (plaz'ma). The noncellular fluid portion of the blood.

platelets (plāt'lets). *plural.* A group of structures making up one of the components of the circulating blood; they are concerned with blood coagulation.

pleura (plūr'a). A thin membrane which both lines the thoracic cavity (**parietal pleura**) and covers the surface of the lungs (**visceral pleura**). (Fig. 24, p. 232)

plexus (pleks'us). A network or mesh of interconnected veins, arteries, lymphatic vessels or nerves (sometimes called a **rete**).

popliteal (pop-lit-ē'al). *adj.* An adjective referring to the posterior part of the knee.

portal vein (port'al). The large vein that collects blood from several abdominal veins and conveys it to the liver. *See* list of veins at the end of the chapter.

pregnancy (preg'nan-sē). The condition resulting from the development of a fertilized **ovum.**

prostate (pros'tāt). A gland making up a part of the male sexual system; it secretes some of the fluid which assists in the transportation of sperm down the urethral canal. (Fig. 25, p. 241; Fig. 26, p. 245)

protein (prō'tē-in). One of a group of nitrogenous compounds found in the body.

protoplasm (prō'tō-plazm). The essential material in all plant and animal cells, and the only known form of matter in which life is exhibited.

pulmonary   (pul'mon-air-ē).   *adj.* PULM=lung. An adjective referring to the lungs and to lung tissue.

pulmonic (pul-mon'ik). *adj.* Pertaining to the pulmonary artery. (Fig. 9, p. 88)

pylorus (pī-lōr'us). The outlet at the terminal end of the stomach which controls the passage of partially-digested food into the first segment of the small intestine (the **duodenum**). (*adj.* – pylor'ic.) (Fig. 5, p. 51)

ramus (rām'us). A branch, particularly of an artery, a nerve or a vein.

rectum (rek'tum). The terminal dilated portion of the intestinal tract (the term does not include the **anus**). (Fig. 12, p. 119; Fig. 19, p. 186; Fig. 20, p. 190; Fig. 26; p. 245)

reflex (rē'fleks). An involuntary muscle or tendon response to a stimulus. (Also used as an adjective.)

renal (rēn'al). *adj.* REN=kidney. Pertaining to the kidneys.

reproduction   (rē-prō-duk'shun).   In medicine, the production of offspring.

respiration (res-pir-ā'shun). The process of breathing; this includes the processes of **inspiration** and **expiration.** (*adj.* – res'piratory.)

rete (rē'tē). A term signifying an interconnected network of nerve fibers, blood vessels, or lymphatic vessels. *See* **plexus.**

rugae (rū'gē). *plural.* Folds or ridges, referring particularly to those of the palate, the lining of the stomach, and the vagina. (Fig. 5, p. 51)

sacro-iliac joint (sāk-rō-il'lē-ak). The slightly movable paired joint between the **sacrum** and the **ilium**. (Fig. 16, p. 143)

saliva (sal-īv'a). The frothy digestive secretion produced by the salivary glands, sometimes called "spit." (*adj.* — sal'ivary.)

salivary glands (sal'i-vair-ē). The several glands that produce saliva (**parotid, sublingual,** and **submaxillary**).

salpinx (sal'pinks). SALPING=fallopian tube. One of the paired fallopian tubes. (*plural* — salpin'ges.)

saphenous vein (saf'e-nus). A large vein of the thigh and leg regions. Due to continuous gravity pressure its valves frequently become inefficient, allowing the formation of **varicose veins.**

scrotum (skrō'tum). The pouch of skin containing the **testicles** and their connected structures. (Fig. 26, p. 245)

semen (sēm'en). SEM=seed. The male reproductive fluid (**seminal fluid**) which contains **spermatozoa.**

seminal vesicles (sem'i-nal ves'i-klz). The paired pockets used for the storage of **spermatozoa** until ejaculation; they are located beneath the base of the bladder. (Fig. 26, p. 245)

septum (sep'tum). A structure which acts as a divider or partition between organs or portions of organs.

serosa (sēr-ō'sa). A general term referring to any **serous membrane.**

serous membrane (sēr'us). The smooth lining of the *closed* body cavities, particularly the abdominal and thoracic cavities. It is often called the serosa and, unlike the mucous membrane, it does not secrete mucus.

serum (sēr'um). The clear, yellowish fluid which separates from clotted blood. The term also refers to the clear fluid which exudes, protectively, in response to injury or some inflammations.

sigmoid colon (sig'moyd). The S-shaped portion of the colon immediately preceding the rectum. The term "sigmoid" is frequently used to designate the sigmoid colon. (Fig. 19, p. 186; Fig. 20, p. 190)

sinus (sīn'us). A specific cavity, recess or hollow. The term generally refers to the **paranasal sinuses** — air spaces found in several of the cranial bones.

skeleton (skel-e-ton). The bony framework of the body.

skull (skull). The bony protective covering of the brain and of the chief sensory organs.

soft palate (pal'et). The muscular tissue partially surrounding the opening from the mouth into the throat. The **uvula** hangs down from the middle of the oval structure.

spermatozoon (sper-ma-tō-zō'on). SPERM=seed. The male seed which fertilizes the **ovum.** (*plural* — spermatozoa.)

sphincter (sfink'ter). A puckering muscle surrounding and closing a tube or orifice.

spinal cord (spīn'al). The prolongation of the stem of the brain; it extends through the vertebral column and gives off both sensory and motor branches.

splanchnic (splank'nik). *adj.* A term referring to the abdominal organs.

spleen (splēn). A large upper abdominal organ whose functions are not completely understood. It is known to be involved in the production (and destruction) of certain blood cells. (Fig. 22, p. 217)

squamous cells (skwām'us). The flat, platelike cells found in the outer layer of the **skin** and of the **mucous membranes.**

stomach (stum'ek). The large upper abdominal organ where most of digestion is initiated. It is situated between the **esophagus** and the **duodenum.** (Fig. 5, p. 51; Fig. 22, p. 217; Fig. 23, p. 230)

50

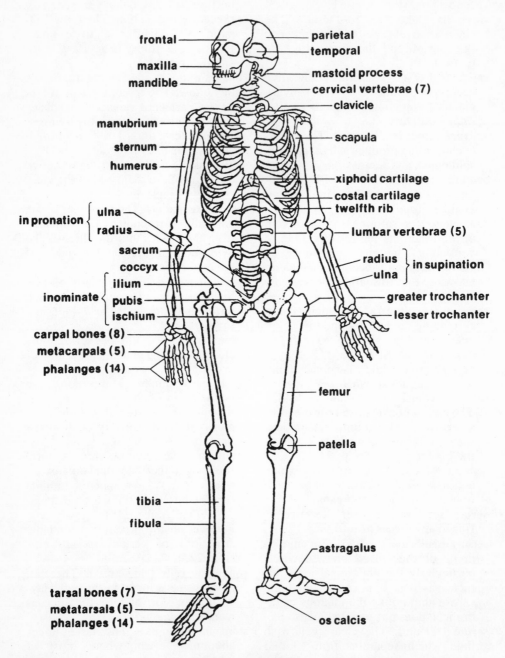

FIG. 4. Skeleton

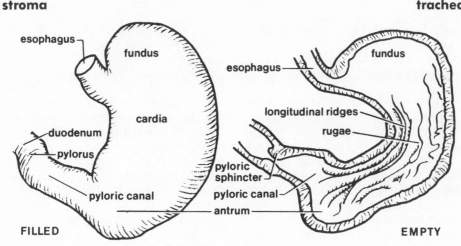

FIG. 5. Stomach

stroma (strōm'a). The supporting tissue framework of the organs of the body as distinguished from the **parenchyma.**

sudoriferous glands (sūd-or-if'er-us). SUD=sweat. The sweat glands, located in the skin.

suprarenal glands (sūp-ra-rēn'al). Another name for the **adrenal glands.**

synovial fluid (sin-ōv'ē-al). A lubricating fluid contained within the capsules of movable **joints** and inside **bursae.**

systolic pressure (sis-tol'ik). The temporary peak of the blood pressure level, produced at the time of maximum heart contraction.

tactile (tak'til). *adj.* Referring to the sense of touch.

tendon (ten'don). The fibrous band into which some muscles narrow down for their attachment to a bone. The bone is then moved when the muscle contracts and shortens. (*adj.* — tend'inous.) *See* the list of tendons at the end of the chapter.

testicle (tes'ti-kl). The paired male genital organ which produces **spermatozoa** and a male sex hormone. It is also called the **testis.** (Fig. 26, p. 245)

testis (tes'tis). Another name for a **testicle.** (Fig. 26, p. 245)

thalamus (thal'a-mus). The brain center which relays sensory impulses to the cerebrum.

thenar eminence (thēn'ar em'i-nens). The fleshy mound on the palm at the base of the thumb.

thigh (thī). The portion of the leg between the knee and the pelvis.

thorax (thōr'aks). The framework of the chest cavity. (*adj.* — thorac'ic.)

thymus (thīm'us). A ductless gland in the neck of infants which normally disappears during early childhood.

thyroid (thī'royd). A ductless gland located in the neck. It produces several secretions intimately concerned with body **metabolism.**

thyroxin (thī-roks'in). One of the hormones secreted by the **thyroid gland.**

tongue (tung). The well-known organ of taste; it also aids in enunciation. (Fig. 18, p. 148)

tonsils (ton'sils). Small encapsulated masses of lymphoid tissue found in each side of the throat.

torso (tor'sō). The trunk of a body.

trachea (trāk'ē-a). The cartilaginous tube which connects the larynx with the two bronchial tubes into which it divides. (Fig. 24, p. 232)

trunk. The body, exclusive of the head and limbs; the **torso.**

trypsin (trip′sin). A protein-digesting **enzyme** produced by the pancreas.

tympanum (timp′a-num). The ear drum. (Also called the tympanic membrane.) (*adj.* — tympan′ic.) (Fig. 17, p. 146)

umbilicus (um-bil′i-kus *or* — bil-ī′kus). The navel — the site of the fetal attachment of the umbilical cord.

urea (yūr′ē-a). One of the constituents of urine and of blood resulting from the breaking down of proteins.

ureter (yūr′e-ter). The paired muscular tube which conveys urine from each kidney *to* the bladder. (*adj.* — uret′eral.) (Fig. 25, p. 241)

urethra (yūr-ēth′ra). The tube which conveys urine outward *from* the bladder. (*adj.* — ureth′ral.) (Fig. 12, p. 119; Fig. 25, p. 241; Fig. 26, p. 245)

urination (yūr-in-ā′shun). The voiding of urine.

urine (yūr′in). The fluid, formed in the kidneys, which conveys waste products, filtered out of the blood, away from the body.

uterus (yūt′er-us). The womb in which the products of conception develop. (Fig. 12, p. 119)

uvula (yūv′yū-la). The part of the **soft palate** which hangs down at the opening to the throat.

vagina (vaj-īn′a). One of the parts of the female genital tract. (*adj.* — vag′inal.) (Fig. 12, p. 119)

vas deferens (vas def′er-enz). The paired tube which conveys spermatozoa from the epididymis to the seminal vesicle on the same side. (*plural* — vas′a deferen′tia) (Fig. 26, p. 245)

vein (vān). A thin-walled blood vessel which carries blood *toward* the heart.

(*adj.* — ven′ous.) *See* the list of veins at the end of the chapter.

vena cava (vēn′a kāv′a). One of the two large venous trunks (**superior** and **inferior**) which convey all unoxygenated blood from the upper and lower parts of the body back *to* the heart. (Fig. 8, p. 85; Fig. 9, p. 88)

ventral (ven′tral). *adj.* An adjective designating the anterior or belly side of the abdomen.

ventricle (ven′tri-kl). Technically any small cavity, but especially referring to one of the two large lower cavities of the heart, or to one of the four cavities of the brain. (*adj.* — ventric′ular.) (Fig. 9, p. 88)

veriform appendix (verm′-i-form appen′diks). A narrow blind tube of varying size which originates from and is continuous with the cavity of the cecum; it is usually referred to simply as the appendix.

vertebra (vert′e-bra). Any one of the 33 bones of the spinal column. Some of these are normally fused together (the **sacral** and the **coccygeal** vertebrae). (*adj.* — verte′bral; *plural.* — vert′ebrae.)

vesicle (ves′i-kl). A general name for a sac or a pocket containing fluid. The term, however, generally refers to the **urinary bladder** or to the **seminal vesicles.** (*adj.* — ves′i-cal.)

viscus (visk′us). Any one of the internal organs of the body. (*plural.* — vis′cera; *adj.* — vis′ceral.)

vocal cords — vocal chords. The membranous bands in the larynx by means of which the voice sounds are produced.

void (voyd). *verb.* To pass urine or fecal material from the body.

vulva (vul′va). A general term applied to the external genital organs of the female.

It seems logical to insert, at this point, condensed lists of the more important arteries, bones, ligaments, muscles, nerves, tendons and veins of the body. Although their pronunciation is shown, the names are not further explained here. Only those terms appear in the Index which are important enough to suggest logical relisting and explaining in connection with a specialty. The other terms are listed for spelling and pronunciation reference.

IMPORTANT ARTERIES

alveolar (al-vē′ō-lr)
aorta (ā-or′ta)
axillary (aks′il-lair-ē)
basilar (bas′i-lr *or* baz′i-lr)
brachial (brā kē-al)
carotid (ka-rot′id) *(4)*
celiac (sēl′ē-ak)
cerebellar (ser-e-bel′lr)
cerebral (ser-rē′bral *or* ser′e-bral)
circumflex (sir′kum-fleks)
colic (kol′ik)
collateral (kol-lat′er-al) *(many)*
coronary (kor′on-nair-ē)
cystic (sis′tik)
digital (dig′i-tl)
dorsalis pedis (dor-sal′is pēd′is)
epigastric (ep-i-gas′trik)
facial (fā′shl)
femoral (fem′ōr-al)
gastric (gas′trik)
gastroepiploic (gas-trō ep-e-plō′ik)
gluteal (glū′te-al *or* glū tē′al)
hemorrhoidal (hem-ōr-royd′al)
hepatic (hē-pat′ik)
hypogastric (hī-pō-gas′trik)
ileocolic (il-ē-ō-kol′ik)

iliac (il′ē-ak)
innominate (in-nom′in-nāt)
intercostal (in-ter-kos′tl) *(many)*
interosseous (in-ter-os′sē-us) *(many)*
mammary (mam′mar-ē)
meningeal (men-in′jē-al)
mesenteric (mes-en-ter′ik)
nutrient (nu′trē-ent)
ovarian (ō-vair′ē-an)
peroneal (per-ōn-nē′al)
popliteal (pop-lit-tē′al)
profunda femoris (prō-fun′da fem′ō-ris)
pulmonary (pul′mon-air-ē)
radial (rād′ē-al)
renal (rēn′al)
spermatic (sper-mat′ik)
splenic (splen′ik)
subclavian (sub-klāv′ē-an)
thyroid (thī′royd)
tibial (tib′ē-al)
ulnar (ul′nar)
uterine (yūt′er-in)
vertebral (ver′te-bral *or* ver-tē′brál)
vesical (ves′i-kl)

IMPORTANT BONES

astragalus (as-trag′a-lus)
atlas (at′las)
calcaneus (kal-kān′nē-us)
calvarium (kal-vair′ē-um) *(composite term)*
carpal (kar′pl) *(16)*
clavicle (klav′i-kl)
coccyx (kok′siks)
cranium (krān′ē-um)
cuboid (kyū′boyd)
cuneiform (kyū-nē′i-form *or* kūn-ē′-i-form)
ethmoid (eth′moyd)
femur (fēm′ur)
fibula (fib′yūl-a)

frontal (frun′tl)
hamate (ham′āt)
humerus (hyūm′er-us)
hyoid (hī-oyd)
ilium (il′ē-um)
innominate (in-nom′i-nāt) *(composite term)*
ischium (is′kē-um)
malleolus (mal-lē′ō-lus)
mandible (mand′i-bl)
maxilla (maks-il′la)
metacarpal (met-a-kar′pl) *(10)*
metatarsal (met-a-tar′sl) *(10)*
nasal (nāz′l)
navicular (na-vik′yūl-ar)

occipital (ok-sip'i-tl)
parietal (par-i'e-tl)
patella (pa-tel'la)
pelvis (pel'vis)
phalanx (fāl'anks)
pubis (pyūb'is)
radius (rād'ē-us)
rib (24)
sacrum (sāk'rum)
scapula (skap'yūl-a)
sesamoid (ses'a-moyd) (several)
sphenoid (sfēn'oyd)
sternum (stern'um)
talus (tāl'us)

tarsal (tar'sl) (14)
temporal (tem'por-al)
tibia (tib'ē-a)
turbinate (turb'in-āt) (6)
ulna (ul'na)
vertebra (vert'e-bra)
cervical (serv'i-kl) (7)
thoracic (thōr-as'ik) (12)
lumbar (lum'bar) (5)
sacral (sāk'rl) (fused) (5)
coccygeal (kok-sij'ē-al) (fused) (4)
vomer (vōm'er)
zygoma (zī-gōm'a)

IMPORTANT LIGAMENTS

annular (or anular) (an'yū-lr) (several)
arcuate (ar'kyū-āt)
broad
collateral (kol-lat'er-al) (many)
costovertebral (kost-ō-vert-ē'brl)
  (several)
cruciate (krū'shē-āt) (4)
falciform (fal'si-form)
gastrohepatic (gas-trō-hē-pat'ik)
hepatic (hē-pat'ik)
Hesselbach's (Hes'el-bahks)

iliofemoral (il-ē-ō-fem'ōr-al)
inguinal (ing'gwin-nl)
intercarpal (in-ter-kar'pl)
interosseous (in-ter-os'sē-us)
nuchal (nū'kl)
pectinate (pek-tin-āt)
Poupart's (Pū-parts')
suspensory (sus-pen'sōr-ē)
Treitz's (trīts'ez)
uterosacral (yūt-er-ō-sāk'ral)
Zinn's (Zinz)

IMPORTANT MUSCLES

abductor (ab-duk'tor) (several)
adductor (ad-duk'tor) (several)
biceps brachii (bī'seps brāk-ē-ī)
biceps femoris (bī'seps fem'or-is)
brachialis (brāk-ē-al'is)
buccinator (buk'sin-ā-tor)
bulbocavernosus (bulb-ō-kav-ern-ō'sus)
ciliary (sil'ē-air-ē)
coracobrachialis (kor-a-kō-brāk-ē-al'is)
deltoid (del'toyd)
diaphragm (dī'a-fram)
digastric (dī-gas'trik)
erector spinae (ē-rek'tor spīn'ē)
extensor (eks-ten'sor) (several)
flexor (fleks'or) (several)
gastrocnemius (gas-trok-nēm'ē-us)
gluteus maximus (glū-tē'us maks'i-
  mus)
gluteus minimus (min'i-mus)
gracilis (gras'il-is)
iliopsoas (il-ē-ō-sō'as)

infraspinatus (in-fra-spin-ā'tus)
intercostal (in-ter-kos'tl) (many)
internal oblique (in-ter'nl ob-lēk')
interosseus (in-ter-os'sē-us) (many)
ischiocavernousus (is-kē-ōkav-ern-ō'
  sus)
latissimus dorsi (la-tis'i-mus dor'sē)
levator ani (lē-vā'tor ān'ē)
levator palpebrae (lē-vā'tor pal-pē'brē)
levator scapulae (lē-vā'tor skap'yū-lē)
longissimus (long-gis'i-mus)
masseter (mas'se-ter)
obturator (ob'tūr-ā-tor)
occipital (ok-sip'i-tl)
orbicularis oculi (or-bik-yū-lair'is ok'
  yū-lē)
orbicularis oris (ōr'is)
pectoralis (pek-tor-al'is)
peroneus (per-ō-nē'us)
platysma (plat-iz'ma)
popliteus (pop-lit-ē'us)

pronator quadratus (prō-nāt'or kwad-rāt'us)

pronator teres (ter'ēz)

psoas major (sō'as māj'or)

pterygoid (ter'i-goyd)

pyramidalis (pir-am-id-al'is)

quadratus lumborum (kwad-rāt'us lum-bōr'um)

quadriceps femoris (kwad'ri-seps fem'or-is)

rectus abdominis (rek'tus ab-dom'i-nis)

sacrospinalis (sāk-rō-spin-al'is)

sartorius (sar-tor'ē-us)

scalenus anterior (skāl-ē'nus)

serratus anterior (ser-rāt'us)

soleus (sōl'ē-us)

sphincter ani (sfink'ter ān'ē)

sphincter vesicae (ves'i-kē)

sternocleidomastoid (ster-nō-klī-dō-mas'toyd)

supinator (sūp'in-ā-tor)

temporal (tem'por-al)

teres major (ter'ēz māj'or)

transversus abdominis (trans-vers'us ab-dom'i-nis)

trapezius (trap-ēz'ē-us)

triceps brachii (trī'seps brāk'ē-ī)

IMPORTANT NERVES

abducens (ab-dūs'ens)

acoustic (a-kūs'tik)

auditory (awd'i-tō-rē)

axillary (aks'il-lair-ē)

ciliary (sil'ē-air-ē)

cutaneous (kyūt-ān'ē-us) (*many*)

facial (fā'shl)

femoral (fem'ōr-al)

glossopharyngeal (glos-ō-fair-inj'ē-al)

hypoglossal (hī-pō-glos'al)

iliohypogastric (il-ē-ō-hī-pō-gas'trik)

infraorbital (in-fra-orb'i-tl)

intercostal (in-ter-kos'tl)

median (mēd'ē-an)

musculocutaneous (mus-kyū-lō-kyūt-ān'ēus)

obturator (ob'tūr-ā-tor)

oculomotor (ok-yūl-ō-mōt'or)

olfactory (ol-fak'tō-rē)

ophthalmic (off-thal'mik)

optic (op'tik)

parasympathetic (pair-a-sim-pa-thet'ik) (*many*)

peroneal (per-on-nē'al)

phrenic (fren'ik)

pudendal (pyū-den'dl)

radial (rād'ē-al)

sacral (sāk'ral)

sciatic (sī-at'ik)

splanchnic (splank'nik)

thoracic (thor-as'ik)

trigeminal (trī-jem'in-al)

trochlear (trōk'lē-ar)

ulnar (ul'nar)

vagus (vāg'us)

vestibular (ves-tib'yūl-ar)

IMPORTANT TENDONS

Achilles (a-kil'lēz)

central

conjoined (kon'joynd')

hamstring (ham'string) (*4*)

supraspinatus (sūp-ra-spin-ā'tus)

patellar (pa-tel'lr)

quadriceps (kwad'ri-seps)

IMPORTANT VEINS

azygos (az'i-gos)

antecubital (an-tē-kyūb'i-tl)

innominate (in-nom'in-nāt)

jugular (jug'yū-lr)

portal (port'al)

saphenous (saf'en-us)

vena cava (vēn'a kāv'a)

Many other veins bear the same name as their arterial counterparts and are not listed here.

*

ⅢⅢ SPECIFIC TERMS
(Related to Medical Specialities)

⑧ Anesthesiology

TIMES HAVE CHANGED since Dr. Crawford Long poured ether over some gauze in Georgia and held it over the patient's nose until he went to sleep. Nowadays **anesthesiologists** administer one of a number of **anesthetic** agents to a patient by one of a number of methods, depending on whether topical, local, regional, or complete **anesthesia** is desired. The patient is being **anesthetized,** and all or part of him becomes **anesthetic** and experiences **anesthesia.** The anesthesiologist continually observes and varies the depth of the anesthesia by adding various components to his anesthetic agent, as the surgical situation requires. And the whole complex, hard-to-pronounce business is still casually referred to by the inelegant expression "giving an anesthetic."

Many localities have no certified anesthesiologist, and in most other locations there are simply not enough to go around when many surgical procedures are being done at the same time. Therefore, it is sometimes necessary for physicians, nurse anesthetists, and technicians who have had training and experience but who are not certified anesthesiologists to administer many anesthetics, particularly those not requiring more complicated methods.

The science of anesthesiology has progressed more rapidly over recent years than most of the other medical specialties. Long and complicated surgical procedures have been made possible by advances in anesthetic techniques and refinements.

The American Board of Anesthesiology requires two years of accredited postgraduate study and training in the field and three years of practice before the applicant can be certified as an anesthesiologist.

CONSULTANTS

Robert W. Churchill, M.D.
Diplomate, American Board of Anesthesiology; Former Associate Professor, Anesthesiology, Stanford University School of Medicine
Santa Rosa, California

James L. Waters, M.D.
Santa Rosa, California

adrenalin (ad-ren′a-lin). A common name for **epinephrine,** a secretion of the adrenal glands; also, a drug produced synthetically, sometimes used to raise the blood pressure during anesthesia.

airway. A composite name for the air passages; also a tube sometimes introduced into the trachea during anesthesia to assure unobstructed breathing.

alveolar air (al-vē′ō-lar). The air contained in the terminal bronchial branches **(alveoli).**

aminophylline (am-i-nof′a-lin *or* am-i-nō-fil′in). A drug sometimes used by anesthesiologists to obtain bronchial and arterial relaxation.

analgesia (an-al-jēz′ē-a). ALG=pain. Absence of the normal sense of pain. (*adj.* — analges′ic.)

analgesic (an-al-jēz′ik). A drug which stops or reduces pain.

Anectine (an-ek′tēn). A proprietary, rapidly acting, muscle relaxant of short duration. (Generic name, **succinylcholine.)**

anesthesia (an-es-thēz′ē-a). ESTHE= feeling. The absence of normal sensation.

anesthesiologist (an-es-thēz-ē-ol′ō-jist). A specialist who practices anesthesiology. *See* introductory paragraphs.

anesthesiology (an-es-thēz-ē-ol′ō-jē). The science and study of anesthesia and anesthetics.

anesthetic (an-es-thet′ik). An agent administered to produce anesthesia. (Also used as an adjective.)

anesthetist (an-es′thet-ist). *See* introductory paragraphs.

anesthetize (an-es′the-tīz). *verb.* To produce a state of anesthesia.

anoxemia (an-oks-ēm′ē-a). OX=oxygen; HEM=blood. A condition characterized by a deficiency of oxygen in the blood.

anoxia (an-oks′ē-a). A deficiency of oxygen in the tissues.

apnea (ap′nē-a *or* ap-nē′a). The cessation of breathing (usually temporary).

atelectasis (at-a-lek′ta-sis). The collapse or incomplete expansion of a lung, or of part of a lung.

atropine (at′rō-pēn). A drug used by anesthesiologists to inhibit secretions which interfere with the proper administration of an anesthetic.

barbiturate (bar-bit′yūr-āt). A general name for any drug derived from barbituric acid. Barbiturates are often used for preanesthetic medications; **Pentothal** is a barbiturate which is used intravenously for rapid induction of anesthesia.

bronchiectasis (brong-kē-ek′ta-sis). Chronic dilatation of the bronchial tubes of the lungs, frequently with **saccule** (small pouch) formation and accumulation of purulent material.

Butesin (Byūt′e-sin). A proprietary drug used for producing topical anesthesia.

cardiac arrest (kard′ē-ak). CARD= heart. Unanticipated cessation of heart action, sometimes encountered during anesthesia or during surgical procedures.

cardiac massage (mas-sazh′). Manual compression of the heart (within the chest cavity) to reestablish circulation during **cardiac arrest.** Although **intrathoracic** massage is still used, the tendency, of late, is toward the use of *external* "cardiac massage."

caudal block (kawd′al). CAUD=tail. A method of anesthetic administration into the caudal canal. In medical jargon, "a caudal"; actually a modification of spinal anesthesia.

cervical plexus block (serv'i-kl pleks'-us). CERV=neck. A method of anesthetic administration by anesthetizing the **cervical plexus** (a nerve network in the neck).

chloroform (klōr'ō-form). A volatile anesthesia-producing liquid administered by inhalation.

cocaine (kō-kān'). A drug which produces local anesthesia; it is administered by topical application.

curare (kyū-rahr'ē or kyū-rahr'a). A drug used to relax muscles during anesthesia; it is relatively long lasting. (Also called **tubocurarine.**).

cyclopropane (sīk-lō-prō'pān). An anesthesia-producing gas; it is very rapid in action.

defibrillation (dē-fib-ril-ā'shun). The reestablishment of normal cardiac rhythm accomplished by electric stimulation of a specific type applied over the heart area.

defibrillator (dē-fib'ril-ā-tor). The electrical apparatus used in **defibrillation.**

divinyl ether (dī-vīn'il ēth'er). A volatile, anesthesia-producing liquid (also known as **Vinethene**); it is very rapid in action.

emphysema (em-fis-ēm'a). In anesthesiology, ballooning of the lung spaces due to the loss of normal elastic tissue, resulting in incomplete expiration of anesthetic gases.

endotracheal (end-ō-trāk'ē-al). adj. Referring to something within the trachea, particularly an airway placed there, under anesthesia, to facilitate breathing.

ephedrine (e-fed'rin). A drug used principally to raise blood pressure during anesthesia.

"epidural" (ep-ē-dūr'al). Medical lingo for a modification of spinal anesthetic administration. (Also used as an adjective.) See **extradural.**

ether (ēth'er). A volatile anesthesia-producing liquid, the vapor of which is administered by inhalation.

ethyl chloride (eth'il klōr'īd). A volatile liquid used as a spray to produce topical anesthesia. Also given by inhalation to produce general anesthesia for short surgical procedures.

ethylene (eth'il-ēn). A gas which produces anesthesia rapidly; it is also highly explosive.

extradural (eks-tra-dūr'al). adj. Referring to something outside the **dura**. (Same as **epidural.**)

field block. The production of anesthesia in a region of the body by the use of an encircling "wall" of injected anesthetic solution which paralyzes the nerves penetrating the "wall."

flowmeter (flō'mēt-er). An apparatus for measuring the flow of gases being administered by the anesthesiologist.

glutethimide (glū-teth'i-mīd). A drug with **hypnotic** qualities. (A proprietary equivalent is **Doriden.**)

halothane (hal'ō-than). A volatile anesthesia-producing liquid. (A proprietary equivalent is **Fluothane.**)

hypercapnia (hī-per-kap'nē-a). The presence of excessive carbon dioxide in the lungs, a condition of deep concern to anesthesiologists.

hyperpnea (hō-perp-nē'a). Respiration which is abnormally increased in rate and depth.

hyperventilation (hī-per-vent-i-lā'shun). Excessive breathing, either accelerated or deepened.

hypnosis (hip-nōs'is). OSIS=condition. An artificially-caused trancelike state during which the patient may follow instructions; it is sometimes used by anesthesiologists, as well as by other clinicians.

hypothermia (hī-pō-therm'ē-a). THERM=heat. Subnormal body temperature, especially one intentionally produced. It is sometimes used for certain surgical procedures, to reduce the depth of anesthesia required, as well as to reduce the amount of oxygen required by brain tissues.

infiltration (in-fil-trā'shun). In anesthesiology, a method of producing local anesthesia by needle-injection of anesthetic solutions.

insufflation (in-suf-flā'shun). In anesthesiology, a method of producing general anesthesia by blowing gases and vapors into the airways.

intracapsular (in-tra-kap'sul-ar). *adj.* Within or into a joint capsule.

intracutaneous (in-tra-kyūt-ān'ē-us). *adj.* CUT=skin. In anesthesiology, an adjective describing the method of producing local anesthesia by injecting an anesthetic liquid into the skin by means of a needle. Similar methods used in other locations are intracap'sular, intradur'al, intramus' cular, intraorb'ital, and intrathec'al.

intradural (in-tra-dūr'al). *adj.* Within the dura.

intramuscular (in-tra-mus'kyūl-ar). *adj.* Within or into a muscle.

intraorbital (in-tra-orb'i-tal). *adj.* Within the orbit.

intrathecal (in-tra-thēk'al). *adj.* Within or into a sheath.

intubation (in-tūb-ā'shun). In anesthesiology, the placing of an endotracheal tube to facilitate breathing.

laryngospasm (lair-ing'gō-spazm). Spasm of the vocal cords, interfering with free respiration.

lidocaine (līd'ō-kān). A drug used to produce local anesthesia. (A proprietary equivalent is **Xylocaine**.)

local anesthesia (an-es-thēz'ē-a). A condition of freedom from pain in a localized portion of the body, induced by infiltration with anesthetic agents through a needle (in medical jargon it is referred to as a "local"). Some commonly used generic solutions are **cocaine, lidocaine** and **procaine**; commonly used proprietary solutions are **Hexylcaine, Metycaine, Novocaine, Nupercaine, Pontocaine** and **Xylocaine.**

morphine (mor'fēn). A pain relieving, habit forming drug derived from opium (sometimes referred to as "morphia").

narcotic (nark-ot'ik). NARC=sleep. A drug given to induce sleep or to relieve pain. The result is a stupor rather than normal sleep. (Also used as an adjective.) Commonly used narcotic drugs are **codeine, Demerol** and **morphine.**

nerve block. Production of anesthesia in a region of the body by injecting anesthetic material around the nerve or nerves supplying that region.

opiate (ōp'ē-āt). Any drug derived from opium. Generally it is sleep inducing, pain relieving, and also habit forming, i.e., a **narcotic.**

oxygen (oks'i-jen). A gaseous element essential to the maintenance of life. It is always administered in conjunction with anesthesia-producing gases and vapors.

Penthrane (pen'thrān). Another proprietary anesthesia-producing vapor given by inhalation.

pentobarbital sodium (pen-tō-barb'i-tal). A sedative drug, frequently given preoperatively. (A proprietary equivalent is **Nembutal.**)

Pentothal sodium (pen'tō-thal). A proprietary drug commonly used in anesthesia. It is usually given intravenously, occasionally by rectum. The generic name is **thiopental sodium.**

peridural (per-ē-dūr'al). *adj.* Referring to a position around the **dura**; in anesthesiology, it is equivalent to **extradural.**

plexus (pleks'us). In anesthesiology, a network of nerve fibers, or nerve centers, controlling sensation in a specific area.

premedication (prē-med-i-kā'shun). Medication given before administering an anesthetic to increase its effectiveness and to protect against certain side reactions.

procaine (prō'kān). Probably the most commonly used of the drugs injected to produce local or regional anesthesia. (**Novocaine** is a common proprietary form.)

reflex. An involuntary muscle reaction occurring in response to a stimulus. Common reflexes bothersome to anesthesiologists are the **"gag reflex"** and **laryngospasm.** Most dangerous, perhaps, is the **"vago-vagal" reflex** which slows, or may even stop, the heart.

regional anesthesia. The loss of sensation in a region of the body by interruption of its nerve supply. It is administered by *field block* and *nerve block.* Other examples of blocks are *caudal block, cervical ganglion block, "saddle block," sphenopalatine ganglion block, spinal block, splanchnic ganglion block, stellate ganglion block,* and *subarachnoid ganglion block.*

relaxant. In anesthesiology, a drug given to produce muscular relaxation.

resuscitation (rē-sus-si-tā'shun). The act of restoring someone to life or consciousness by physical measures such as **"artificial" respiration** and **"cardiac massage."**

"saddle block". Medical jargon for a low-spinal anesthetic. The area anesthetized corresponds to that which would be in contact with a saddle.

scopolamine (skōp-ol'a-mēn). A drug frequently employed to diminish preoperative apprehension and to protect against possible side effects and/or undesirable reflexes.

sedative (sed'a-tiv). A general name for "a calmer downer" drug, sometimes called a tranquilizer. Also used as an adjective. Commonly used examples are **Equanil** and **Valium.**

"spinal". Medical jargon for the injection of an anesthetic solution into the **subdural space,** to temporarily anesthetize the spinal cord below that level.

thiopental sodium (thī-ō-pen'tal). *See* **Pentothal sodium** (proprietary).

tidal exchange. The amount of air involved in each normal respiratory cycle. (Also called **tidal air.**)

topical anesthesia. The production of anesthesia of the surface of an area or organ by swabbing, painting, or spraying the area with a particular anesthetic agent. Commonly used agents for producing topical anesthesia are **Benzocaine, Butesin, cocaine, ethyl chloride,** and **Xylocaine.**

trachea (trāk'ē-a). The cartilaginous air passage starting beneath the larynx and terminating in the two bronchial tubes. (Fig. 24, p. 232)

tranquilizer. An inclusive name for any "quit worrying" drug. (Probably the most overused class of drugs.)

tribromoethanol — tribromethanol (trī-brōm-ō-eth'an-ol, trī-brōm-eth'an-ol). A sleep-inducing drug. (A proprietary equivalent is **Avertin.**)

Trilene (trī'lēn). A commonly used proprietary anesthesia-producing volatile liquid; it is frequently self-administered by inhalation of the vapor.

vasodepressor (vāz-ō-dē-pres'or). Any one of a number of drugs which lower the blood pressure; they are also called vasodilators. (A drug producing the opposite effect is called a **vasopressor.**)

Vinethene (vīn'e-thēn). A proprietary form of divinyl ether.

⑨ Dentistry

ALTHOUGH DENTISTRY is not a branch of medicine, it seems proper to include a list of dental terms in this book. There is no connection between the American Dental Association and the American Medical Association. Dentistry is a separate profession which has its own rules and regulations and sets its own strict requirements for licensure and practice.

Although dentistry may seem to be a rather narrow profession, it has many branches and subspecialties. Each of these requires additional postgraduate training courses, generally two years in length. An **exodontist** specializes in the extraction of teeth. An **endodontist** specializes in the care of pulpless or no longer vital teeth. A **pedodontist** is interested in the special dental problems of children. A **periodontist** cares for the bony and soft tissues surrounding the teeth. An **orthodontist** focuses his attention on the proper spacing and alignment of teeth for the best aesthetic and functional result. A **prosthodontist** specializes in the proper replacement of teeth. An **oral surgeon** does surgery of the jaws and oral cavity.

There is considerable interchange between the professions of medicine and dentistry. Dentists realize and carry out their responsibility to refer cases of cancer, systemic infections, congenital abnormalities, etc. to physicians. Medical men, by the same token, refer more and more of their suspected cases of dental infection and dental problems to dentists. Oral surgeons and orthodontists are frequently consulted by plastic and other surgeons.

A **dental assistant** is generally trained in a dental assisting course at the community college level, or by the dentist she assists. She does not require a special license. A **dental hygienist,** on the other hand, must be licensed. She is allowed to do work in the oral cavity of patients but generally restricts her activity to dental prophylactic care. A **dental techni-**

cian generally works in a dental laboratory where he (or she) assists in preparing dental prostheses, inlays and dentures from casts or molds obtained by the dentist.

In order to obtain a degree in dentistry—generally D.D.S., (but D.M.D. in Oregon)—an individual must complete a four-year course in a dental college. From two to four years of preliminary college work is required for admission to a dental college.

CONSULTANT

Robert S. Tuttle, D.D.S.
Santa Rosa, California

abrasion (a-brā′zhun). In dentistry this term refers to the wearing down of teeth from the continuous wear and tear of use in **mastication.**

abutment (a-but′ment). In dentistry, the tooth that provides the point of anchorage and support for a bridge or other orthodontic appliance.

acrylic resin (a-kril′ik rez′in). Plastic material usually used in fabricating dentures or crowns, or occasionally as a restorative filling material.

A.D.A. Abbreviation for the name of the American Dental Association.

alloy (al′loy). The product when two or more metals are fused by heat. Technically, the result is a mixture and not a chemical compound. The term is generally used to designate silver filling material.

alveolar process (al-vē′ō-lar). The part of the bone which projects above the surface of the mandible or the maxilla, supporting the teeth and forming their sockets.

alveolus (al-vē′ō-lus). In dentistry, the tooth socket in the **alveolar process.** (*plural* — alve′oli.)

anaerobe (an′er-ōb). AER=air. A microorganism which can grow in the absence of oxygen — in fact, exposure to air generally destroys the organism. (*adj.* — anaerob′ic.)

anodontia (an-ō-don′sha). DONT= tooth. Absence of teeth, due either to their natural absence (lack of formation or failure of eruption) or subsequent loss. (*adj.* — anodon′tik.)

antisialogogue (an-tē-sī-al′ō-gog). Medication which reduces the flow of saliva.

apex (ā′peks). In dentistry, this term refers to the tip of the root of a tooth. (*adj.* — ap′ical.) (Fig. 6, p. 67)

aphthous ulcer (af′thus). *See* **aphthous stomatitis.**

apical foramen (āp′i-kl for-ā′men). The foramen in the end of a root through which the dental nerve enters the tooth. (Fig. 6, p. 67)

apical curettement (kyūr-et′ment). Surgical removal of infectious material surrounding the apex of a root, but not involving removal of the root.

apicoectomy (āp-i-kō-ek′tō-mē). Surgical removal of the apex of a tooth root.

articulate (ar-tik′yūl-āt). *verb.* To adjust the relationship of natural or artificial teeth in one jaw to those of the opposite jaw for proper mastication.

articulator (ar-tik′yūl-ā-tor). An instrument for holding models or casts of a patient's dental arches and teeth in proper relationship to facilitate acquiring proper occlusion with the teeth of the opposite jaw.

artifact — or **artefact** (art′i-fakt). A false image *or* shadow on an x-ray film due to unnatural mechanical factors, and therefore of no significance.

aspirate (as′pir-āt). *verb.* To remove or withdraw by suction.

aspirator (as′pir-ā-tor). A piece of equipment consisting of a hose and suction nozzle used to aspirate debris, saliva and water from the patient's mouth during dental treatment.

bicuspid (bī-kusp′id). A tooth having two **cusps.** There are two bicuspids in each quadrant of the mouth. They are located between the **cuspids** and the **molars.** (Fig. 7, p. 69)

bitewing radiograph (bīt′wing). A specific type of dental x-ray that shows, on one film, the crowns of upper and lower teeth and their supporting tissues. A bitewing film is generally taken to disclose interdental decay.

"bleeder." A general term applied to a patient with coagulation problems. This is important in dentistry because of the frequent inaccessibility of the bleeding point.

bridge work. A general term indicating dental prostheses which support a tooth or teeth, and which replace missing teeth. The ends of a bridge are generally anchored to firm teeth on either side of the missing tooth.

bruxism (bruks'izm). Grinding or clenching the teeth, generally occurring when asleep or when under severe nervous strain.

buccal (buk'kl). *adj.* Pertaining to the cheek. The buccal surface of a tooth is that one located next to the cheek.

bur—burr. A small rotary cutting instrument of steel operated in a dental drill. A bur is used for cutting teeth, cement or metal.

burnishing (bur'nish-ing). Polishing by friction.

candidiasis (kan-did-ī'a-sis). A mouth infection due to fungi of the genus candida.

canine (kān'īn). A name sometimes given to the two cuspid teeth of the upper jaw. *See* **cuspid.**

"canker sore" (kang'ker). *See* **aphthous stomatitis.**

caries (kair-ēz). Decay in tooth structure. (*adj.*—carious.)

cavity (kav'i-tē). A hollow or hole in a tooth produced by dental caries. Cavities may involve one or more surfaces of a tooth.

cementum (sē-ment'um). The hard bone-like substance that covers the **dentine** of the roots of the teeth. (Fig. 6, p. 67)

cervical line (serv'i-kl). The barely visible line of junction between the **enamel** (covering the crown) and the **cementum** (covering the root) of a tooth. (Fig. 6, p. 67)

compound. A name frequently given to a wax-like product used in dental offices. It can be molded when warmed.

condyle (kon'dīl). In dentistry, the projecting knob at the end of the **mandible** which articulates with the rest of the skull.

crown. The part of a tooth which is normally visible in the mouth and which is covered with enamel. An artificial crown is a cap of plastic or metal that acts as a restoration for the natural crown. (Fig. 6, p. 67)

cusp (kusp). A marked elevation or projection on the **masticating** surface of a tooth.

cuspid (kusp'id). A tooth with one **cusp.** There are four cuspids, one in each quadrant, located between the **incisors** and the **bicuspids.** The upper cuspids are sometimes called canines or eye teeth. (Fig. 7, p. 69)

D.D.S. Abbreviation for Doctor of Dental Surgery, the degree awarded at the completion of four years of formal study in an accredited dental college. In some states the degree awarded is D.M.D. (Doctor of Dental Medicine).

deciduous teeth (dē-sid'yū-us). The twenty teeth of childhood which are normally replaced by permanent teeth. Other names are milk teeth, primary teeth and baby teeth.

dental assistant. DENT=tooth. *See* introductory paragraphs.

dental hygienist (hī-jē-en'ist). *See* introductory paragraphs.

dental plaque (plak). A tenacious mat of microbial colonies that forms on tooth surfaces. There is a close relationship between plaque formation and dental caries.

"dental stone." A variation of plaster of Paris (much harder and stronger) used for making dies and models from which crowns, inlays, and other dental appliances can be fabricated in a dental laboratory.

dental surfaces. The various surfaces of a tooth:

labial surface (lāb'ē-al). The surface of a tooth facing the lips.

lingual surface (ling'gwal). The surface of a tooth facing the tongue.

buccal surface (buk'kl). The surface of a tooth facing the cheek.

occlusal surface (ok-klūz'al). The chewing or biting surface of a tooth.

facial surface. A term designating the buccal and labial surfaces of the teeth, collectively.

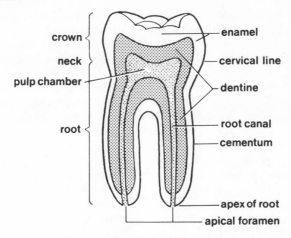

crown

neck

pulp chamber

root

enamel

cervical line

dentine

root canal

cementum

apex of root

apical foramen

FIG. 6. Structure of a Tooth

dental technician. *See* introductory paragraphs.

dentifrice (dent'i-fris). Tooth paste or tooth powder.

dentine (dent'in). The tissue of a tooth beneath the enamel. It comprises the greater bulk of a tooth and is somewhat softer than tooth enamel. (Fig. 6, p. 67)

dentition (den-tish'un). A name used to designate the general character and arrangement of the teeth taken as a whole.

denture (dent'chur). An artificial substitute for missing teeth.
 immediate denture. A prosthesis which is inserted into the mouth immediately following the extraction of teeth.
 partial denture. A replacement for one or more lost teeth.
 complete denture. A dental prosthesis that replaces all the upper or lower teeth.

edentulous (ē-dent'yūl-us). *adj.* Without teeth.

enamel (en-am'el). The hard tissue that covers the dentine of the crown portion of the teeth. Tooth enamel is the hardest natural material in the body. It varies in thickness, being thickest over the chewing and biting surfaces of the teeth. (Fig. 6, p. 67)

endodontics (end-ō-dont'iks). A branch of dentistry which deals with the care of **pulpless teeth** (teeth no longer vital).

endodontist (end-ō-dont'ist). *See* introductory paragraphs.

engine. In dentistry this refers to the power plant which activates various pieces of dental equipment.

epulis (ep'yūl-is). A fibrous tumor of the gums, usually attached to the jaw bone. It is usually benign.

eruption (ē-rup'shun). In dentistry, the progression of a new tooth into the mouth from its place of formation.

exodontics (eks-ō-dont'iks) — **exodontia.** A branch of dentistry that deals with the extraction of teeth.

exodontist (eks-ō-dont'ist). *See* introductory paragraphs.

exostosis (eks-os-tōs'is). OS=bone. In dentistry, an outgrowth from the root of a tooth.

expectorate (eks-pek'tor-āt). *verb.* To spit.

explorer. A strong, thin instrument with a sharp point which comes in various shapes. It is used to test the surface of the teeth for cavity formation.

extraction. The removal of a tooth from the mouth ("pulling a tooth").

eye tooth. A name sometimes given to either of the two cuspid teeth of the upper jaw.

floss. Nylon or silk cord which has been waxed; it is used to clean the spaces between the teeth.

fluoridation (flūr-i-dā'shun). Introduction of fluoride into the water supply as a preventive measure against dental caries.

fluoride (flūr'īd). A chemical sometimes introduced into the water supply to prevent or retard dental caries.

foramen (for-ām'en). A hole or channel, particularly in bone, through which nerves and blood vessels pass. (*plural*—foramina.)

forceps (for'seps). In dentistry, any one of several kinds of pliers-like instruments for grasping teeth. Various designs of the forceps' jaws accommodate to different teeth in different locations in the mouth.

fossa (fos'sa). A round or angular depression or pit on the surface of a tooth. Fossae occur most commonly on the lingual surface of the **incisors** and on the occlusal surfaces of the **bicuspids** and **molars**. (*plural*—fossae.)

gingiva (jin'jiv-a). The gum. Technically, that part of the oral mucous membrane which covers the necks of the teeth and the alveolar process. (*plural*—gingivae.)

gingivitis (jin-jiv-īt'is). Inflammation involving the gum tissue only.

gingivoglossitis (jin-jiv-ō-glos-sīt'is). Simultaneous inflammation of the gums and tongue.

gingivostomatitis (jin-jiv-ō-stōm-a-tīt'-is). Inflammation involving both the gums and the mucous lining of the mouth.

impacted tooth (im-pak'ted)—**impaction.** Generally, a tooth that has been prevented from erupting because of being inbedded in the soft or bony tissues of the jaw in an abnormal manner.

impression. A "negative" likeness of teeth or of the jaws, produced by a dentist by allowing a suitable material to "set" in the mouth. When set, the impression is used to make a "positive" cast or model of the original structures.

incisor (in-sīz'er). One of the four teeth in the middle of each jaw, two in each quadrant. The incisors are cutting teeth. The four nearest the middle of the jaw are called the central incisors; those next are called the lateral incisors. (Fig. 7, p. 69)

inlay (in'lā). A dental inlay is a filling made outside of the mouth from a model or mold of the cavity into which it will be cemented to restore the missing tooth.

interdental space (in-ter-dent'al). The space between two adjacent teeth.

investment. A plaster like material in which inlays, crowns and dentures are enclosed during casting, soldering and curing.

leukoplakia (lūk-ō-plāk'ē-a). White patches in the mouth, sometimes seen by dentists but not generally due to dental conditions.

Ludwig's angina (Lud'wigz anj-ī'na). A specific inflammation of the floor of the mouth sometimes seen by dentists but generally not due to dental conditions. (The unusual use of the term **angina** suggests that it really hurts!)

malocclusion (mal-ok-klū'zhun). Deviation from the normally acceptable contact of the teeth of the upper jaw with those of the lower jaw.

mandible (mand'i-bl). The horseshoe shaped bone forming the lower jaw. (*adj.*—mandibular.)

masticate (mast'i-kāt). *verb.* To chew. (*noun*—mastica'tion.)

maxilla (maks-il'la). The upper jawbone. (*adj.*—maxillary.)

mental foramen. The aperture in each side of the **mandible** through which the mental nerve emerges to join the mandibular nerve.

molar (mol'ar). A grinding tooth. There are three molars in each dental quadrant. They are the teeth farthest from the midline and are designed to perform the grinding part of mastication.

The third molar is sometimes called the "wisdom tooth" and generally does not erupt until the patient is well into his teens. (Fig. 7, p. 69)

moniliasis (mōn-i-lī′a-sis). A disease affecting the lining of the mouth, sometimes seen by dentists. Another name is "thrush."

occlusion (ok-klū′zhun). The natural fitting together of the upper and lower teeth when the mouth is closed. Occlusion is also important during the movements of the lower jaw involved in the act of chewing.

odontalgia (ō-dont-alj′ē-a). Toothache!

odontology (ō-dont-ol′ō-jē). A synonym for dentistry, especially in Europe where dentistry is starting to be regarded as a branch of medicine.

operative dentistry. That branch of dentistry concerned with the care and restoration of carious or damaged teeth as compared, for example, with **orthodontic** dentistry.

oral surgeon. A dentist who specializes in surgery of the oral cavity. An oral surgeon generally also does extractions.

orthodontics (orth-ō-dont′iks) — **orthodontia.** That branch of dentistry which deals with the causes, prevention and treatment of irregularities in the position of the teeth.

orthodontist (orth-ō-dont′ist). *See* introductory paragraphs.

palate (pal′at). The roof of the mouth. *See* **soft palate.**

pedodontics (pēd-ō-dont′iks) — **pedodontia.** The branch of dentistry that deals with dental conditions in children.

pedodontist (pēd-ō-dont′ist). *See* introductory paragraphs.

periapical abscess (per-ē-āp′i-kl). An abscess which develops around the root of a tooth.

periodontics (per-ē-ō-dont′iks) — **periodontia.** The branch of dentistry that deals with the prevention and treatment of disease of the bone and the soft tissues surrounding the teeth.

periodontist (per-ē-ō-dont′ist). *See* introductory paragraphs.

permanent teeth. The second set of teeth (32 in number) as distinguished from the **deciduous teeth** (20 in number). See Fig. 7, below.

phenol (fēn′ol). Carbolic acid, sometimes used to cauterize a cavity or as a disinfectant and germicide.

plaster of Paris. Roasted calcium sulphate powder which hardens when mixed with water. It is used by dentists to make casts and impressions. *See* **dental stone.**

prophylaxis (prō-fil-aks′is). In dentistry the term generally refers to the removal of tartar and stains from the

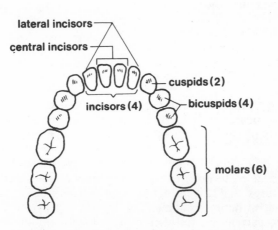

lateral incisors
central incisors
cuspids (2)
incisors (4)
bicuspids (4)
molars (6)

FIG. 7. Permanent Lower Teeth

surfaces of the teeth. It also refers to fluoride treatment of water supplies. (*adj.* – prophylac'tic.)

prosthesis (dental) (pros-thēs'is). Any replacement for natural dentition, such as a denture, bridge, partial denture, etc.

prosthodontics (pros-thō-dont'iks). The branch of dentistry that deals with the planning and fitting of partial and complete dentures. A synonym is prosthodontia.

prosthodontist (pros-thō-dont'ist). *See* introductory paragraphs.

pulp. The soft tissue found in the central cavity of a tooth (**pulp chamber**). It contains the nerve, blood vessels and lymphatic vessels which connect the tooth with the rest of the body.

pulp chamber. The central cavity of the tooth. It lies in the crown of the tooth and continues down the dental roots. It contains the blood vessels and nerves of the tooth. (Fig. 6, p. 67)

pulpitis (pulp-ī'tis). Inflammation of the dental pulp.

pulpectomy (pulp-ek'tō-mē). The complete surgical removal of the pulp of a tooth.

pulpotomy (pulp-ot'ō-mē). The removal of part of the pulp of a tooth. It is sometimes used in children's dentistry.

pumice (pum'is). Powdered volcanic ash used in cleaning and polishing teeth or dentures.

ramus (rām'us). In dentistry, the part of the mandible which is in back of the posterior teeth.

R.D.H. Abbreviation for Registered Dental Hygienist.

resorption (rē-sorp'shun). In dentistry, the gradual disappearance of the root of a tooth, particularly the root of a **deciduous tooth.**

restoration (rest-or-ā'shun). A broad term sometimes used to refer to the artificial structures that are used to replace missing structures: fillings, inlays, bridges, partial and full dentures, etc.

retainer. *See* space maintainer.

root. The portion of a tooth which is fixed in the tooth socket. Roots are covered with **cementum.** (Fig. 6, p. 67)

root canal. The continuation of the pulp chamber which traverses the length of the root of a tooth. It contains pulp tissue and ends at the apical foramen at the end of the root. (Fig. 6, p. 67)

rouge (rūzh). Iron oxide, used in cake or stick form, as a mild abrasive to polish certain teeth.

rubber dam. A thin sheet of very lively rubber which a dentist perforates and fits over the tooth or teeth on which he is working in order to isolate the area from the rest of the oral cavity.

saddle. The part of the base of a denture (partial or complete) which distributes the stress of mastication to the alveolar ridge. It usually carries replacement teeth.

scaling (skāl'ing). A dental procedure carried out to remove tartar and necrotic tissue from around the neck and roots of the teeth. It is commonly performed in the "cleaning" of the teeth.

sialadenitis (sī-al-ad-en-īt'is). Inflammation of a salivary gland which is sometimes detected by dentists.

soft palate. The horseshoe-shaped muscle forming the top and sides of the opening of the mouth into the throat. The **uvula** hangs down from the middle of the oval structure.

space maintainer (not container or retainer). An appliance constructed to prevent teeth from encroaching upon a space from which teeth have been lost prematurely. It is used by orthodontists to prevent malocclusion.

spatulation (spat-yūl-ā'shun). Mixing by means of a flat blunt instrument.

stomatitis (stōm-a-tīt'is). A general term referring to ulceration in the mouth.

sublingual (sub-ling'gwal). *adj.* LINGUA=tongue. Beneath the tongue.

submaxillary (sub-maks'il-lair-ē). *adj.* Beneath the mandible.

supernumerary tooth (sūp-er-nūm'er-air-e). A tooth in excess of the normal number.

synthetic (sin-thet'ik). A substance formed (synthesized) by artificial means as opposed to having been formed by natural processes. In dentistry the term generally designates a tooth colored filling material, "synthetic porcelain."

tartar (tar'ter). A hard deposit on the teeth, more properly called "salivary calculus." It is most common on those dental surfaces nearest the salivary ducts.

"trench mouth." A name sometimes given to **Vincent's angina.**

trituration (trit-tūr-ā'shun). The mixing of two or more constituents by grinding or rubbing.

ulcerative stomatitis (ul'ser-ā-tiv stōm-a-tīt'is). Discrete ulcers of the mouth, gums, and cheeks which are sometimes seen by dentists.

Vincent's angina. A specific disease of the gums, mouth or tonsils which is often seen by dentists.

"wisdom teeth." A name sometimes applied to the four third molars which normally erupt in the late teens.

10 Dermatology

THE FIELD OF DERMATOLOGY encompasses the diagnosis and treatment of diseases of the skin and the diagnosis of internal disorders manifested by changes in the skin. Dermatology might more concisely be described as cutaneous medicine. Diseases of the skin and its related mucous membranes represent probably ten percent of the practice of medicine. This may be explained by the fact that the skin is the largest organ of the body, weighing approximately ten pounds. The terminology of dermatology is difficult because it has retained more Latin nomenclature than the other specialties.

The scope of dermatology becomes apparent when we consider the many functions of the skin; the many systemic disorders which have cutaneous signs and symptoms; the many drug reactions which involve the skin; the daily contact of the skin with potential irritants and allergens; its vulnerability to injury; its tendency to produce tumors, both benign and malignant; and the social and industrial importance of even one skin symptom like itching. The complex perfection of its strong, dense, elastic, waterproof, thermal proof, almost puncture proof construction is nothing short of phenomenal.

Certification of a doctor by the American Board of Dermatology specifies three to four years of specialty training preceding appropriate written and personally conducted examination interviews by members of the Board.

CONSULTANTS

Walter E. Weber, M.D.
Diplomate, American Board of Dermatology; Former Associate Clinical Professor, Dermatology, Stanford University School of Medicine
Santa Rosa, California

Warren K. Hanson, M.D.
Diplomate, American Board of Dermatology; Assistant Professor, Dermatology, Stanford University School of Medicine
San Francisco, California

Paul M. Crossland M.D.*
Diplomate, American Board of Dermatology; Former Assistant Professor, Dermatology, Stanford University School of Medicine
Santa Rosa, California
*deceased

acanthosis (a-kan-thō′sis). Thickening of the prickle cell layer of the skin. (*adj.*—acanthot′ic.)

acne (ak′nē). A skin condition involving inflammation of the **sebaceous glands.** (*adj.*—acne′ic, acne′iform.)

acne vulgaris (vul-ga′ris). The usual type of acne, most common among teen-agers.

actinic (ak-tin′ik). *adj.* Relating to the rays of the electromagnetic spectrum (ultraviolet rays, x-rays, etc.).

allergen (al′er-jen). A substance capable of producing an allergic reaction (sometimes a **dermatitis**). (*adj.*—allergen′ic.)

allergy (al′er-jē). The state of being hypersensitive to an agent, condition or situation. (*adj.*—aller′gic.)

alopecia (al-ō-pē′shē-a *or* al-ō-pē′sha). Total or partial baldness.

alopecia areata (a-rē-a′ta). Baldness occurring in spots and generally appearing suddenly.

angioma (an-jē-ō′ma). ANG=blood vessel. An abnormal, **benign** skin tumor consisting mostly of blood vessels. (*adj.*—angiom′atous.)

angioma cavernosum (kav-er-nō′sum). An angioma in which the blood vessels are relatively large and deep.

angioma, strawberry. A strawberry colored birthmark, sometimes seen in infants, consisting of an enlargement of the superficial blood vessels.

angioneurotic edema (an-jē-ō-nū-rot′ik e-dē′ma). A disorder generally involving the superficial blood vessels and sometimes called "giant urticaria." It may also include swelling of other areas, particularly the larynx.

anhidrosis (an-i-drō′sis). HIDR=sweat. An abnormal partial or complete inability to excrete sweat. (*adj.* anhidrot′ic.)

antifungal (an-tē-fung′gal). An agent used to combat fungus infection. (Also used as an adjective.)

antipruritic (an-tē-prū-rit′ik). PRUR= itch. An agent used to relieve or prevent itching. (Also used as an adjective.)

aphtha (af′tha). A characteristic mouth lesion due to one of several causes (generally called "canker sore"). (*adj.*—aph′thous; *plural*—aph′thae.)

aphthous stomatitis (af′thus stōm-a-tī′tis). STOMA=mouth. A characteristic disease of the lining of the mouth ("canker sores").

atopic dermatitis (ā-top′ik derm-a-tī′tis), DERM=skin. A characteristic skin condition that sometimes occurs in hypersensitive individuals (those susceptible to allergies like the eczema–hay fever–asthma complex).

autoeczematization (aw-tō-ek-zem-it-i-zā′shun). A characteristic skin condition apparently brought on by sensitization to a person's own skin allergens.

basal cell epithelioma (ep-i-thēl-ē-ōm′a). A particular type of skin cancer related to the basal cells of the epidermis.

blepharitis (blef-ar-ī′tis). BLEPH=eyelid. An inflammatory condition of the eyelid margins.

bulla (bul′la). A large blister. (*adj.*— bul′lous.)

Burow's solution (Bur′rōz). An agent commonly used in preparing wet dressings for certain skin disorders.

calcinosis cutis (kal-sin-ō′sis kyūt′is). CALC=stone. A broad term referring to a condition in which calcium is deposited in the skin in abnormal amounts.

callus (kal′lus). A localized hardened, thickened area of skin, generally the result of repeated friction or pressure (sometimes called a **callos′ity**).

carbuncle (kar′bung-kl). A specific, extensive, deep type of bacterial inflammation of the skin and subcutaneous tissues.

chancre (shang′ker). The primary, ulcerated lesion of **syphilis** occurring at the site of inoculation. Chancres are also characteristic of tuberculosis of the skin, and of anthrax.

chancroid (shang′kroyd). A venereal, genital infection which is not syphilitic.

cheilitis (kīl-ī′tis). CHEIL=lips. A broad term describing any inflammatory process of the lips.

chloasma (klō-as′ma). A patchy (generally brownish) discoloration of the skin. Although the cause is not known, it is frequently associated with pregnancy.

chondritis (kon-drī′tis). CHONDR= cartilage. A term denoting an inflammatory condition of **cartilage.** Dermatology is concerned only when the affected cartilage lies directly beneath the skin.

clavus (klāv′us). A nice name for a corn.

collagen disease (kol′la-jen). A broad term including those conditions in which **collagen** (the connective tissue portion of the true skin and of other organs) is disturbed. Examples are **lupus erythematosus** and **scleroderma.**

comedo (kō-mē′dō). The dried secretion of an oil gland in the skin; a "blackhead." (*plural*—comedon′es.)

condyloma acuminatum (kon-dil-ōm′a a-kyūm-in-a′tum). A particular kind of wartlike growth (sometimes venereal) seen on the genito-anal regions. Like all warts, it is due to a **virus.** (*plural*—condyl′mata acumina′ta.)

corium (kōr′e-um). The true skin or **dermis** located beneath the epidermis.

cryotherapy (krī-ō-ther′a-pē). CRYO= cold; THERAP=treatment. Treatment of skin conditions with the application of refrigerants, such as carbon dioxide, liquid nitrogen and liquid oxygen.

curettage (kyūr-e-tahzh′). In dermatology, the procedure of cleansing the bottom of an excavated lesion by scraping.

cutaneous (kyūt-ā′nē-us). *adj.* CUT= skin. Relating to the skin.

cuticle (kyūt′i-kl). The **epidermis** (the outer layer of the skin) surrounding a nail.

cyanosis (sī-an-ō′sis). A bluish discoloration of the skin and **mucous membranes,** particularly that caused by deficient oxygen content in the blood (brought on by venous congestion).

dandruff (dan′druf). Who doesn't know about dandruff? *See* **seborrhea.**

decubitus ulcer (dē-kyūb′i-tus). Ulceration caused by prolonged external pressure ("bedsore").

depigmentation (dē-pig-men-tā′shun). The removal, absence or loss of natural or inplanted pigments from the skin.

depilatory (dē-pil′a-tō-rē). PIL=hair. An agent used for removing hairs. (Also used as an adjective.)

dermabrasion (derm-a-brā′zhun). DERM=skin. The surgical removing of the outer layer of the skin in any desired thickness by any one of several methods.

dermatitis (derm-a-tī′tis). A very generalized term used to refer to "inflammation of the skin."

dermatitis artefacta   **epidermis**   **75**

dermatitis artefacta (ar-te-fak'ta). Skin injury which is generally self-inflicted.

dermatitis herpetiformis (her-pet-i-form'is). A specific disease characterized by small blisters.

dermatitis medicamentosa (med-i-ka-men-tōs'a). A reaction resulting from drugs taken internally.

dermatitis seborrheica (seb-ō-rē'i-ka). An inflammatory disease characterised by greasy scaling of the skin.

dermatitis venenata (ven-e-na'ta). An acute allergic inflammation caused by contact with an irritant or a contact allergen, such as poison oak, poison ivy, etc.

dermatologist (derm-a-tol'ō-jist). A specialist who practices dermatology.

dermatology (derm-a-tol'ō-jē). *See* introductory paragraphs.

dermatomycosis (derm-a-tō-mī-kō'sis). MYCO=fungus. A general term which covers any skin infection due to a **fungus.**

dermatophytosis (derm-a-tō-fī-tō'sis). A superficial **fungus** infection of the skin due to one of several species of fungi. A common form is "athlete's foot." *See* **epidermophytosis.**

dermatosis (derm-a-tō'sis). A broad term covering any abnormal skin condition. Skin tumors, whether benign or malignant, are not included in the term.

dermis (derm'mis). The layer of the skin between the epidermis (the outer layer) and the subcutaneous fat; the true skin, also called the **cutis.**

dermographia (derm-ō-graf'ē-a). GRAPH=write. A skin condition in which light strokes or pressure produce temporary hive reaction. (Also called **dermographism** and **dermatographism.**)

desiccation (des-i-kā'shun). SIC=dry. In dermatology, a procedure in which skin tissue is dried to an extreme degree by means of a high frequency electrode ("electric needle").

It is often used in connection with **curettage.**

desquamation (des-kwa-mā'shun). The act of shedding or peeling off of the outer layers of the skin, as after sunburn.

detritus (dē-trī'tus). Scales, crusts, and loosened skin. (*adj.*—detrit'ic.)

discoid (dis'koyd). *adj.* A term referring to skin lesions that are well demarcated and resemble a disk.

disseminated (dis-sem'i-nāt-ed). *adj.* Of widespread distribution on the skin; or, accompanied by internal lesions.

"dry ice". The vernacular name for solid carbon dioxide, sometimes used in treating skin conditions.

ecchymosis (ek-i-mō'sis). Escaped blood in the skin or in the superficial tissues (a "black and blue spot"). (*adj.*—ecchymot'ic; *plural*—ecchy-mo'ses.)

ecthyma (ek-thīm'a *or* ek'thim-a). A particular type of skin eruption due to bacteria. The lesion is deeper than **impetigo,** which it resembles.

eczema (ek'ze-ma). A widely inclusive term covering a superficial skin disease which has many forms. (*adj.*—eczem'atous.) (**Eczematoid**=eczema-like.)

eczema, infantile (in'fan-tīl). A broad term sometimes used to refer to several types of **dermatitis** seen in infants.

eczema, nummular (num'yūl-ar). An eczema with coin-shaped lesions.

electrodesiccation, (e-lek-tro-des-i-kā'shun). Another name for **desiccation.**

electrolysis (ē-lek-trol'i-sis). LYS=destroy. An electrical process sometimes used to destroy hair roots. (*adj.*—electrolyt'ic.)

emollient (ē-mol'yent). MOL=soft. An agent (generally an ointment) used to soften the skin. (Also used as an adjective.)

ephelis (e-fēl'is). A fancy name for a freckle. (*plural*—ephel'ides.)

epidermis (ep-i-derm'is). The outer layer of the skin. (*adj.*—epiderm'al.)

epidermophytosis (ep-i-derm-ō-fīt'ō-sis). PHYT=yeast. A skin disorder caused by fungi or yeasts which involves only the **epidermis.**

epilation (ep-i-lā'shun). The removal of the hairs by the roots from an area of the skin.

epithelioma (ep-i-thēl-ē-ōm-a). A skin tumor originating from the **epithelium.** Present usage prefers the term basal cell epithelioma, squamous cell epithelioma, etc. (*adj.* — epitheliom'atous *or* epithel'ioid.)

erysipelas (er-e-sip'e-las). A (**streptococcal**) skin disease frequently accompanied by severe constitutional symptoms (happily, now seldom seen).

erythema (er-i-thēm'a). ERYTH=red. A name applied to many types of redness of the skin which are due to many causes. (*adj.* — erythem'atous.)

erythema multiforme (mul'ti-form-ē). A skin disease with peculiar circular and annular patterns, as the term indicates.

erythema nodosum (nō-dōs'um). A condition characterized by the formation of small reddish nodules, generally on the front of the leg. It may be due to systemic involvement of some sort.

erythroderma — erythrodermia (e-rēth-rō-derm'a). A broad term used to designate any condition in which the skin is reddened.

eschar (es'kar). The crust or scab caused by a burn from exposure to either heat or chemicals.

exanthem (eks-an'them). A particular type of skin eruption. (*adj.* exanthem'atous.)

excoriation (eks-kōr-ē-ā'shun). Loss of the superficial skin layer resulting from scratching or picking.

follicle (fol'i-kl). A structure in the skin from which a hair grows.

folliculitis (fol-lik-yū-lī'tis). Inflammation of the hair follicles.

fulguration (ful-gyū-rā'shun *or* ful-gū-rā'shun). In dermatology, a synonym for **electrodesiccation.**

fungicide (fun'ji-sīd *or* fung-i-sīd'). An agent that kills fungi. (*adj.* — fungicid'al.)

fungus (fung'gus). A primitive form of plant life which may cause skin infections as well as infection of other organs. (*adj.* — fung'gous; *pl.* — fung'gi.)

furuncle (fyū'rung-kl *or* fur'ung-kl). A medical term designating a boil.

furunculosis (fur-ung-kyū-lō'sis). Multiple, simultaneous, or recurring boils.

fusiform (fyūs'i-form). *adj.* Spindle shaped.

glabrous (glā'brus). *adj.* Referring to smooth skin, that is, without coarse hair.

granuloma annulare (gran-yū-lō'ma an-yū-lair'e). A skin disease usually arranged in a ring around a normal-appearing center.

grenz rays (grenz). One of the kinds of x-rays used by dermatologists in treating skin conditions.

hemangioma (hēm-an-jē-ōm'a). HEM= blood. *See* angioma.

herpes (her'pēz). An inflammatory (viral) skin disease characterized by successive blister formations. (*adj.* — herpet'ic.)

herpes progenitalis (pro-jen-it-tāl'is). Herpes simplex limited to the genital regions.

herpes simplex (sim'pleks). "Fever blisters" or "cold sores."

herpes zoster (zos'ter). "Shingles," caused by the chickenpox-zoster virus.

hirsutism (hēr'sūt-izm). Abnormal hairiness, particularly of females.

hordeolum (hor-dē'ō-lum). Inflammation of one or more of the sebaceous glands at the edge of the eyelid. (A nice name for a **sty.**)

hyperesthesia (hī-per-es-thēz'ē-a). ESTHE=feeling. Excessive sensitivity of the skin. (*adj.* — hyperesthet'ic.)

hyperkeratosis (hī-per-ker-a-tō'sis). KERAT=horn. Excessive development of the horny layer of the skin.

hypertrichosis (hī-per-trik-ō'sis). — **hypertrichiasis** (hī-per-trik-īa'sis). TRICH=hair. Excessive hairiness. (*adj.* hypertrichōt'ic.)

ichthyosis (ik-thē-ō'sis). A specific series of diseases characterized by rough, dry, scaly skin due to decreased number or diminished function of sweat glands or oil glands.

icterus (ik'ter-us). Jaundice; a yellow skin color most commonly associated with certain liver or gallbladder conditions. (*adj.* — icter'ic.)

impetigo contagiosa (im-pe-tī'gō kon-tāj-ē-ō'sa). A bacterial inflammatory skin disease which is contagious. It is characterized by crusting.

induration (in-dūr-ā'shun). DUR=hard. A state of extreme hardness. (*adj.* — in'durated.)

intertrigo (in-ter-trī'gō). Dermatitis of apposed skin surfaces (under the arms, in the groin, etc.). "Athlete's foot" is the most common type. (*adj.* — intertrig'enous.)

intracutaneous (in-tra-kyūt-ā'ne-us). *adj.* Within the skin. (Same as **intradermal.**)

intradermal (in-tra-derm'al). *adj.* DERM=skin. Within the **dermis.** (Same as **intracutaneous.**)

inunction (in-unk'shun). The rubbing of an oil or ointment into the skin. (Also noun, the material used.)

irradiation (ir-rād'ē-ā-shun). The process of applying or exposing to electromagnetic energy, such as ultraviolet light or x-ray exposure.

keloid (kēl'oyd). An abnormal, heavy, raised scar formation, generally due to unknown causes.

keratin (ker'a-tin). A chemical constituent of the outer skin, hair and nails.

keratolysis (ker-a-tol'i-sis). Separation or destruction of the outer, horny skin layer. (*adj.* — keratolyt'ic.)

keratosis (ker-a-tō'sis). An abnormal horny overgrowth of the outer layer of skin. (*adj.* — keratot'ic.)

kraurosis (kraouw-rōs'sis). A dry, shriveled condition of the skin, generally referring to that of the external genitalia of elderly females.

leonine facies (lē'ō-nīn fā'sēz *or* fā'shēz). A facial condition which imparts a lion-like expression. It is sometimes seen in **leprosy.**

leprosy (lep'rō-sē). A chronic bacterial disease exhibiting many varied features. It is also called **Hansen's disease** and has many skin manifestations.

leukoderma — **leukodermia** (lūk-ō-derm'a). LEUK=white. A condition in which small areas of the skin are abnormally white.

leukoplakia (lūk-ō-plāk'ē-a). In dermatology, a chronic (sometimes precancerous) disease of the mucous membranes which show flattened, white, thickened patches. (*adj.* — leukoplak'ic)

lichen chronicus simplex (lī'ken kron'ikus sim'pleks). A chronic, localized, itchy, papular eruption generally seen about the ankles, elbows, and neck; the skin is generally thickened from scratching.

lichenification (lī-ken-i-fi-kā'shun). A leathery, thickened condition of the skin generally due to chronic irritation.

lichen planus (lī'ken plān'us). A characteristic skin disease with flat, purplish, papular-like lesions.

liquid nitrogen (nīt'rō-jen). A liquid refrigerant used in the treatment of some skin diseases.

liquid oxygen. Another liquid refrigerant used in the treatment of certain skin diseases.

lotio alba (lō'shē-ō alb'a). A compound sulfur solution used in treating some skin diseases.

lunula (lūn'yū-la). The "moon" of a fingernail.

lupus erythematosus (lūp′us er-i-them-a-tō′sus). A **collagen** disease often characterized by special reddish lesions and a "butterfly" rash on the face.

lupus vulgaris (vul-ga′ris). A skin disease due to **tuberculosis,** but often resembling one type of **lupus erythematosus.**

maceration (mas-er-ā′shun). In dermatology, a water-logged condition of the skin resulting from prolonged or repeated wetting, giving a whitish, wrinkled appearance.

macula (mak′yūl-ah)—**macule.** A discolored skin spot which is not elevated above the surface.

maculopapular (mak′yūl-ō-pap′yūl-ar). *adj.* Describing a skin eruption consisting of both **macules** and **papules.**

matrix (mā′triks). The area from which development takes place. In dermatology, the bed from which the nail keeps growing, or the root from which a hair develops.

melanoma (mel-a-nōm′a). MELA= black. A malignant tumor, often black.

mole (mōl). A term frequently used by lay people to designate a raised skin blemish. Many of them are pigmented.

molluscum contagiosum (mol-lus′kum kon-tā-jē-ōs′um). A disease characterized by firm, scattered, umbilicated papules. It is caused by a virus and is contagious and chronic.

moniliasis (mōn-i-lī′a-sis). A general term used to designate any one of a group of conditions caused by the organism Candida (Monilia).

mucocutaneous (myūk-ō-kyūt-ā′nē-us). MUCO=mucus. *adj.* Referring to that line or area where the mucosa lining a body cavity and the external skin meet.

mycosis (mī-kō′sis). A general name for any skin condition caused by a **fungus.**

mycosis fungoides (fung-goy′dēz). A specific, chronic, itchy, skin condition which sometimes ends in malignancy. The term has no relation to fungus infection.

neurodermatitis (nūr-ō-derm-a-tī′tis). NEURO=nerve. A broad term referring to those skin conditions brought on by a disturbance of the cutaneous nerves or of the nervous system.

nevus (nēv′us). A congenital or hereditary skin blemish. (*plural*—nev′i.)

nummular (num′yūl-ar). *adj.* Describing skin lesions resembling a coin.

onychia (ō-nik′ē-a). Inflammation of the nailbed of a finger or toe.

onycholysis (on-ik-ō-lī′sis). The separation or loosening of a nail from the nail bed.

osteoma cutis (os-tē-ōm′a kyūt′is). OS= bone. A bony formation within the skin.

papilloma (pap-il-lōm′a). In dermatology, a skin swelling or tumor or tag resembling a nipple and having a broad base.

papule (pap′yūl). A small, solid skin elevation. (*adj.*—papular.)

paronychia (pa-ron-ik′ē-a). Inflammation around the periphery of a nail.

pediculosis (ped-ik-yū-lō′sis). Infestation with lice.

pediculosis capitis (kap′i-tis). Infestation of the hair of the head with lice.

pediculosis corporis (korp′or-is). Infestation of the body with lice.

pediculosis pubis (pyūb′is). Infestation with crab lice in the pubic hair ("crabs").

pemphigoid (pem′fi-goyd). An eruption which resembles pemphigus but is not pemphigus.

pemphigus (pem′fi-gus). A skin disease, often serious, characterized by large blisters.

periungual (per-ē-ung′gwal). *adj.* Around a nail.

petechia (pe-tē′kē-a). A pinpoint hemorrhage in the skin. It often indicates deeper lying disorders. (*plural,—* pete'chiae.)

photodermatitis (fō-tō-derm-a-tī'tis). An inclusive word referring to any of the inflammatory conditions of the skin caused by exposure to light. (Some photodermatitis may be caused by fluorescent light!)

photosensitive (fō-tō-sen'sit-iv). *adj.* Sensitive to light.

pityriasis rosea (pit-e-rī'a-sis rōs'ē-a). A skin condition characterized by fine, branny, scaling plaques.

plantar (plan'tar). *adj.* Referring to the sole of the foot.

plantar wart. A painful area of skin which develops on the sole of the foot at a pressure point.

pruritus (prūr-ī'tus). A nice word for itching. (*adj.*—prurit'ic.)

psoriasis (sōr-ī'a-sis). A specific, annoying, unpredictable, hard-to-treat skin disease of unknown cause. It is characterized by thickened plaques with white scales.

pulicosis (pul-i-kōs'is). The skin condition resulting from having flea bites.

punch biopsy (bī'op-sē). The flat specimen of skin obtained for microscopic examination when a **punch** (a tubular tool with a sharp edge) is used.

purpura (purp'er-a). A purplish discoloration of the skin resulting from **hemorrhage** into tissue.

pustule (pust'yūl). A pus-containing skin elevation. (*adj.*—pustular.)

pyoderma—pyodermia (pī-ō-derm'á). PYO=pus. Any skin disease characterized by pus formation.

radiodermatitis (rād-ē-ō-derm-a-tī'tis). A term designating a skin reaction or inflammation resulting from overexposure to x-rays, radium, or other radioactive sources.

"ringworm". An old vernacular term designating a contagious, fungus-caused skin disorder often exhibiting ring-like patches.

rosacea (rō-zā'sē-a *or* rō-zā'shē-a). A chronic skin condition involving the

nose, forehead and cheeks (sometimes called **acne rosacea**).

rubella (rū-bel'la). "German measles."

rubeola (rū-bē-ō'la). "Regular measles."

salicylic acid (sal-i-sil'ik). A chemical often used by dermatologists to remove excessive **epidermis.**

sarcoidosis (sar-koid-ō'sis). A skin disease exhibiting various kinds of internal and cutaneous lesions, all characterized by a specific arrangement of the **epithelioid** cells.

scabies (skā'bēz). A skin disease due to a parasite commonly called the itch mite; the disease is often called "the itch" or the "seven-year itch."

scarlatina (skar-la-tēn'a). An old name for a mild form of **scarlet fever.**

scleroderma (skler-ō-derm'a). SCLER= hard; DERM=skin. A chronic skin condition characterized by hardening of the skin.

seborrhea (seb-ō-rē'a). SEB=oil. A condition of abnormal activity of the sebaceous skin glands.

seborrhea oleosa (ō-lē-ōs'a). A seborrhea characterized by oiliness of the skin (oily dandruff).

seborrhea sicca (sik'a). A seborrhea characterized by dryness of the skin, sometimes with scaling (dry dandruff).

sebum (sēb'um). The oil secretion of the sebaceous skin glands.

senile keratosis (sēn'īl ker-a-tō'sis). A dry, persistent, localized scaling of the skin frequently seen in elderly people; it is generally due to excessive sun exposure, and occasionally becomes malignant. A more acceptable term is **actinic keratosis.**

slough (sluff). A cast-off mass of skin, generally accompanied by other dead tissue. (Also used as a verb.)

solar dermatitis (sōl'ar). A general term applying to any one of several skin affections due to exposure to the sun's rays.

squamous cells (skwā'mus). The flat epidermal cells of the skin.

squamous cell carcinoma (kar-sin-ōm′a). A malignant deterioration of some of the squamous cells of the skin.

stasis dermatitis (stā′sis). A skin condition, particularly of the lower legs, supposedly related to the excess venous congestion of the area often associated with **varicose veins.**

stomatitis (stōm-a-tī′tis). STOM= mouth. Inflammation of the lining of the mouth.

subcutaneous (sub-kyūt-ān′ē-us). *adj.* An adjective indicating a position just beneath the skin.

sudoriferous (sūd-or-if′er-us). *adj.* SUDOR=sweat. Referring to the "sweat glands" of the skin.

syphilide (sif′il-ēd)—**syphilid.** A cutaneous manifestation of **syphilis.** (*plural.*—syphil′ides.)

syphilis (sif′il-is). A venereal disease which has systemic effects if it is untreated.

telangiectasis (tel-an-jē-ek′ta-sis). A group of dilated, tiny surface blood vessels. (*plural.*—telangiec′tases.)

tetracycline (tet-ra-sī′klēn). The generic name of an antibiotic widely used in the treatment of skin infections.

tinea (tin′ē-a). A superficial skin infection caused by a **fungus.**

tinea capitis (kap′i-tis). A fungus infection of the scalp.

tinea cruris (krūr′is). A fungus infection of the upper thigh or the genital areas.

tinea pedis (ped′is). A fungus infection of the foot, generally located between the toes.

tinea versicolor (ver-si-kōl′or). A fungus infection characterized by a change of color in the skin, notably white patches.

Treponema pallidum (Trep-ō-nēm′a pal′li-dum). The organism which causes **syphilis.**

Trichophyton (Trī-kof′i-ton). A particular kind of **fungus,** often responsible for skin conditions.

trichophytosis (trik-ō-fi-tō′sis). The result of **Trichophyton** infection. (*plural.*—trichophyto′ses.)

trichosis (trīk-ō′sis). A general term designating any abnormal condition of hair.

trophic ulcer (trof′ik ul′ser). An ulcer resulting from poor nerve or blood supply.

urticaria (urt-i-kair′ē-a). A raised, itchy skin reaction ("hives"). (*adj.* urticar′ial.)

variola (va-rī′ō-la). Smallpox.

verruca (ver-rūk′a). A wart. (*plural.*—verru′cae.)

verruca acuminata (a-kyūm-in-a′ta). A particular, multi-pointed wart, usually seen in the genital or anal regions.

verruca vulgaris (vul-ga′ris). The "garden variety" of wart.

vesicant (ves′i-kant). An agent used to produce blisters.

vesicle (ves′i-kl). A small blister.

vitiligo (vit-il-ī′gō). A skin condition marked by the formation of smooth, light-colored patches.

wart. *See* **verruca.**

wen. An old term applying to a cyst originating from epidermal cells or sebaceous glands.

wheal (wēl). A raised area of skin which is transitory, usually whitish, and generally itchy (a "hive").

xanthelasma (zan-thel-az′ma). A condition characterized by soft yellowish spots on the eyelids due to cholesterol deposits.

xanthoma (zan-thō′ma). A yellowish skin nodule, also due to deposited cholesterol.

xeroderma (zē-rō-derm′a). XERO=dry. A skin condition characterized by abnormal dryness, somewhat similar to **ichthyosis.**

xerosis (zer-ō′sis). A generic term indicating abnormal dryness of the skin.

11 Internal Medicine

INTERNAL MEDICINE INCLUDES the care and treatment of most of the nonsurgical diseases, especially those of the internal organs. It is probably the most extensive specialty of all. Since it includes no surgery, the internist refers his operative patients and then resumes charge of them after their recovery from surgery.

In times past, when medicine consisted of the three specialties — medicine, surgery, and obstetrics — the internist was the "medical doctor." He still represents the medical side of the triad, and although various subspecialties have appeared — allergy, arthritis, endocrinology, hematology, to name a few — the internist is still the central point of medical diagnosis and treatment. His activities probably cover a wider field than any other specialty.

The advances in the care of coronary disease attacks have led to the establistment of "coronary care units" in most hospitals. These units are invariably in charge of internists. Emergency treatment by special ambulance crews, the special knowledge of the nursing staff who receive the patients, and the electronic equipment which allows exact, continuous, visual observation of the patient's progress have notably improved the immediate and long-term mortality rate of coronary disease. Similar improvements have taken place in the recognition and surgical care of cardiac abnormalities, vascular malformations, and pulmonary diseases. Many of these improvements have been initiated by physiologically oriented internists.

The American Board of Internal Medicine requires a three-year approved residency before admitting candidates to examination for certification. The American College of Physicians additionally issues a fellowship degree (F.A.C.P.) to selected approved applicants who exhibit special interest and competence in the nonsurgical specialties.

CONSULTANT

John F. Stegeman, M.D., F.A.C.P.
Diplomate, American Board of Internal Medicine
Athens, Georgia

abeyance (a-bā′ans). A state of temporary inactivity of a disease process.

abort (a-bort′). To check or halt a disease process. *See* "Obstetrics and Gynecology" chapter.

acetone (as′e-tōn). A chemical found in large quantities in the urine of diabetics. It often gives rise to **acidosis.**

acetonemia (as-e-tōn-ēm′ē-a). The presence of large amounts of acetone in the blood, as in diabetic **acidosis.**

acetonuria (as-e-tōn-ūr′ē-a). The presence of large amounts of acetone in the urine. Also called **ketonuria.**

acetylsalicylic acid, (a-set′il-sal-i-sil′ik). Aspirin.

achlorhydria (ā-klor-hid′rēa). CHLOR= hydrochloric acid. The absence of hydrochloric acid from the stomach secretions.

acholuria (ā-kōl-ūr′ē-a). CHOL=bile. The absence of liver bile in the urine. The term generally refers to the absence of this pigment even though jaundice is present.

acid-fast. *adj.* Not readily decolorized by acid or other means when stained. Generally refers to a characteristic posessed by the tubercle bacillus, the organism that causes tuberculosis.

acidosis (as-i-dō′sis). A disorder caused when the body fluids have an abnormally high acid content, as in uncontrolled **diabetes mellitus** and in **uremia.**

acrocyanosis (ak-rō-sī-an-ō′sis). Blueness of the hands and feet due to a disturbance in blood circulation. It is usually a functional disorder of the superficial vessels and does not involve deeper circulation.

ACTH. Abbreviation for **adrenocorticotrophic hormone (corticotropin),** a secretion of the pituitary glands that stimulates the adrenal cortex to secrete **cortisone.**

actinomycosis (ak-tin-ō-mī-kō′sis). A fungus disease usually affecting the mouth and jaws.

Adams-Stokes disease (or syndrome). Transient loss of consciousness due to **asystole** of several seconds' duration. Consciousness usually returns immediately upon reestablishment of normal heart beat.

Addison's anemia (a-nēm′ē-a). *See* **pernicious anemia.** (*adj.* –addison′in.)

Addison's disease. A disease of the adrenal glands in which the glands fail to secrete sufficient hormone to regulate sodium metabolism and thus sustain normal blood pressure.

adenoma (ad-e-nōm′a). A usually **benign** tumor affecting glandular tissue. (*adj.* – adenom′atous.)

adenopathy (ad-en-op′a-thē). A general term denoting any enlargement of the lymphatic glands.

adrenalin (ad-ren′a-lin). A common name for **epinephrine**, a secretion of the adrenal medulla. *Adrenalin chloride* is a medicinal agent with the same properties as natural epinephrine. It is usually given by injection.

adrenocorticotropic hormone (ad-rēn-ō-kort-i-kō-trōp′ik). A secretion of the pituitary gland that stimulates the adrenal cortex to secrete **cortisone.** *See* **ACTH.**

adrenogenital syndrome (ad-rēn-ō-jen′i-tal). A disorder characterized by masculine physical and mental traits in females. It is caused by the oversecretion of hormones by the adrenal glands.

aerobacter (air′ō-bak-ter). A genus of organisms occurring normally in the intestines but capable of causing infection if other organs or tissues are contaminated. It is now called **enterobacter.**

aerophagia (air-ō-fāj-a) – **aerophagy** (air-ō-fajē). PHAG=swallow. The usually involuntary swallowing of air. Aerophagia is displayed by some nervous patients, and may be a cause of belching.

afebrile (ā-fēb'ril). *adj.* Without fever.

agglutination (ag'glūt-in-ā'shun). A clumping by **antibodies** of organisms or cells in a fluid, thus precipitating and neutralizing them. In the laboratory specific diseases can be identified by the presence of antibodies in the patient's blood. They cause clumping of known organisms or cells in a test tube.

agraphia (ā-graf'ē-a). GRAPH=write. Inability to write thoughts, as occurs after certain types of strokes.

ague (ā'gyū). (1) **Malaria.** (2) Any **neuralgia.**

air hunger. Shortness of breath; craving for air.

akinesis (ā-kin-ē'sis). Loss of muscle function. (*adj.* – akinet'ic.)

albino (alb-īn'ō). A person lacking in normal skin, hair and eye pigment.

albumin – albumen (al-byūm'in). An essential protein fraction found in blood and tissues. In a healthy individual, albumin does not usually cross the kidney barrier; it is therefore considered abnormal when it is found in urine.

albuminuria (al-byūm-in-ur'ē-a). The presence of albumin in the urine. It is preferably called **proteinuria.**

alcoholic (al-kō-hol'ik). A person addicted to drinking alcohol.

alcoholism (al'kō-hol-izm). Chronic illness caused by acute or repeated indulgence in alcoholic liquors.

aldosterone (al-dō-ster-ōn' *or* al-dost'er-ōn). A hormone produced by the adrenal cortex. It is involved with electrolyte balance.

aleukemic (a-lūk-ēm'ik). LEUK=white. *adj.* Without leukocytes. It is usually applied to a form of leukemia in which the leukocytes are abnormally low in quantity (instead of increased as in other leukemias).

alexia (a-leks'ē-a). Inability to read, as occurs after certain types of **strokes.**

algesia (al-jēz'ē-a). ALG=pain. Sensitivity to pain.

alimentary canal (al-i-men'ta-rē). The digestive tract from the mouth to the anus.

alkali (al'ka-lī). An agent that neutralizes acid, especially one used for correction of excessive stomach acidity. (*adj.* – al'kaline.)

alkalizer (al'ka-līz-er). **Antacid.**

alkalosis (al-ka-lōs'is). A disorder caused by an abnormally high **alkaline** (basic) content in the blood and in the tissues.

allergy (al'er-jē). An abnormal reaction to an agent due to being oversensitive to it. (*adj.* – aller'gic.)

alopecia (al-ō-pē'sha). Baldness.

alveolitis (al-vē-ō-lī'tis). Inflammation of the alveoli. In pneumonia only localized segments of lung tissue are involved.

amaurosis (am-aw-rō'sis). Blindness due to disturbance of the brain or of the optic nerve, rather than to a defect within the eye itself. (*adj.* amaurot'ic.)

ambulatory (am'byūl-a-tō-rē) – **ambulant** (am'byūl-ant). *adj.* Able to walk; not confined to bed.

amebicide (a-mēb'i-sīd). An agent that destroys **amebas.** (*adj.* – amebicid'al.)

amebic dysentery (a-mēb'ik). Inflammation of the intestines caused by **amebas** that invade intestinal walls.

amenorrhea (ā-men-or-rē'a). Absence of **menstruation.**

ampulla of Vater (am-pul'la of Vat'er). An enlarged portion of the common bile duct and the pancreatic duct at the point where they enter the intestine.

amyloid (am'i-loyd). A starch like substance sometimes abnormally deposited in various organs.

anabolic agent (an-a-bol'ik). An agent which aids in the building up of tissues through its capacity to create a positive nitrogen balance.

anaerobe (an'er-ōb). AER=air. An organism that thrives best in oxygen-deficient surroundings, such as in deep puncture wounds. (*adj.* anaerob'ic.)

anaphylactic shock (an-a-fil-ak'tik). A shock produced by **anaphylaxis.**

anaphylaxis (an-a-fil-aks'is). A severe reaction to a substance, due to being oversensitive to it; a severe allergic reaction involving the whole system.

anasarca (an-a-sar'ka). An abnormal accumulation of fluid within tissues, usually large in amount.

anemia (an-ēm'ē-a). A condition caused by a deficiency of red blood corpuscles or of **hemoglogin.** *See* **Cooley's anemia, megaloblastic anemia, pernicious anemia, Mediterranean anemia,** and **sickle cell anemia.**

   primary anemia. Anemia resulting from a deficiency of blood-forming elements.

   secondary anemia. Anemia produced by a deficiency of iron due to chronic blood loss.

aneurysm — anurism (an'yūr-izm). A bulge in an artery caused by a thinning, stretching, or weakening of its wall.

angiitis (anj-ē-ī'tis). ANG=blood vessel. Inflammation in the wall of a blood vessel.

angina (an-jīn'a). Pain. (*adj.* — an'ginal *or* angi'nal.)

angina pectoris (pek'tor-is). A disease in which sudden chest pains occur, due to narrowing or spasm of one or more coronary arteries, depriving the heart muscle of adequate blood flow during periods of physical or mental stress.

angiogram — angiography (an'jē-ō-gram) (an-jē-og'ra-fē) ANG=blood vessel. X-ray visualization of a blood vessel which has been previously filled with dye to enhance visualization.

angioma (an-jē-ōm'a). A tumor (generally **benign**) made up of blood vessels or lymph vessels.

anorexia (an-or-rek'sēa). Loss of appetite.

antacid. An agent that neutralizes acid. It is usually prescribed to relieve stomach hyperacidity.

antecubital fossa (an-tē-kūb'i-tl fos'sa). The area in front of the elbow joint.

anthelmintic (an-thel-mint'ik). An agent that kills **parasitic** worms.

anticoagulant (an-tē-kō-ag'yū-lant). An agent that inhibits blood coagulation, such as **heparin** or **coumarin** compounds.

antihypertensive (an-tē-hī-per-ten'siv). An agent which counteracts high blood pressure.

antipyretic (an-tē-pī-ret'ik). PYR=heat. An agent that diminishes fever.

antistreptomysin titer (an-tē-strep-tō-mī'sin tī'ter). A laboratory procedure used to help determine whether a patient has been exposed to the bacteria **streptococci.**

antithyroid agent (an'tē-thy-royd). An agent that counteracts the effect of excess thyroid hormones.

antitussive agent (an-ti-tus'siv). A cough reliever.

anuria (an-ūr'ē-a). The absence of urinary secretion. (*adj.* — anur'ic.)

aortitis (ā-or-tī'tis). Inflammation of the wall of the aorta.

aortogram — (ā-ort'ō-gram). — **graphy** (–tog'ra-fē). X-ray of the aorta after distending it with opaque material.

apex. The pointed end of the heart; also the uppermost part of the lung. (*adj.* — ap'ical.)

aphagia (a-fāj'ē-a). Inability to swallow.

aphasia (a-fāz'ē-a *or* a-fāzh'ya). Diminution or loss of one of the powers of expression or understanding, such as inability to speak because of a stroke; *auditory aphasia,* inability to understand words. (*adj.* — aphas'ic.)

aphonia (a-fōn'e-a). PHON=speak. Loss of voice. (*adj.* — aphon'ic.)

aplastic anemia (a-plas'tic). Anemia due to failure of development of red blood cells.

arachnodactyly (a-rak'nō-dak'til-ē). A condition, usually inherited, a characteristic of which is elongation of the fingers.

arrest In medicine, to slow down or to stop, particularly as related to the course of a disease or illness.

arsenical (ar-sen'i-kl). A name given to any agent containing arsenic.

arteriosclerosis (ar-tēr-ē-ō-skler-ō'sis). SCLER=hard. Degenerative hardening of the arteries, often resulting in deficient blood supply to tissues and organs.

arthritis (arth-rīt'is). Inflammation in one or more joints. It is classified into many types.

asbestosis (as-bes-tō'sis). Lung disease caused by inhaling asbestos particles. It is an occupational disease.

ascites (a-sīt'ēz). The abnormal accumulation of fluid in the abdominal cavity, generally due to obstructive liver disease or to cardiac malfunction. (adj.—ascit'ic.)

aspirate (as'pir-āt). (1) To accidentally suck liquids or solids into the trachea (windpipe); (2) to withdraw fluid from a cavity, by suction.

aspirin (as'pir-in). An analgesic **antipyretic** agent. (See **acetylsalicylic acid.**)

asthma (az'ma). A condition characterized by wheezing respiration, due to constriction or spasm of the bronchial tubes. (adj.—asthmat'ic.)

asthmatic (as-mat'ik). A person who suffers from asthma.

astringent (a-strin'jent). An agent that contracts tissues.

asystole (a-sist'ō-lē). Failure of the ventricle to contract at the time of the expected heart beat.

atabrine (at'a-brēn). A drug used prophylactically and actively in the treatment of malaria.

atrium (āt'rē-um) — auricle (awr'i-kl). One of the two upper of the four heart chambers. (See **auricle.**) (Fig. 8, below; Fig. 9, p. 88)

aura (aw'ra). A sensation, usually visual, that sometimes precedes an epileptic attack.

auricle (awr'i-kl). An older term applying to the **atrium.**

auscultate (aws'kul-tāt). verb. To examine by listening, usually with a stethoscope.

auscultation (aws-kul-tā'shun). The act of listening to diagnostic sounds, usually with a stethoscope.

autoagglutination (aw-tō-ag-glūt-i-nā'shun). Clumping of one's blood corpuscles by one's own serum, caused by certain chronic diseases.

avascular (a-vas'kyūl-ar). adj. Without blood.

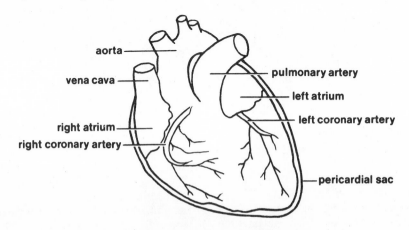

FIG. 8. External View of the Heart

avitaminosis (a-vīt-a-min-ō'sis). A term referring to any one of a number of conditions due to lack of vitamins.

azotemia (ā-zō-tēm'ē-a). The abnormal accumulation of nitrogenous waste products in the blood due to failure of the kidneys to excrete these materials at a satisfactory rate.

Babinski's reflex (Ba-bin'skēs). An abnormal reflex (extension and separation of the toes) when the lower surface of the foot is stimulated.

bacteremia (bak-ter-ēm'ē-a). The presence of **bacteria** in the blood stream.

bactericidal (bak-ter-i-sīd'al). *adj.* Lethal to **bacteria.**

barbital (barb'i-tal). One of the barbiturates.

barbiturate (barb-it'yūr-āt). A composite term including any sleep-producing salt of barbituric acid.

barbiturism (barb-bit'tyūr-izm). A condition caused by taking **barbiturates** habitually or in excessive doses.

basal metabolism (bās'l met-ab'ōl-izm). A term designating the energy expended by a resting person. It is measured in terms of oxygen consumption.

basilar (bās'i-lar). *adj.* Pertaining to the base part of an organ.

"bends." Caisson disease.

beriberi (ber'ē ber'ē). A disease caused by deficiency of Vitamin B_1 in the food intake.

berylliosis (ber-il-ē-ōs'is). A disease caused by exposure to beryllium (usually found in neon fixtures).

bicarbonate (bī-karb'i-nāt). Any salt of carbonic acid. The commonly used sodium salt, soda bicarbonate (baking soda), gives a strongly alkaline reaction.

bigeminy (bī-jem'in-ē). A pulse irregularity characterized by paired beats followed by a short pause, then another round of paired beats, short pause, and so on.

biliary cirrhosis (bil-ē-air'ē sir-rōs'is). A liver disease caused by the backing up of bile into the liver tissue due to

obstruction in the bile ducts. It may cause destruction of liver cells.

blastomycosis (blas-tō-mī-kōs'is). An uncommon disease caused by infection with the fungus Blastomyces.

Boeck's sarcoid (Beks sark'oyd). *See* **sarcoidosis.**

botulism (bot'yūl-izm). Food poisoning usually caused by foods improperly canned. It may seriously affect the central nervous system.

bradycardia (brad-ē-kard'ē-a). BRADY=slow; CARD=heart. Slow heartbeat, a term ordinarily reserved for heart rate below 50 beats per minute.

Bright's disease (Brīts). A common name for nephritis, particularly referring to the chronic, noninfectious type.

Brill's disease (Brilz). An infection resembling typhus fever which is caused by a rickettsial organism.

bromism (brōm'izm). Poisoning caused by overdosage or habitual usage of bromide salts.

bronchiectasis (brong-kē-ek'ta-sis). A chronic inflammatory disease of the lungs in which the walls of a number of alveoli and bronchioles have been destroyed. Such a situation predisposes to chronic infection of the involved portion of the lungs.

bronchiospasm — bronchospasm (brong' kē-ō-spazm) (brong'kō-spazm). Narrowing of the bronchial tubes due to allergy or infection.

bronchitis (brong-kīt'is). BRON=lung. Inflammation of the bronchial tubes.

bronchopneumonia (brong-kō-nū-mōn' ē-a). PNEUM=air. Inflammation of the lungs which arises in the terminal part of the bronchial tubes and is usually due to infection with a specific organism.

Brucella (Brūs-el'la). A genus of bacteria that causes undulant fever **(brucellosis).**

brucellin (brūs-el'lin). A preparation injected into the skin to aid in the diagnosis of undulant fever.

brucellosis (brūs-el-lō′sis). A chronic febrile illness caused by the Brucella organism, usually contracted from infected milk or meat. *See* **Bang's disease** and **undulant fever.**

Brudzinski's sign (Brud-zin′skēz). A diagnostic sign due to inflammation of the meninges. It aids in the diagnosis of **meningitis.**

bruit (brū′ē). A certain abnormal sound sometimes heard when a stethoscope is placed over a blood vessel. It may indicate any one of several conditions.

Buerger's disease (Burg′erz). A disease caused by obliteration of arteries, often leading to gangrene of the parts of the body which are ordinarily supplied by the arteries involved. It is sometimes called thromboangiitis obliterans, and is most often seen in the lower extremities.

bulbar (bulb′ar). *adj.* Referring to the bulb of the brain where vital centers are located.

bundle of His (Hiss). The nerve pathway of the heart that. supplies the impulse for the cardiac muscle to contract.

bursitis (burs-ī′tis). Inflammation of or in a **bursa.**

caisson disease (kās′son). A disease of deep-sea divers and others working under high atmospheric conditions. *See* **"bends."**

cancerogenic (kan-ser-ō-jen′ik). *adj.* Capable of producing **cancer.**

cancerophobia (kan-ser-ō-fōb′ē-a). An obsessive fear of cancer.

capillary (kap′il-lair-ē). The smallest of the blood vessels. They connect arteries to veins.

carboxyhemoglobin (kar-box-ē-hēm′ō-glōb-in). A compound formed by carbon monoxide and hemoglobin in cases of carbon monoxide poisoning.

carboxyhemoglobinemia (karb-oks-ē-hēm-ō-glōb-in-ēm′ē-a). The presence of **carboxyhemoglobin** in the blood due to carbon monoxide poisoning.

carcinogenic (kar-sin-ō-jen′ik). *adj.* Capable of producing **carcinoma** or **cancer.** *See* **cancerogenic.**

carcinoid (kar′sin-oyd). A tumor of low grade malignancy which is often found in the intestines and which produces unusual systemic symptoms.

carcinoma (kar-sin-ōm′a). **A malignant** tumor of epithelial cell derivation.

carcinomatosis (kar-sin-ōm-a-tō′sis). The presence of cancer throughout the body.

cardiac (kard′ē-ak). *adj.* Pertaining to the heart; also, a noun meaning a person suffering from heart disease.

cardiac arrhythmia (a-rith′mē-a). Defect in the rhythm of the heart beat which is often accompanied by a dangerous increase in heart rate.

cardiac cycle (kard′ē-ak sīk′l). The cardiac movements that occur in the heart from the beginning of one heart beat until the beginning of the next beat.

cardiac edema (ē-dēm′a). Edema or swelling due to failure of the heart to circulate the blood properly.

cardiogram (kard′ē-ō-gram). – **cardiograph** (– ō-graf) – **cardiography** (– og′ra-fē). *See* **electrocardiogram**, – ograph, – graphy.

cardiologist (kard-ē-ol′ō-jist). A heart specialist.

cardiology (kard-ē-ol′ō-jē). The study of heart disease.

cardiomegaly (kard-ē-ō-meg′a-lē). Enlargement of the heart.

cardiospasm (kard′ē-ō-spazm). Spasm of the circular muscle at the lower end of the esophagus, often leading to chest pains and **dysphagia.**

cardiovascular (kard-ē-ō-vas′kyūl-ar). *adj.* Pertaining to the heart and the blood vessels.

carditis (kard-ī′tis). Inflamation of any one of the three layers of the heart. *See* **pericarditis, endocarditis, myocarditis.**

caries (kā′rēz). Decay, especially tooth decay (**dental caries**).

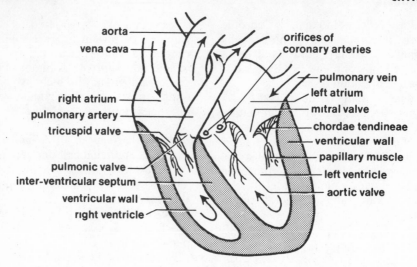

FIG. 9. Internal View of the Heart

Labels in figure:
aorta, vena cava, orifices of coronary arteries, pulmonary vein, left atrium, mitral valve, chordae tendineae, ventricular wall, papillary muscle, left ventricle, aortic valve, right atrium, pulmonary artery, tricuspid valve, pulmonic valve, inter-ventricular septum, ventricular wall, right ventricle

carminative (kar-min′a-tiv). A preparation that relieves distress from gas.

carotenemia (kair-ō-ten-ēm′ē-a) — **carrotemia** — **carotinemia.** The presence of abnormal quantities of yellow pigment, derived from vegetables (especially carrots), in the blood, sufficient to discolor the skin yellow. Also called **carotenosis.**

caseous (kās′ē-us). *adj.* Cheese like; of semisoft consistency and containing irregular cavities.

catabolism (ka-tab′ō-lizm). Breaking down of tissue as opposed to **annabolism,** the building up of tissue, in the metabolic process. (*adj.* — catabol′ic.)

catharsis (ka-thar′sis). Cleansing of the lower alimentary canal by the use of laxatives.

cellulotoxic (sel-yūl-lō-toks′ik). *adj. See* **cytotoxic.**

cervical (serv′i-kl). *adj.* Pertaining to the neck or to the cervix uteri.

Cheyne-Stokes respiration (Chān-Stōks). A type of respiration caused by brain disease, characterized by rapid deep respirations followed by a period of diminished or absent respiration.

cholera (kol′er-a). An acute, often fulminating, intestinal disease which occurs principally in Asiatic countries.

cholesterol (kō-les′ter-ol). A fat-like substance found in all animal tissue. It occurs in the blood stream of humans normally; if present in excess, it may cause a deposit of excess fatty material in the walls of blood vessels. It also forms the substance of a common type of **gallstones.**

chorea (kōr-e′a). A disorder of the nervous system characterized by involuntary and purposeless muscular movement. Also called **St. Vitus dance.**

choreiform (kōr-ē′i-form). *adj.* Muscular movements resembling chorea or caused by **chorea.**

Chvostek's sign (Voz′teks). The reflex movement of the jaw muscles when the facial nerve is stimulated.

cinchonism (sin′kon-izm). Poisoning by quinine or its related compounds.

cirrhosis (sir-rō′sis). (**portal** *or* **Laennec's**). Hardening of the liver, due to degeneration of liver cells. When caused by chronic alcoholism, it is also referred to as *alcoholic cirrhosis.*

claudication (klawd-i-kā'shun). Lameness or pain in a limb brought on by exercise. *See* **intermittent claudication.**

clonus (klōn'us). A series of rhythmic muscular spasms, especially as a response to certain stimuli.

coagulant (kō-ag'yūl-ant). An agent which causes blood clotting.

coccidioidomycosis (kok-sid-ē-oyd-ō-mī-kō'sis). An infectious fungal disease involving various organs. Also called **San Joaquin fever.**

coli (kōl'ē). A group of **bacteria** occurring normally within the intestinal tract, but capable of producing disease in the other tissues when they become contaminated with the organism.

coli, Escherichia (Esh-er-ik'ē-a). Commonly referred to as E. coli, one of the specific members of the coli group.

coliform (kōl'i-form). *adj.* Bacteria resembling those ordinarily found in the intestinal tract.

colitis (kōl-ī'tis). Inflammation of the large intestine, usually giving rise to diarrhea.

collagen disease (kol'la-jen). One of a group of chronic diseases affecting the connective tissue as well as multiple joints and organs.

comatose (kōm'a-tōs). *adj.* In a state of **coma.**

concretio cordis (kon-kresh'ē-ō kord'is). Constriction of the heart muscle due to a diseased adherent **pericardium.**

conus, pulmonary (kōn'us pul'mon-air-ē). PULM=lung. A bulge in the heart shadow as seen on an x-ray film, that corresponds with the pulmonary artery outlet of the right ventricle.

Cooley's anemia (Kūl'ēz an-ēm'ē-a). *See* **thalassemia.**

coronary (kor'ō-nair-ē). *adj.* Pertaining to the blood vessels of the heart muscle; noun, "coronary," a contraction for **coronary occlusion** or **thrombosis.**

coronary arteries. *plural.* Those arteries supplying the heart muscle with blood. (Fig. 8, p. 85)

coronary disease. Disease caused by hardening of the coronary arteries.

coronary insufficiency. Inadequate circulation through the coronary arteries, generally due to arteriosclerosis.

coronary occlusion (ok-klū'zhun). A blockage of a coronary artery, ordinarily known as a "heart attack."

cor pulmonale (kor pul-mon-al'). COR=heart. Insufficiency and dilatation of the right ventricle of the heart due to back pressure within the pulmonary blood circuit created by diseased lungs.

corpuscle, blood (kor'pus-el). A cell that is part of the solid portion of the blood. *Red* blood cell—the cell that transports hemoglobin, the oxygen-carrying agent of the blood. *White* blood cell—the colorless cell of the blood that is used by the body in combating infection.

crenated (krē'nāt-ed). *adj.* Notched appearance of cells that have been damaged by an abnormal environment, particularly referring to the red corpuscles whose cell walls have been damaged by lowered osmotic pressure in the fluid surrounding the cells.

crepitant (krep'i-tant). *adj.* A dry crackling sound heard in certain lung conditions or diseases when a stethoscope is placed over the involved area.

croup (krūp). Laryngitis accompanied by a harsh cough and difficult respiration.

cusp (kusp). One of the triangular segments of a heart valve. They prevent the return flow (escape) of blood when the heart contracts.

cystitis (sist-ī'tis). Inflammation of the urinary bladder.

cytotoxic (sī-tō-toks'ik). *adj.* CYTO=cell. Destructive to cells, especially as applied to agents that destroy or inhibit cancer cells.

decerebrate rigidity (dē-ser′ē-brāt). Muscular rigidity caused by extensive brain damage.

decompensation, cardiac (dē-kom-pen-sā′shun). Failure of the heart muscle to function efficiently, resulting in congestion of the lungs and of other organs and tissues. Also called **congestive heart failure.**

dengue (deng′gē). A mosquito-borne infectious disease characterized by fever and aching.

depressant. (1) A medicine which reduces vital energy, functional activity, and muscular relaxation; (2) A situation or circumstance which tends to create mental depression in a patient.

desensitize (dē-sen′si-tīz). *verb.* To render insensitive to contact with an agent that has previously caused an allergic reaction.

dextrocardia (deks-trō-kard′ē-a). The presence of the heart on the right side of the chest due to a developmental anomaly.

diabetes (dī-a-bēt′es). A name given to each of two diseases in which excessive water is eliminated from the kidneys.

diabetes insipidus (in-sip′i-dus). A disease of pituitary gland insufficiency, causing great loss of water through the kidneys. Chronic thirst is an accompanying symptom.

diabetes mellitus (mel′i-tus). A disease caused by insufficient production of insulin by the endocrine portion of the pancreas. As a result carbohydrates are poorly absorbed and stored, and sugar is lost in the urine. Juvenile diabetes is a severe type which usually begins in childhood or in the teens.

diabetic (dī-a-bet′ik). One who suffers from **diabetes.**

diaphoretic (dī-a-fōr-et′ik). An agent that produces sweating.

diaphragmatic hernia (dī-a-frag-mat′ik hern′ē-a). Protrusion of a portion of the stomach into the chest cavity through a weakened segment of the diaphragm. Also called **hiatus hernia.** (Fig. 23, p. 230)

diastole (dī-as′tō-lē). The resting stage of the heart, before and after contraction, during which the heart is completely distended with blood. (*adj.*— diastol′ic.)

diastolic pressure (dī-as-tol′ik). The measurement of blood pressure taken while the heart is in its resting stage, as opposed to the higher systolic pressure which is measured during the contraction of the heart.

diathesis (dī-ath′e-sis). A constitutional condition causing a predisposition to contract certain diseases.

dicrotic pulse (dī-krot′ik). A double beat, especially the double beat of a single pulse in which two distinct impulses are **palpable.** *See* **bigeminy.**

dietetic (dī-e-tet′ik). *adj.* Pertaining to food or diet. Sometimes the term is used to refer to special foods for special needs.

digital examination (dij′i-tl). Examination performed with one or more fingers.

digitalis (dij-i-tal′is). Dried leaves of the foxglove plant which is used, in many forms, as a heart stimulant.

digitalization (dij-i-tal-i-zā′shun). The process of administering digitalis, or its related compounds, until full therapeutic effect of the drug has been reached.

diphasic (dō-fāz′ik). *adj.* Occurring in two phases or directions. Various diphasic waves are graphically recorded on an **electrocardiogram.**

diplegia (dī-plēj′ē-a *or* –ja′). Paralysis on both sides of the body.

disorientation (dis-ōr-i-en-tā′shun). Mental confusion, especially of time and place.

diverticulitis (dī-vert-ik-yūl-ī′tis). Inflammation of a diverticulum, or of two or more diverticula.

dorsalis pedis (dor-sal′is pēd′is). The artery near the top of the foot, the pulsation of which can normally be palpated.

dosage (dōs′āj). The amount of medicine to be given at one time, generally including the time of administration or the interval between successive administrations.

dram. An apothecary system measurement of fluid, roughly equivalent to 4 or 5 cc, or one teaspoonful.

dullness. A term applied to a nonresonant percussion note in an area where a resonant note is ordinarily expected.

dysarthria (dis-arth′rē-a). Abnormal speech characterized by difficulty with articulation.

dyscrasia (dis-krāz′ē-a). Abnormal makeup, particularly of the blood, leading to loss of function or to disease.

dysentery (dis′en-ter-ē). Diarrhea accompanied by blood or mucus, or both.

dyskinesia (dis-kin-ēz′ē-a). Loss or partial loss of power or function.

dyspepsia (dis-pep′sē-a). A general term equivalent to "indigestion." (*adj.* —dyspep′tic.)

dysphonia (dis-fōn′ē-a). Difficulty in speaking.

dyspnea (disp′nē-a). Shortness of breath. (*adj.* —dyspne′ic.)

dystrophy (dis′trō-fē). Faulty or defective growth or nutrition.

edema (e-dēm′a). The accumulation of excessive serous fluid in the tissues. It is generally due either to cardiac insufficiency or to kidney malfunction. (*adj.* —edem′atous.)

edentulous (ē-dent′yūl-us). *adj.* Without teeth.

electrocardiogram (ē-lek-trō-kard′ē-ō-gram). A tracing of the electrical current involved in the various cycles of the heart beat.

electrolyte (ē-lek′trō-līt). A compound which, when dissolved in liquid, becomes a conductor of electricity and

is broken down by the passage of the current.

electrolyte balance. The relative proportion in which various vital body electrolytes are normally present in the blood.

elephantiasis (el-e-fant-tī′a-sis). Huge swelling of tissues or organs caused by obstruction of the lymph flow.

elixir (ē′liks-er). An alcoholic solution often used as a solvent for medicine.

embolus (em′bol-us). A clot or other material that plugs a blood vessel and is brought by the blood stream from some other location in the vascular system.

emetic (ē-met′ik). An agent taken by mouth that induces vomiting.

emphysema, pulmonary (em-fi-sēm′a pul′mon-air-ē). A chronic disease of the lungs in which enough functional units (**alveoli**) have been destroyed by disease to prevent proper exchange of gases within the units. As a result, new air in the lung spaces cannot be efficiently utilized for oxygenation purposes.

empyema (em-pī-ēm′a). A collection of pus within a cavity, especially the chest cavity.

encephalitis (en-sef-a-lī′tis). CEPH= head. Inflammation of the brain.

endarteritis (end-ar-ter-ī′tis). Inflammation of the inner lining of an artery.

endocarditis (end-ō-kard-ī′tis). Inflammation of the inner lining of the heart, including the heart valves.

endocrine gland (end′ō-krin). Any one of a number of ductless glands which secrete hormones and other agents directly into the blood stream.

endocrinologist (end-ō-krin-ol′ō-jist). A doctor who specializes in **endocrinology.**

endocrinology (end-ō-krin-ol′ō-jē). The study of the ductless glands and their secretions.

enteric (en-ter′ik). *adj.* Pertaining to the intestinal tract.

enteritis (en-ter-ī′tis). Inflammation of

the intestinal tract, especially the small intestine.

enterococcus (en-ter-ō-kok′kus). A form of streptococcus which exists innocently within the intestinal tract but which is capable of producing disease when other organs or tissues are contaminated with it.

eosinophilia (ē-ō-sin-ō-fil′ē-a). A collection in the blood of an unusually large number of **eosinophiles,** suggesting certain possible diseases.

epigastrium (ep-i-gast′rē-um). The upper region of the abdomen, above the navel.

epilepsy (ep-i-lep′sē). A nervous disorder resulting from a brain disturbance causing transient loss of consciousness, with or without convulsions. When accompanied by convulsions, it is sometimes called **grand mal. Petit mal** (momentary blackouts) may or may not be on an epileptic basis.

epileptic (ep-i-lep′tik). *adj.* Pertaining to **epilepsy**; also, noun, a person afflicted with epilepsy.

epileptiform (ep-i-lep′ti-form). *adj.* Referring to an attack resembling **epilepsy.**

epinephrine (ep-i-nef′rin). The active ingredient of the secretion of the inner portion of the adrenal (suprarenal) gland.

epistaxis (ep-i-taks′is). Nosebleed.

eruption. A breaking out of the skin.

esophagitis (ē-sof-a-jī′tis). Inflammation of the esophagus.

exanthem (eks-an′them *or* egs-an′them). Any rash, especially one accompanied by some other manifestation of disease.

expectorant (eks-pek′tō-rant). An agent that promotes the coughing up of mucus from the respiratory tract.

facies (fā′shēz). The characteristic appearance or expression of the face which often accompanies and suggests a condition or disease. Some examples are *abdominal, adenoid,*

cardiac, leonine, Parkinson's, and *acromegalic.*

febrile (fēb′rīl). *adj.* Feverish.

fibrillation (fib-ril-ā′shun). Twitching of heart muscle tissue rather than normal contraction (*auricular fibrillation*—affecting the auricles; *ventricular fibrillation*—involving only the ventricles).

filaria (fil-air′ē-a). A family of parasitic worms.

filariasis (fil-a-rī′a-sis). A disease due to infestation with parasites (**filaria**) which block the local lymph channels and cause swelling. *See* **elephantiasis.**

flatus (flāt′us). Gas or air in the stomach or intestines.

fluke (flūk). A parasitic worm which sometimes causes severe liver damage in the host.

functional murmur. A cardiac murmur not associated with valvular defects. It generally has little significance.

gall (gawl). Another name for **bile**, the liver secretion.

gallstone. A concretion sometimes found in the gallbladder. Gallstones generally contain cholesterol.

gastric juice. The digestive fluid secreted by the stomach.

gastritis (gas-trī′tis). Inflammation of the wall of the stomach, often due to irritants such as alcohol.

gastroscope (gas′trō-skōp). A lighted instrument allowing **visual examination** of the interior of the stomach.

gastroscopy (gas-tros′ko-pē) Examination of the interior of the stomach with the **gastroscope.**

gavage (ga-vazh′). Feeding by means of a stomach tube; also used as a verb, to perform gavage.

geriatrics (jer-i-at′riks). The science of the treatment of the aged and aging.

gingivitis (jinj-i-vī′tis). Inflammation of the gums.

glanders (gland′ers). A fungus disease transmitted from horses to man.

glaucoma (glaow-kōm′a). A disease of the eye caused by increased pressure within the eyeball.

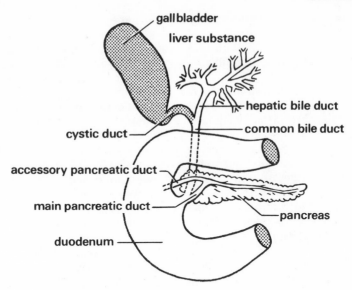

gall bladder
liver substance
hepatic bile duct
cystic duct
common bile duct
accessory pancreatic duct
main pancreatic duct
pancreas
duodenum

FIG. 10. Biliary System

globulin (glob′yūl-in). One of the principal ingredients of protein.

globus hystericus (glōb′us his-ter′i-kus). The sensation of having a lump in the throat, generally due to nervousness.

glomerulonephritis (glom-er′yūl-ō-nef-rī′tis). Inflammation of the kidney in which the **glomeruli** (filtering units) are involved.

glomerulus (glom-er′yūl-us). The small capillary tuft which makes up the first part of each functioning unit of the kidneys. The blood wastes are filtered through the glomerulus into the urine.

glossitis (glos-sī′tis). GLOSS=tongue. Inflammation of the tongue.

glossodynia (glos-ō-din′ē-a). Painful tongue.

glucose (glū′kōs). A name given to **dextrose,** one of the commonly used nutriments. It is generally administered intravenously.

glycosuria (glī-cōs-yūr′ē-a). The presence of sugar in the urine.

goiter — goitre (goy′ter). An enlargement of the thyroid gland which may be caused by its overactivity. *Exophthalmic goiter* is one type of over-

activity accompanied by toxic symptoms (including bulging of the eyes, which gives it its name).

gonadotropic (gōn-ad-ō-trōp′ik) — **gonadotrophic** (gōn-ad-o-trōf′ik). *adj.* In general, having an influence on the male or female sex glands, specifically by those hormones excreted by the pituitary gland which stimulate the testes and ovaries.

gout (gowt). A form of recurrent arthritis caused by the presence of excess uric acid in the blood. (*adj.* — gout′y.)

grain (grān). A unit of the apothecary system of medical weights and measures, amounting to 0.065 grams. (The use of the apothecary system is gradually being discontinued in many localities.)

gram. A unit of the metric system of weights and measures. One gram equals approximately 15 grains. *See* **grain.**

grand mal (grahn mahl). *See* **epilepsy.**

granulocytopenia (gran-yūl-ō-sīt-ō-pēn′ē-a). A deficiency of **granulocytes** in the blood.

Graves' disease. Another name for *exophthalmic goiter. See* **goiter.**

gumma (gum'ma). A soft, gummy, degenerative tissue occurring in some organs. It may be caused by chronic infectious diseases, especially by syphilis.

gynecomastia (gīn-e-kō-mast'ē-a). MAST=breast. Abnormally large size of the male breasts or swelling of the male nipple. It is often seen when malignancy of the prostate is being treated with female sex hormone, and sometimes transiently in healthy normal males during puberty.

heart block. The interruption of normal electrical connection between the auricle and the ventricle, usually classified as first, second, or third degree. In the latter form, also called complete heart block, all connection is lost and the ventricles contract independently of the auricles.

heartburn. An indefinite symptom complex consisting of a burning in the throat, and of the regurgitation of sour stomach contents into the throat.

heart failure, congestive. The accumulation of fluid in body tissues due to the inability of the failing heart to return the blood to circulation.

heat exhaustion. Collapse due to loss of fluid and salts from oversweating. Also called **heat prostration.**

heat stroke. Sometimes used as a synonym for heat exhaustion, but more frequently refers to severe and sustained rise in fever due to the failure of the body-heat-regulating mechanism after severe exposure to the sun and elevated temperatures.

heliotherapy (hē-lē-ō-ther'a-pē). HELI=sun. Bathing in the sun or under ultraviolet lamps for therapeutic effect.

hemagglutination (hēm-ag-glūt-in-ā'shun). HEM=blood. Clumping of the blood corpuscles due to the influence of certain noxious agents or diseases.

hemagglutinin (hēm-ag-glūt'in-in). An agent that causes clumping of blood corpuscles.

hematemesis (hēm-a-tem'e-sis). Vomiting of blood.

hematocrit (hēm-at'ō-krit). A laboratory test in which the red blood cells are **centrifuged** and separated from the blood serum, and expressed as percentage of the total volume of blood.

hematology (hēm-a-tol'ō-jē). A study of the blood and of blood diseases.

hemiplegia (hem-i-plēj'ē-a). Paralysis of one lateral half of the body. (*adj.*— hemipleg'ic.)

hemochromatosis — hemachromatosis (hēm-ō-krōm-a-tō'sis). CHROM= color. A disease characterized by discoloration of skin and tissues, due to congestion with iron pigments from the blood. Also called "bronze diabetes."

hemoglobin (hēm-ō-glōb'in). The oxygen carrying pigment of the red blood cells, which gives blood its red color.

hemoglobinuria (hēm-ō-glōb-in-ūr'ē-a). The presence of free **hemoglobin** in the urine, a result of **hemolysis** in certain disease states, such as severe forms of **malaria.**

hemolysis (hēm-ol'i-sis). LYS=destroy. Breakdown of the wall of red blood cells with the escape of **hemoglobin** into the blood serum.

hemolytic (hēm-ō-lit'ik). *adj.* Productive of **hemolysis.**

hemophilia (hēm-ō-fil'ē-a). A congenital or hereditary tendency toward easy or frequent bleeding, due to a deficient clotting mechanism. (*adj.*— hemophyl'iac.)

hemophiliac (hēm-ō-fil'ē-ak). A person suffering from **hemophilia.**

hemoptysis (hēm-op'ti-sis). A coughing up or spitting up of blood.

hemosiderosis (hēm-ō-sid-er-ō'sis). A condition in which excessive iron pigment is stored in tissues.

hemothorax (hēm-ō-thōr'aks). Blood in the chest cavity.

Henoch's purpura (Hen'oks purp'er-a). **Purpura** of allergic origin, accompanied by other symptoms.

heparin (hep'ar-in). A naturally occurring substance that interferes with the synthesis of blood clots. In cases of threatened arterial obstruction due to blood clots arising in veins and on the walls of diseased hearts, extracts of heparin are given by injection to prevent these blood clots.

heparinize (hep'ar-in-īz). *verb*. To prevent clotting by the injection of **heparin.**

hepatic (hē-pat'ik). HEPAR=liver. *adj*. Pertaining to the liver.

hepatitis (hep-a-tīt'is). Inflammation of the liver. It is usually the result of infection by a transmissible virus and often causes jaundice.

hepatoma (hep-a-tōm'a). A tumor of the liver.

hepatosplenomegaly (hē-pat-ō-splen-ō-meg'a-lē) MEG=large. Simultaneous enlargement of the liver and the spleen.

hernia (hern'ē-a). Protrusion of part of an organ beyond its normal confines, through an abnormal opening. *See* **hiatus hernia** or **diaphragmatic hernia.**

heterophil antibody test (het'er-ō-fil an'ti-bod-ē). A blood test employing sheep cells to aid in the diagnosis of **mononucleosis.**

histamine (hist'a-min). A fluid substance produced by the body in certain allergic reactions; also, a commercially produced chemical used in laboratory testing, and also to desensitize allergic patients.

histoplasmosis (his-tō-plaz-mō'sis). A disease caused by Histoplasma, a germ of the fungus type.

hives (hīvz). A common name for **urticaria.**

Hodgkin's disease (Hoj'kinz). One of a group of malignant tumors of the lymph glands, known as **lymphomas.**

hookworm. A parasitic worm in the intestine that enters the body through the skin.

hormone (hor'mōn). A substance produced by **ductless glands** (secreted directly into the blood stream) which exerts control over many of the body processes. An *inhibitory hormone* is one which neutralizes the effect of another hormone.

hydropneumothorax (hī-drō-nūm-ō-thōr'aks). A simultaneous collection of fluid and air in the chest cavity resulting from lung disease or penetrating injuries of the chest wall.

hypalgesia (hip-al-jēz'ē-a) — **hypalgia** (hip-al'jē-a). ALG=pain. Diminished sensitivity to pain.

hyperalgesia (hī-per-al-jēz'ē-a). An increased sensitivity to pain.

hypercholesterolemia (hī-per-kōl-est-er-ol-ēm'ē-a). An excessive amount of **cholesterol** in the blood.

hyperemesis (hī-per-em'e-sis). Excessive vomiting.

hyperglycemia (hī-per-glī-sēm'ē-a). GLY=sweet. An excessive amount of sugar in the blood.

hyperinsulinism (hī-per-in'sul-in-izm). Too much insulin in the system, caused either by injection or by oversecretion of the pancreas leading to an abnormally low blood sugar. *See* **hypoglycemia.**

hyperkalemia (hī-per-kal-ēm'ē-a). KAL=potassium. An excess of potassium in the blood. Also called **hyperpotassemia.**

hypernatremia (hī-per-nāt-rēm'ē-a). NAT=sodium. An excess of sodium in the blood.

hyperparathyroidism (hī-per-par-a-thī'royd-izm). Oversecretion of the parathyroid glands which may cause softening of the bones and kidney complications, due to excessive calcium in the blood stream.

hyperproteinemia (hī-per-prō-tin-ēm'ē-a). An excess of protein in the blood.

hyperpyrexia (hī-per-pī-reks'ē-a). Elevation of the body temperature; fever.

hypersplenism (hī-per-splen'izm). Increased activity (and often enlargement) of the spleen leading to abnormal destruction of blood cells and/or platelets.

hypertension. High blood pressure.

hypertension, essential. High blood pressure due to unknown causes.

hypertension, malignant. A severe progressive form of essential hypertension leading to damage to the kidneys, eyes, heart, and other organs.

hyperthyroidism (hī-per-thī′royd-izm). *See* **thyrotoxicosis.**

hyperuricemia (hī-per-yūr-i-sēm′ē-a). Excessive uric acid in the blood.

hyperventilation (hī-per-vent-i-lā′shun). Overbreathing which is sometimes seen in hysterical persons. It leads to transient **alkalosis,** and sometimes produces uncontrollable muscle contractions, tingling, and other alarming (but harmless) symptoms.

hypnotic (hip-not′ik). *adj.* Pertaining to sleep or hypnosis-induced unconsciousness. Also used as a noun, meaning an agent that dulls the senses or induces sleep.

hypnotism (hip′nō-tizm). The art of artificially producing sleep or a trance-like state by mental suggestion.

hypochondriasis (hī-pō-kon-drī′a-sis). Mental suffering from imaginary ailments caused by anxiety over one's health.

hypochromic anemia (hī-pō-krōm′ik an-ēm′ē-a). Anemia characterized by the presence in the blood of red cells which are lacking in iron pigment and give a pale appearance under the microscope.

hypoglycemia (hī-pō-glī-sēm′ē-a). A chronic condition of a too low blood sugar level due to an easily-stimulated overproduction of **insulin.**

hypothyroidism (hī-pō-thī′royd-izm). A condition resulting from paucity of thyroid secretion. It is sometimes characterized by lethargy, slowness of speech and puffiness of the face. *See* **myxedema.**

hysteria (his-tēr′ē-a). An illness resulting from emotional conflict caused by anxiety or fear, and frequently char-

acterized by attention-seeking, impulsive demonstrations.

ileitis (il-ē-ī′tis). Inflammation of the **ileum,** the terminal portion of the small intestine. Regional, or terminal, ileitis involves only the most distant segment of the ileum.

immunization (im-mūn-i-zā′shun). The process of rendering a patient resistant to a specific disease by the administration of certain agents.

immunization, active. Immunization in which the patient's own antibodies are stimulated by the introduction of vaccine.

immunization, passive. Immunization in which antibodies that have been developed in the serum of animals, principally horses, are injected directly into the patient, rendering temporary immunity.

impetigo (im-pe-tīg′ō). A spreading skin infection consisting of small pus pockets.

incompetence. Inadequate function, especially in regard to heart valves. *See* **insufficiency.**

infarct (in′farkt). A segment of dead tissue resulting from lack of blood supply.

infarction (in-fark′shun). The development of one or more **infarcts.**

influenza (in-flū-en′za). An acute epidemic disease of viral origin which is generally of short duration and usually causes fever, headache, and inflammation of the respiratory and/or digestive system. It is frequently called **"flu."**

infusion (in-fūs′zhun). The **intravenous** or **subcutaneous** administration of fluid into the tissues, using a needle.

inoculate (in-ok′yūl-āt). *verb.* To administer immune substances such as vaccine; to introduce bacteria or other organisms into laboratory animals, or onto a culture plate.

insufficiency. In cardiology, a term denoting inadequacy to perform a function, particularly referring to the inability of the heart to perform its ordinary duty (**cardiac insufficiency**). Other specific insufficiencies are those of the aortic, mitral and tricuspid valves.

insulin (in'sūl-in). A natural pancreatic hormone involved with the metabolism of sugar in the body and so with the presence and treatment of diabetes. Diabetic persons unable to secrete proper amounts of their own insulin are often dependent upon injections of insulin extracted from the pancreas of animals.

intensive care unit. A section of the hospital where intensively ill patients are concentrated and treated.

interatrial defect (in-ter-āt'rē-al) — **interauricular defect** (in-ter-awr-ik'yūl-ar). A persistent communication between the **atria** (**auricles**) after birth due to developmental failure of the **septum** between the two chambers to close. This permits a stream of blood to flow abnormally between the chambers, diverting it from the normal channel flow. *See* **foramen ovale.**

interlobar (in-ter-lōb'ar). *adj.* Between the lobes of the lung.

intermittent claudication (clawd-i-kā'shun). Pain, usually in the calves, which is due to insufficient circulation and is brought on by walking. It is usually relieved by resting.

internist (in'tern-ist). A specialist in the field of **internal medicine,** which includes the diagnosis and treatment of disease, especially of the internal organs.

intraventricular septal defect (in-traven'trik'yūl-ar sept'al). A persistent opening in the wall between the heart's two ventricles due to the developmental failure of the septum between the two chambers to close. The defect allows abnormal mixing of blood between the two chambers, leading to complications.

isotonic solution (ī-sō-ton'ik). A solution having the same percentage of salts and electrolytes as the blood, and therefore suitable for intravenous injection without danger of altering the chemical balance of the blood.

jaundice (jawn'dis). Yellowness of the skin and the whites of the eyes due to excess bile in the blood, secondary to liver dysfunction or bile duct obstruction.

ketonemia (kē-tōn-ēm'ē-a). The presence of acid bodies (**ketones**) in the blood.

ketonuria (kē-tōn-ūr'ē-a). The presence of acid bodies (**ketones**) in the urine.

ketosis (kē-tō'sis). **Acidosis** caused by the presence of excess acid bodies (**ketones**) in the system.

Kimmelstiel-Wilson disease (Kim'melstēl). **Nephritis** caused by the damaging action of **diabetes mellitus** on the kidneys.

Koplik's spots (Kop'liks). Minute particles resembling grains of salt found just within the mouth of patients with measles (**rubeola**). It is often the earliest diagnostic sign of measles.

Kussmaul respiration (Kūs'mawl). Excessively deep breathing, such as is seen in acidosis.

labyrinthitis (lab-ir-in-thī'tis). A disturbance in the inner ear mechanism that leads to nausea, dizziness, and to a loss of the sense of balance. *See* **Meniere's syndrome.**

leptospirosis (lep-tō-spir-ō'sis). *See* **Weil's disease.**

leukemia (lūk-ēm'ē-a). LEUK=white. A malignant overgrowth of the blood-forming organs resulting in the overproduction of white corpuscles and the eventual destruction of other blood and blood-forming elements. (*adj.* — leukem'ic.)

leukemoid (lūk-ēm'oyd). *adj.* Resembling leukemia.

leukocytosis (lūk-ō-sīt-ō'sis). CYT= cell. Increase in the total number of white corpuscles in the blood, such as occurs in most infections.

leukopenia (lūk-ō-pēn′ē-a). Decrease in the number of white corpuscles below the normal standard.

leukoplakia (lūk-ō-plāk′ē-a). A potentially premalignant condition characterized by the presence of white patches on the surface of certain mucous membranes, principally inside the mouth and on the floor of the bladder.

lipemia (lip-ēm′ē-a). LIP=fat. The presence of abnormal amounts of fatty substances in the blood stream.

lithiasis (lith-ī′a-sis). LITH=stone. The formation of concretions or stones.

lobar pneumonia (lōb′ar). Inflammation of the lung that is confined to one or more particular lobes.

lupus erythematosus (lūp′us er-rith-them-a-tōs′us). A chronic disease of unknown origin affecting many organs and tissues.

lymphadenitis (limf-ad-en-ī′tis). ADEN=gland. Inflammation of the lymph glands.

lymphadenopathy (limf-ad-en-op′a-thē). PATH=disease. Swelling of the lymph glands.

lymphangitis (limf-anj-ī′tis). ANG= blood vessel. Inflammation of the lymph vessels.

lymphogranuloma inguinale (limf-ō-gran-yūl-ōm′a ing-gwin-al′ē). *See* lymphopathia venerea.

lymphoma (limf-ōm′a). A malignant tumor of one or more lymph glands.

lymphopathia venerea (limf-ō-path′ē-a ven-ēr′ē-a). An uncommon venereal disease characterized by swelling of the lymph glands of the groin.

lysin (līs′in). An antibody that dissolves or destroys cells.

lysis (līs′is). (1) General lessening of the severity of a disease; (2) destruction of cells by lysins.

malaria. A parasitic disease transmitted by the bite of an infected mosquito.

Marie Strumpell disease (Strump′el). Arthritis of the spine, generally resulting in fusion of the vertebrae.

measles. *See* rubeola and rubella.

Meckel's diverticulum (mek′lz dī-ver-tik′yūl-um). A projection or pocket which arises from the small intestine and may become acutely inflamed. It is the result of an unobliterated rudimentary fetal structure.

Mediterranean anemia. *See* thalassemia.

megaloblastic anemia (meg-a-lō-blas′tik). MEG=large. Anemia characterized by the presence of large immature red blood corpuscles.

melena (mel-ēn′a). Bloody discharge from the bowels.

Meniere's syndrome (Men-ē-ārz′ sin′ drōm). *See* labyrinthitis.

metabolism (me-tab′ō-lizm). The sum of the energy expended in the building up and breaking down of tissue. (*adj.* – metabol′ic.)

methemoglobin (met-hēm-ō-glōb′in). An abnormal form of hemoglobin formed by certain chemicals, contained in certain drugs.

migraine (mīg′rān). Headache of nervous or allergic origin, usually one-sided and often accompanied by nausea and vomiting.

mitral insufficiency (mīt′ral). Incompetence of the mitral valve.

mitral stenosis (sten-ō′sis). Hardening and narrowing of the mitral valve.

mitral valve. A name given to the valve between the left auricle and the left ventricle. (Fig. 9, p. 88)

mononucleosis, infectious (mōn-ō-nūk-lē-ō′sis). An acute, self-limiting, infectious disease caused by a virus. It is characterized by a fever, enlarged lymph glands (particularly those of the neck) and a characteristic blood picture.

multiple myeloma (mī-el-ōm′a). A malignant tumor of the bone marrow which occurs in many areas of the skeleton.

multiple sclerosis (skler-ō′sis). SCLER= hard. A disease of the spinal cord resulting in the loss of various functions of the involved nerves and muscles. It is usually progressive but with intermittent periods of improvement and exacerbation.

murmur. A blowing or musical sound heard through a stethoscope, especially during examination of the heart; sometimes, but not always, it signifies a disease of the heart valve. Occasionally it signifies the presence of an abnormal opening in the partition between the two sides of the heart.

murmur, functional. A murmur that is harmless and is unrelated to any structural abnormality.

myasthenia gravis (mī-as-thēn'ē-a grav' is). A chronic disease characterized by muscular weakness, generally without **atrophy** of the muscles.

myelitis (mī-el-ī'tis). A word referring to infection in two divergent locations, the spinal cord and the bone marrow.

myeloma, plasma cell (mī-el-ōm'a). A malignant tumor of the bone marrow, often multiple, and characterized by the presence of a specific type of cell.

myocardial infarction (mī-ō-kard'ē-al in-fark'shun). CARD=heart. The usual "heart attack" caused by loss of circulation to a segment of heart muscle resulting fron plugging of a coronary artery.

myocarditis (mī-ō-kard-ī'tis). Inflammation of the heart muscle, usually due to infectious agents.

myxedema (miks'e-dēm-a). A condition caused by underfunctioning of the thyroid gland. It is characterized by boggy swelling of the face and hands.

nematodes (nem'a-tōds). *plural.* Parasitic worms.

nephritis (nef-rī'tis). Inflammation or degeneration of one or both kidneys. (*adj.*—nephrit'ic.)

glomerulonephritis (glom-er'yūl-ō-nef-rī'tis). Nephritis characterized by degeneration of the functional units (glomeruli).

pyelonephritis (pī-el-ō-nef-rī'tis). Nephritis generally caused by bacterial invasion of the collecting struc-

tures of the kidney (pelvis and calices).

nephrosis (nef-rō'sis). Disease of a portion of the kidney tubules, usually causing the presence of a large amount of **albumin** in the urine. (*adj.*—nephrot'ic.)

neurasthenia (nūr-as-thēn'ē-a). NEUR= nerve. A group of symptoms, generally on a psychogenic basis, resulting in extreme fatigue or weakness not necessarily related to exertion.

neurosyphilis (nūr-ō-sif'il-is). Disease of the nervous system due to **syphilis.**

neutropenia (nūt-rō-pēn'ē-a). A paucity of white blood corpuscles.

node (nōd). A localized swelling, especially that of a lymph node.

nystagmus (nis-tag'mus). A repeating, involuntary movement of the eyeball, generally taking place in one plane (slow, with a fast return). It is often seen in disturbances of the inner ear as well as in certain neurological diseases.

opisthotonos (op-is-thot'ō-nos). A spasm or stiffening of the back and neck muscles causing the head to be bent backward.

orthostatic albuminuria (or-thō-stat'ik al-būm-in-ūr'ē-a). Albuminuria present only when the patient is in a standing position, tending to clear up when he lies down.

orthostatic hypotension (hī-pō-ten' shun). Low blood pressure present only when the patient is in a standing or upright position.

osteoarthritis ((os-tē-ō-arth-rī'tis). OS= bone; ARTH=joint. Inflammation of the bones and joints with formation of bone spurs around the joints. It is usually found in older people.

osteoporosis (os-tē-ō-pōr-ō'sis). Softening of the bone due to loss of mineral deposits, as is often seen in older people (particularly in women past the menopause).

oxyuriasis (oks-i-yūr-ī'a-sis). Infestation with pinworms.

Oxyuris (Oks-i-yūr'is). A parasitic worm generally called a pinworm.

palpation (pal-pā'shun). The act of examining by feeling with the hands or fingers.

palpitation (pal-pi-tā'shun). Rapid, vigorous action of the heart, often in proportions which disturb the patient. *See* **paroxysmal tachycardia.**

palsy (pawl'zē). Paralysis.

pancarditis (pan-kard-ī'tis). Inflammation of the entire wall of the heart and its membranes, most commonly caused by rheumatic fever.

pancreatitis (pan-krē-a-tī'tis). Inflammation of the pancreas.

paralysis agitans (par-al'i-sis aj'i-tanz). Parkinson's disease.

paralytic ileus (il'ē-us). Paralysis of the bowel wall with resulting loss of peristalsis and of bowel function.

Parkinson's disease (Park'in-sonz). A condition caused by hardening of the arteries of the brain or by encephalitis which results in muscular rigidity and tremor. Also called **parkinsonism** or **paralysis agitans.**

paroxysmal tachycardia (par-oks-siz' mal tak-i-kard'ē-a). Tachycardia occuring suddenly, without warning.

percussion (per-kush'un). The act of detecting the presence of abnormal fluid or masses by tapping with the fingers; a resonant note suggests hollowness or an air-filled organ, while a dull note suggests the presence of fluid or a solid mass.

periarteritis nodosa (per-i-art-er-ī'tis nōd-ōs'a). Swelling and inflammation of the walls of arteries producing nodules and often accompanied by severe systemic symptoms. The cause is unknown.

pericarditis (per-i-kard-ī'tis). Inflammation of the pericardial sac, the membrane enclosing the heart.

periorbital (per-i-orb'i-tl). *adj.* ORB= eye. Around the eye socket.

peristalsis (per-i-stawl'sis). The wavelike contractions of the wall of the bowel that propel the food along the digestive tract. (*adj.*—peristal'tic.) *See* **ureteral peristalsis.**

pernicious (per-nish'us). *adj.* Severe, malignant, or tending to be fatal if unchecked.

pernicious anemia. A now controlled (formerly fatal) type of primary **anemia** caused by a deficiency of Vitamin B_{12}.

pertussis (per-tus'sis). A contagious disease, usually of childhood, which causes inflammation of the throat and bronchial tubes. This inflammation causes the characteristic "whoop" sound. Also called **whooping cough.**

phlebitis (fleb-i'tis). PHLEB=vein. Inflammation of the wall of a vein.

phlebothrombosis (fleb-ō-throm-bōs'is). **Occlusion** of a vein by a blood clot.

plethora (pleth'or-a). A condition marked by an increased quantity of blood in the system and by a full pulse. It may cause a tendency to nosebleed and a feeling of pressure in the head. (*adj.*—pleth'oric.)

plethoric (pleth'or-ik). *adj.* Flushed or red-faced, due to the presence of increased blood flow to the face.

pleurisy (plūr'i-sē). Inflammation of the **pleura**.

pleuritis (plūr-ī'tis). **Pleurisy.**

pleurocarditis (plūr-ō-kard-ī'tis). Simultaneous **pleurisy** and **pericarditis.**

pleurodynia (plūr-ō-din'ē-a). Pain in the muscles separating the ribs. Epidemic pleurodynia (**Bornholm's disease**) is caused by viral inflammation of the involved muscles and is often accompanied by fever and malaise.

pneumococcus (nūm-ō-kok'us). The organism, generally a diplococcus, that causes pneumonia and a number of other diseases.

pneumoconiosis (nūm-ō-kōn-i-ō'sis). A chronic lung disease caused by long-term inhalation of coal and other dusts.

pneumonia (nūm-ōn'ē-a). Inflammation of one or both lungs.

bronchopneumonia (brong'kō-nū-mōn-ē-a). Pneumonia concentrated about the bronchi and their divisions.

lobar pneumonia (lōb′ar). Pneumonia involving a single lobe of the lung, rarely two or more lobes.

primary atypical pneumonia. Pneumonia characterized by patchy areas of inflammation in one or both lungs, caused by a virus-like organism.

virus pneumonia. Pneumonia caused by one of the virus families.

poliomyelitis (pōl-ē-ō-mī-el-ī′tis). Inflammation of the gray substance of the spinal cord, often resulting in paralysis of the muscles supplied by the nerves affected.

polyarthritis (pol-ē-arth-rī′tis). Inflammation of several joints at the same time.

polycythemia (pol-ē-sī-thēm′ēa). An excess of red corpuscles in the blood.

presystolic (prē-sis-tol′ik). *adj.* Occurring just before **systole** (therefore, late in **diastole**) and generally referring to a particular heart sound or murmur.

prodrome (prō′drōm). An early symptom forecasting the onset of disease. (*adj.* – prodrom′al.)

prognosis (prog-nōs′sis). Outlook as to the expected course of a disease. (*adj.* – prognos′tic; *verb* – prognosticate.)

proteinuria (prō-ten-ūr′e-a). The presence of protein in the urine.

psychomotor epilepsy (sīk-ō-mōt′or ep′ i-lep-sē). Epilepsy with a strong psychic factor in its causation.

pylorospasm (pī-lōr′ō-spazm). Spasm at the lower end of the stomach, tending to obstruct the flow of food through it and often causing pain and vomiting.

pyrogen (pīr′ō-jen). PYR=fire, fever. A fever-producing agent sometimes occurring as a contaminant found in intravenous fluid.

pyrosis (pīr-ōs′is). A fancy name for heartburn.

Queckenstedt test (kwek′en-stet). A test of the spinal fluid pressure to determine whether a block exists which interferes with the free flow of spinal fluid.

rabies (rāb′ēz). An infectious disease, usually fatal, transmitted to humans by the bite of an infected animal.

rale (ral). A rattly sound heard with a stethoscope in the presence of abnormal fluid in the lungs.

regional ileitis (il-ē-ī′tis). *See* **ileitis.**

rheumatic fever. A febrile disease, most often of childhood and young adulthood, characterized by inflamed joints and often by cardiac complications.

rheumatism (rūm′a-tizm). A broad term referring to inflammation of the joints and associated connective tissues.

Rickettsia (Rik-et′sē-a). A genus of virus-like organisms that cause such diseases as **typhus** and **Rocky Mountain spotted fever**.

salmonellosis (sal-mon-el-lōs′is). A severe intestinal infection transmitted to man by infected food or by contact with the excreta of.infected animals and pets.

sarcoidosis (sark-oyd-dōs′is). A chronic disease characterized by the presence of multiple, benign, tumor like nodules in the lungs and in various other tissues. Also called **Boeck′s sarcoid**.

scarlet fever. An acute, contagious disease associated with a rash, caused by a variety of streptococcus. It may have kidney complications.

schizophrenia (skitz′ō-fren-ē-a). A mental breakdown in which there is a complete disassociation with reality.

scleroderma. (skler-ō-derm′a). SCLER=hard; DERM=skin. A disease characterized by hardening of the skin.

sclerosis (skler-ōs′is). Hardening.

scurvy (skurv′ē). A nutritional disease characterized by capillary hemorrhages, due to a deficiency of Vitamin C.

sedation. A drowsy effect produced by the taking of a sedative.

sedative. An agent which produces calm, and inhibits nervousness.

seizure. (1) a sudden attack by a disease process; (2) a muscular spasm or convulsion.

septicemia (sep-ti-sēm′ē-a). "Blood poisoning"; the presence of **bacteria** in the blood stream.

serum sickness. An acute illness produced by the injection of horse serum which is used in the prevention and treatment of certain diseases.

Shigella (Shig-el′a). A genus of bacteria, some members of which produce dysentery.

shock. Prostration accompanied by a dropping blood pressure and a resulting circulatory deficiency.

sickle cell anemia. A hereditary disease of the Negro race in which there are sickle-shaped erythrocytes in the blood stream. It may have other characteristic features.

sicklemia (sik-lēm′ē-a). The presence of sickle cells in the bloodstream. *See* **sickle cell anemia.**

silicosis (sil-i-kōs′is). A chronic occupational inflammation of the lungs due to the inhalation of stone dust.

smallpox. · An acute, communicable, eruptive disease, now rarely seen · because of the widespread practice of vaccination. Also called **variola.**

sphygmomanometer (sfig-mō-man-om′e-ter). An instrument for measuring arterial blood pressure. There are many forms of the instrument.

sporotrichosis (spōr-ō-trik-ōs′is). An infection by a fungus, characterized by abscesses beneath the skin.

sprue (sprū). An intestinal disorder in which there is a failure to digest fats.

Staphylococcus (Staf-il-ō-kok′kus). A genus of bacteria found especially in skin infections such as boils. Some staphylococci become resistant to antibiotics and are then difficult to eradicate. (*adj.*—staphylococ′cal.)

stasis (stās′is). A slowing or stopping of the flow of blood.

status angina. Rapidly recurring episodes of **angina pectoris** without apparent provocation.

status asthmaticus (as-mat′i-kus). An unabating or persistent form of **asthma.**

status epilepticus (ep-i-lep′ti-kus). Rapidly repeating **epileptic** seizures, one so closely following the other that there seems to be no rest period.

steatorrhea (stē-at-or-rē′a). The presence of excessive fat in the stool.

sternopuncture (stern-ōpunk′tchur). The introduction of a needle into the **sternum** (breastbone) for the purpose of obtaining bone marrow for study.

Stokes-Adams syndrome. *See* **Adams-Stokes syndrome.**

stoma (stōm′a). In gastroenterology, an opening artificially made between the stomach and the small intestine, to allow passage of food.

stomatitis (stōm-a-tī′tis). Inflammation of the lining of the mouth.

Streptococcus (Strep-tō-kok′kus). A genus of **bacteria** which causes many acute forms of disease. Streptococcal sore throat is one type. (*adj.*—streptococ′cal.)

stroke. A term generally referring to a sudden paralytic attack, due to blockage of an artery, or to a hemorrhage in the brain.

subacute bacterial endocarditis (end-ō-kard-ī′tis). A bacterial infection of heart valves which often causes **septicemia** by feeding the organisms directly into the blood stream. It may follow **rheumatic fever.**

subarachnoid hemorrhage (sub-a-rak′noyd). A hemorrhage occurring beneath the middle layer (**arachnoid**) of the brain's coverings.

subdural hematoma (sub-dūr′al hēm-a-tōm′a). A blood clot located just beneath the outer covering (**dura**) of the brain.

sulfonamide (sul-fon′a-mēd). Any one of that group of drugs often called "sulfa" drugs which combat bacteria through chemical action.

Sydenham's chorea (Sid′en-hamz kōr-ē′a). **St. Vitus' dance.** *See* **chorea.**

syndrome (sin'drōm). A combination of symptoms and signs occurring simultaneously that is suggestive of a certain disease process.

syphilis (sif'i-lis). A contagious venereal disease, the manifestations of which, if untreated, may affect one or more of the body systems of tissues, especially the heart and central nervous system. (*adj.* — syphilit'ic.)

systole (sist'ō-lē). The contraction or beat of the heart.

systolic pressure (sis-tol'ik). The peak of pressure in the vascular system at the time of systole (ventricular contraction).

tachycardia (tak-i-kard'ē-a). Rapid heart beat.

tachypnea (tak-ip'nē-a). Excessively rapid, shallow respiration.

Taenia (Tēn'ē-a). A genus of tapeworm.

tamponade (tam-pon-ahd'). In cardiology, the interference with the function of the heart due to pressure caused by a collection of fluid (often blood) within the **pericardial sac.**

tapeworm. A flat, segmented, parasitic worm found in the intestines of infected persons.

telangiectasia — telangiectasis (tel-anj-i-ek-tāz'ē-a) (tel-anj-i-ek'ta-sis). A discolored (generally reddened) area of skin, caused by the local dilatation of the capillaries and minute arteries of the area.

tendinitis (ten-din-ī'tis). Inflammation of a tendon or of tendons.

tenesmus (ten-ez'mus). Uncomfortable straining in attempting to evacuate the bowel or the bladder.

testosterone (tes-tost'er-ōn). The male hormone. It is also produced synthetically for use in treating certain conditions.

tetanus (tet'a-nus). An infectious disease causing spasm of certain muscle groups. It is generally secondary to an infected puncture wound. (Also called "lockjaw.")

tetany (tet'a-nē) Intermittent muscle spasms and twitchings due to abnormal calcium metabolism.

tetralogy of Fallot (tet-ral'ō-jē of Fal'lō'). A congenital defect of the heart made up of four abnormalities.

thalassemia (thal-a-sēm'ē-a). **Primary anemia** occurring in persons of Mediterranean origin.

thromboangiitis (throm-bō-anj-ē-ī'tis). THROMB=clot; ANG=vessel. Inflammation of the inner walls of an artery, often with clot formation.

thromboangiitis obliterans (ob-lit'er-anz). A type of thromboangiitis causing obstruction of the involved artery and thus leading to gangrene of the area supplied by the artery.

thrombophlebitis (throm-bō-flēb-ī'tis). Inflammation of the wall of a vein with clot formation.

thrombosis (throm-bō'sis). The forming of a blood clot within a blood vessel.

thyroiditis (thī-royd-ī'tis). Inflammation of the thyroid gland, usually a self-limiting benign disease.

thyrotoxicosis (thī-rō-toks-i-kōs'is). A disease caused by overactivity of the thyroid gland; also called **hyperthyroidism,** which produces accelerated metabolism.

tic (tik). A quick, sudden muscle spasm, often of a recurring nature.

tic douloureux (dūl'ū-rū). Sudden facial pain, often occurring in paroxysms caused by **neuralgia.**

toxicity (toks-is'i-tē). The potential of a drug or agent to poison the system, or to cause adverse effects, in addition to the therapeutic effects.

tracheitis (trāk-ē-ī'tis). Inflammation of the trachea.

transudate (trans'ū-dāt). Any *noninflammatory*, watery substance which has diffused through a membrane, or through pores of tissues, and collected in a pocket. It is opposed to **exudate,** a collection of inflammatory fluid.

Trichinella (Trik-in-nel'a). A genus of **nematode** parasites responsible for **trichinosis.**

trichinosis (trik-in-ōs'is). Infestation with Trichinella, generally due to the eating of raw or rare pork. It is often fatal. Also called **trichiniasis.**

Trichomonas (Trik-ō-mōn'as). A genus of parasitic protozoa.

Trichomonas vaginalis. A species of Trichomonas most often found in vaginal secretions, leading to inflammation of the vaginal wall.

tricuspid valve (trī-kus'pid). A name given to the valve between the right auricle and the right ventricle. (Fig. 9, p. 88)

tubercle (tūb'er-kl). The basic lesion, nodule or granuloma caused by **tuberculosis.**

tubercle bacillus (ba-sil'lus). The **bacillus** which causes **tuberculosis.**

tuberculin test (tūb-erk'yūl-in). A skin test used in screening for the presence of **tuberculosis.**

tuberculosis (tūb-erk-yūl-ō'sis). A chronic disease which has a special affinity for the lungs and which may occur in a number of tissues and organs.

tularemia (tūl-ar-ēm'ē-a). A chronic disease transmitted to man from rabbits or other rodents, generally through handling of the carcass.

typhoid fever. A severe contagious disease accompanied by fever and prostration, caused by infection with typhoid bacilli.

typhus fever. A febrile infection transmitted by the bite of a rat flea in this country, and usually by the louse in European and other countries.

ulcer. An open sore that excavates the underlying tissue.

   duodenal ulcer (dū-ō-dēn'al *or* dū-od'e-nal). An ulcer that occurs in the first segment of the small intestine.

   gastric ulcer (gast'rik). An ulcer occurring in the wall of the stomach, of special importance because of its occasional degeneration into cancer.

   peptic ulcer (pep'tik). A broad term covering either a gastric or a duodenal ulcer.

ulcerative colitis (ul'ser-ā-tiv cōl-ī'tis). Inflammation of the wall of the large intestine, characterized by multiple small ulcers and ordinarily accompanied by diarrhea or **dysentery.**

undulant fever (und'yūl-ent). *See* **brucellosis.**

uremia (yūr-ēm'ē-a). The presence of excessive nitrogenous wastes in the blood stream due to failure of the kidneys to excrete them into the urine.

urobilinogen (yūr-ō-bil-in'ō-jen). A pigmented substance formed from bile, the presence of which in the urine is important in determining the cause of jaundice.

valvulitis (valv-yūl-ī'tis). Inflammation of a heart valve.

varicella (vair-i-sel'a). Chickenpox.

variola (vair-i'ō-la). Smallpox.

vasoconstriction (vā-zō-kon-strik'shun). Diminution in the caliber of blood vessels. It may be due to certain diseases or be caused by drug action.

vasoconstrictor (vā-zō-kon-strik'tor). An agent causing vasoconstriction.

vasodilator (vā-zō-dī-lā'tor). An agent that causes an increase in the caliber of blood vessels, producing greater blood flow to the part involved.

vasospasm (vā'zō-spazm). Localized, temporary constriction of a vessel.

vermifuge (verm'i-fyūj). An agent which rids the body of worms.

vertigo (vert'i-gō). A type of dizziness, particularly characterized by the sensation of whirling. It may be caused by a number of conditions.

viremia (vīr-ēm'ē-a) — **virusemia** (vīr-us-ēm'ia). The presence of viruses in the blood stream.

vitiligo (vit-il-ī'gō). Smooth, light colored patches on the skin. The cause is undetermined.

Weil's disease (Wīlz). A febrile illness spread by the excreta of rats.

Wenckebach's phenomenon (Wenk'e-bahks fē-nom'e-non). A form of incomplete heart block in which the auricles and ventricles contract in a constant pattern, independently of each other.

whooping cough. The commonly-used name for **pertussis.**

Zenker's diverticulum (Zeng'kerz dī-vert-ik'yūl-um). An outpocketing off the esophagus which may trap food and lead to difficulty in swallowing.

12 Neurology and Neurosurgery

NEUROLOGY IS THAT branch of medicine involved with disturbances of the physical nervous system. Neurology deals with the care and diagnosis of affections of the central and peripheral nervous systems, such as pain and loss of motion, and with affections of the autonomic nervous system which controls involuntary, internal functions.

The neurologist functions mainly as a diagnostician. He performs no surgery, but he is often responsible for the care of patients with cerebrovascular diseases, migraine, epilepsy, multiple sclerosis, muscular dystrophy, and brain and spinal cord tumors. The increasing availability and accuracy of elaborate electronic equipment has helped to make neurologic diagnosis more precise.

By contrast, a neurological surgeon performs surgery on the brain and spinal cord, and on the peripheral and autonomic nerves. Necessarily the scope of neurosurgery includes the bones covering these nervous system structures, so that surgical lesions of the skull and spinal column which compress the brain, spinal cord, or spinal nerves, also fall within the province of the neurosurgeon. Head and spinal injuries incurred in traffic accidents are treated by the neurosurgeon, and, with the improvements in the recognition and treatment of brain and spinal cord tumors, cerebrovascular disease in now also treated by neurosurgeons working with vascular surgeons.

The American Board of Psychiatry and Neurology still certifies neurologists as well as psychiatrists. The Board requires a neurologist to have completed two years of residency and two years of practice before he can apply for certification. The American Board of Neurosurgery requires four years of approved residency and two years of practice before admitting applicants to examination.

CONSULTANTS

Donald Macrae, M.D., M.R.C.P.,
F.R.F.P.S.
*Diplomate, American Board of Psychiatry and Neurology (Neurology);
Professor and Chairman of Neurology,
University of California Medical
Center
San Francisco, California*

Lawrence H. Arnstein, M.D.
*Diplomate, American Board of Neurosurgery
Palo Alto, California*

David G. Scheetz, M.D.
*Diplomate, American Board of Neurosurgery
Santa Rosa, California*

abducens nerve (ab-dūs'ens). The sixth
cranial nerve (paired) which controls
outward movement of the eyeball.

Achilles reflex (A-kil'lēz). Involuntary
contraction of the calf muscles when
the heel tendon is struck sharply,
causing the foot to turn downward.

acoustic nerve (a-kūs'tik). ACOU=
hear. The eighth cranial nerve
(paired) which is involved with the
sense of hearing and with balance.

afferent (af-fer'ent). *adj.* In neurology,
referring to the direction of an impulse proceeding *toward* the cell
body of the neuron. *See* **efferent.**

agnosia (ag-nōs'ē-a). GNO=know.
Inability to recognize by touch, hearing, sight, smell or taste, though not
blind nor deaf.

agraphia (ā-graf'ē-a). GRAPH=write.
Inability to write one's thoughts due
to a brain lesion.

akinesia (ā-kin-ēz'ē-a *or* −zha)−**akinesis.** Inability to make primary automatic movements.

alexia (a-leks'ē-a). Inability to read,
because of a brain lesion.

algesia (al-gēz'ē-a). Sensitivity to pain.

amaurotic family idiocy (am-awr-ot'ik).
A slowly progressive, familial, hereditary, fatal disease sometimes seen in
infants. It usually goes on to blind-

ness and idiocy before death supervenes.

amnesia (am-nē'zha). Loss of memory
for a period of time.

amyotrophic lateral sclerosis (ā-mī-ō-trof'ik sklēr-ō'sis). Slow degeneration of motor cells in the brain and
the spinal cord, resulting in muscle
wasting and weakness.

anamnesia (an-am-nē'zha *or* −zē-a)−
anamnesis (an-am-nē'sis). A scientific name for memory.

anarthria (an-arth'rē-a). Inability to articulate words clearly because of a
brain or muscle disturbance.

aphasia (a-fāz'ē-a). Inability to express one's self by speech, writing or
sounds, or to comprehend speech,
due to injury or disease of the brain
centers.

aphonia (a-fōn'ē-a). PHON=speak.
Inability to make a vocal sound.

arachnoid (a-rak'noyd). One of the
three layers of the **meninges.** The
arachnoid, mostly a web of blood
vessels, lies between the **dura mater**
and the **pia mater.**

astereognosis (as-tēr-ē-og-nōs'is).
STER=solid; GNO=know. Inability
to identify an object by touch.

asynergia (ā-sin-erj'ē-a *or* −ja). In neurology, a disturbance of coordination
of the several muscular actions involved in executing a planned, purposeful act.

ataxia (ā-taks'ē-a) Inability to accomplish muscular coordination. It may
affect the limbs or gait.

atonia (ā-tōn'ē-a)−**atony** (at'o-nē).
TON=tension. Lack of normal tone
or strength (flaccidity).

auditory nerve (awd'i-tō-rē). AUD=
hear. The eighth cranial nerve
(paired). Its two branches are involved with the sense of hearing and
with balance. (Also called the **acoustic nerve.**)

autonomic nervous system (awt-ō-nom'
ik). The involuntary division of the
nervous system, which supplies automatic innervation for the internal ac-

tivities of the body necessary for the continuance and adjustments of life. (Also called the **involuntary,** the **sympathetic,** or the **vegetative nervous system.**)

Babinski's reflex (Ba-bin'skiz). The backward bending response of the great toe upon stroking the bottom of the foot. Important conclusions regarding the integrity of certain motor pathways can be drawn from the toe's response.

basal ganglia (bās'al gang'gli-a). A group of important brain centers.

Bell's palsy (pawl'zē). Facial paralysis due to malfunction of the peripheral part of the seventh (facial) nerve.

Brown-Sequard syndrome (Brown-Sē' kward sin'drōm). A condition resulting from damage to half of the spinal cord. Due to the crossing over of certain nerve fibers, it results in loss of pain and temperature sensation on one side and weakness on the other side, below the level of damage.

bulb. The **medulla oblongata.** (*adj.* — bulb'ar.)

bulbar palsy (bulb'ar pawl'zē). A syndrome characterized by dysfunction of the muscles of the lip, tongue, mouth, pharynx and larynx.

burr hole A hole made in a bone, particularly the skull, with a small drill, for surgical purposes.

catecholamines   (kat-a-kōl'a-mēnz). *plural.* The end products of some of the secretions of the adrenal gland. Certain of them, notably **epinephrine** and **norepinephrine** influence nervous system activity. They are also the transmitter substances that pass the nerve impulse along at the synapse, from one neuron to the next neuron.

cauda equina (kawd'a ē-kwīn'a). CAUD=tail; EQUI=horse. The bundle of nerve roots into which the spinal cord divides in the lower end of the spinal canal—like a horse's tail.

caudate nucleus (kawd'āt nūk'lē-us). An important part of the gray matter of the brain; part of the basal ganglia.

causalgia (kawz-alj'ē-a). ALG=pain. A state of distorted sensation, usually burning pain following an injury to a sensory nerve. It is often associated with a glossy skin over the afflicted area.

cephalgia — cephalalgia (sef-alj'ē-a, sef-al-al'ja). Headache.

cerebellum (ser-e-bel'lum). A special part of the brain at the back of the skull, with two functions: control of the movements of the limbs, and control of equilibrium.

cerebrospinal fluid (ser-ē-brō-spīn'al). The fluid contained within the cerebral ventricles, the subarachnoid space, and the central canal of the spinal cord. (Also called **spinal fluid.**)

cerebrum (ser-ēb'rum). The larger, upper portion of the brain which predominantly controls thought and voluntary action. It consists of the right and left cerebral hemispheres.

Chvostek's sign (vos'teks). A reflex movement of the facial muscles when the facial nerve is stimulated by tapping. It is often seen with disturbed calcium metabolism, but more often with hypoventilation. **Chvostek-Weiss sign** is another name.

cisterna magna (sis-tern'a mag'na). The large **subarachnoid space** between the cerebellum and the medulla. It contains cerebrospinal fluid and tapping it is called a **cisterna puncture.**

cochlea (kōk'lē-a). The spiral organ in the inner ear which contains the auditory nerve endings.

cochlear nerve (kōk'lē-ar). The name for the hearing portion of the eighth cranial nerve.

concussion (kon-kush'un). Loss or alteration of consciousness from a direct, closed head injury.

cordotomy — chordotomy (kord-ot'ō-mē). Surgical division of the pain tracts in the spinal cord in order to relieve intractable pain.

corpus callosum (korp'us kal-lō'sum). CORPUS=body. A group of fibers connecting the two cerebral hemispheres.

cranial nerves (krān'ē-al). The twelve (paired) nerves which supply sensitivity and motor power to the head and neck.

craniotabes (krān-ē-ō-tāb'ēz). Spotty thickening of a baby's skull, usually from rickets or inherited syphilis.

craniotomy (krān-ē-ot'ō-mē). An opening made surgically for entry into the cranial vault.

cremasteric reflex (krēm-as-ter'ik). A reflex raising of the testicle on stimulation of the thigh. It indicates integrity of the spinal roots at the upper lumbar level.

Crutchfield tongs (Krutch'fēld). A device used in applying skeletal traction to the head in certain situations, such as fractured cervical vertebrae.

Cushing's sign (Kūsh'ingz). A neurological sign suggesting the possibility of tumor at the base of the brain.

decompression. A lowering of pressure by surgical procedure. It generally refers to relief of intra-cranial pressure by removing part of the cranium or some fluid or mass.

degeneration (dē-jen-er-ā'shun). In neurology, the distally-progressing deterioration of a nerve that has been cut or damaged.

dura (dūr'a). A common abbreviation for the **dura mater** — the thick, outermost covering of the brain and the spinal cord.

efferent (ef-fer'ent). *adj.* In neurology, referring to the direction of an impulse proceeding *away* from the cell body of the neuron. See **afferent.**

encephalomalacia (en-sef-a-lō-mal-ā' sha). MALAC=soft. A slow, widespread cerebral softening, usually arising from **arteriosclerosis.**

encephalomyelitis (en-sef-a-lō-mī-el-i tis). Concurrent inflammation of both the brain and the spinal cord.

epidural (ep-i-dūr'al). *adj.* Referring to a position upon or outside of the **dura.**

epigastric reflex (ep-i-gast'rik). GAST= stomach. An abdominal reflex used to determine nerve-pathway continuity, or lack of it.

epilepsy (ep'i-lep-sē). A disturbance of the brain resulting in muscle spasm seizures or loss of consciousness. Convulsions sometimes accompany an attack.

equilibration (ē-kwil-i-brā'shun). The maintenance or restoration of normal equilibrium.

equilibrium (ē-kwil-ib'rē-um). The state of body balance in which opposing forces equalize each other. Neurologically, this involves the semicircular canals, the eighth cranial nerve, the cerebellum, and head-neck muscles.

Erb's paralysis. A characteristic paralysis of the upper arm and part of the chest wall.

extradural (eks-tra-dūr'al). *adj.* Referring to a position outside of or around the **dura.**

facial diplegia (dī-plē'ja *or* −jē-a). PLEG=paralysis. Paralysis involving both sides of the face.

facial nerve. The seventh cranial nerve (paired) which innervates most of the facial muscles.

filum terminale (fīl'um term-in-al'ē). TERM=end. A thin fibrous band which anchors the end of the spinal cord to the **coccyx.**

foot drop. A condition in which the foot drops when walking, due to paralysis of muscles, as seen in a lesion of the peroneal nerve.

ganglion (gang'glē-on). A collection of nerve cells along the course of a nerve pathway which initiates or reinforces nerve impulses. (*plural.* − ganglia.) Prominent ganglia are the geniculate, the sphenopalatine, the gasserian and the stellate.

Gigli's saw (gig'liz). A flexible wire saw frequently used in performing **craniotomy.**

glioma (glī-ōm′a). A common type of neurological tumor arising from the supporting cells of the nervous system.

globus pallidus (glōb′us pal′li-dus). The inner part of the lenticulate nucleus of the brain.

glossopharyngeal nerve (glos-sō-far-inj′ē-al). GLOSS=tongue; PHARYN= throat. The ninth cranial nerve (paired) supplying sensory innervation to the posterior third of the tongue and to the throat.

gluteal reflex (glūt′ē-al). A reflex involving the skin and muscles of the buttocks.

gray matter. The more cellular portion of the brain and spinal cord. It is differentiated from the white matter which it mostly surrounds.

gyrus (ji-rus). Any one of the many tortuous folds of the outer layer of the brain.

hematomyelia (hēm-a-tō-mī-ēl′ē-a). HEM=blood; MYEL=nerve. An enlargement of the central canal of the spinal cord produced by hemorrhage and bleeding.

hemiparesis (hem-ē-pair-ē′sis *or* hem-ē-pair′e-sis). Muscular weakness limited to one side of the body.

hiccup (hik′kup). The well-known spasm of the diaphragm, the cause of which is frequently unexplainable. The technical name is **singul′tus.**

hippocampus (hip-pō-kam′pus). A projection on the floor of the lateral ventricle of the brain. It is involved in the **olfactory** (smelling) process.

hydrocephalus (hī-drō-sef′a-lus). HYDR=water; CEPH=head. Distension of fluid spaces within or over the surface of the brain. In children it results in enlargement of the head.

hypoglossal nerve (hī-pō-glos′sl). The twelfth cranial nerve (paired) supplying the muscles of the tongue.

hypophysectomy (hī-pof-e-sek′tō-mē). Surgical resection of the **hypophysis** (pituitary gland).

hypophysis (hī-pof′e-sis). The pituitary gland.

innervation (in-ner-vā′shun). A term implying both the distribution of nerves to a part and the supplying of nervous impulses for that part.

intercostal nerve (in-ter-kost′al). COST=rib. One of the nerves (paired) which lie at the lower edge of the ribs. It supplies skin sensations and contributes to muscle movement of the chest wall.

intracerebral hemorrhage (in-tra-ser-ēb′ral hem′or-ij). Hemorrhage into the cerebral tissue.

involuntary nervous system. *See* **autonomic nervous system.**

jacksonian epilepsy (jak-sōn′ē-an). A specific pattern of involuntary movements coming from a focal irritation of the motor cells in the cerebral cortex.

Kernig's sign (Kurn′igs). A sign generally diagnostic of the presence of **meningitis.**

labyrinth (lab′i-rinth). In neurology, it refers to the internal ear. made up of the cochlea, the vestibule, and the semicircular canals.

laminectomy (lam-in-ek′tō-mē). Surgical excision of the posterior arch of a vertebral body, generally done to allow examination of the spinal canal and its contents or to relieve pressure on a spinal nerve.

lateral ventricle (vent′ri-kl). One of the two large cavities in the cerebrum. The two lateral ventricles connect and are continuous with the third and fourth ventricles of the medulla and spinal cord. All of them contain spinal fluid.

lemniscus (lem-nis′kus). A band of nerve fibers in the brain stem.

lenticulate nucleus (len-tik′yūl-āt nūk′lē-us)—**lenticulate body.** An important (paired) nerve center located near the base of the brain.

leptomeningitis (lep-tō-men-in-jī′tis). Inflammation of the meninges, limited to the pia mater and the arachnoid layers.

Litten's sign (Lit'tnz). An occasionally-seen sign indicating paralysis of the diaphragm.

Little's disease. A congenital, spastic stiffness of the limbs due to brain and spinal-cord deficiencies.

lobotomy (lō-bot'ō-mē). An incision made into the white matter of the brain to interrupt certain nerve pathways to the frontal lobe and thereby promote changes in mood or behavior.

lymphokinesis (lim-fō-kin-ē'sis). Movement of the fluid (**endolymph**) in the semicircular canals and therefore vital to balance and equilibrium.

medulla oblongata (mēd-ul'la ob-long-gaht'a). That portion of the nervous system connecting, consisting of, and continuous with, the brain and spinal cord. (Generally called the medulla.)

Meniere's syndrome (Men-i-airz') — **Meniere's disease.** — A condition of varying degrees of deafness, dizziness, and noise in the ears (tinnitus) due to abnormality within the labyrinth.

meninges (men-in'jēz). *plural.* A composite term for the three membranes that cover the brain: the dura mater, the pia mater, and the arachnoid.

meningioma (men-in-jē-ōm'a). OMA= tumor. A tumor arising from the meningeal brain covering, usually the dura mater.

meningismus (men-in-jiz'mus). Stiffness of the neck produced by irritation of the **meninges.**

meningitis (men-in-jī'tis). Inflammation of the **meninges.**

meningocele (men-inj'jō-sēl *or* men-ing' gō-sēl). Hernial protrusion of the **meninges** through a defect of the skull or spinal column.

migraine (mīg'rān). A syndrome characterized by periodic headaches (often one-sided), nausea, vomiting, and other sensory disturbances. It is thought to be vascular in origin.

monoplegia (mōn-ō-plēj'ya). Paralysis of one limb or of a single part.

motor aphasia (a-fāzh'ya). Inability to verbalize words because of a lesion of the cerebral cortex. There is no paralysis of the muscles of speech.

multiple sclerosis (sklēr-ō'sis). An incurable disease marked by sclerosis in varying patches throughout the nervous system. It is characterized by weakness, incoordination, and many other signs of cerebral or spinal cord involvement.

muscular dystrophy (dis'tro-fē). Progressive atrophy and weakness of the muscles which is often hereditary. It does not involve the spinal cord.

myasthenia gravis (mī-as-thēn'ē-a grav' is). A chronic, generally progressive paralysis of the muscular system, secondary to failure of nerve stimulus to cross the myoneural junction.

myelin sheath (mī'e-lin). The characteristic, fat-like covering or sheath of some nerve fibers.

myelitis (mī-el-ī'tis). In neurology, inflammation of the spinal cord.

myelocele (mī'el-ō-sēl). Posterior protrusion of parts of the spinal cord through a congenital defect in the wall of the spinal canal.

myoneural junction (mī-ō-nūr'al). The joining point between a nerve and the muscle it innervates.

narcolepsy (nark-ō-lep'sē). NARC= sleep. A condition marked by an episodic uncontrollable desire for sleep, usually accompanied by **catalepsy.**

Negri bodies (Nāg'ri). Certain microscopic cells present in the cerebellum of animals or humans dying from **rabies.** Their presence is characteristic of the disease.

neuralgia (nūr-alj'ē-a). NEUR=nerve; ALG=pain. Pain in or along the course of one or more nerves. Types of neuralgia are distinguished according to the part affected, or to the cause, such as intercostal, trigeminal, obturator, pudendal, occipital, etc.

neurectomy (nūr-ek'tō-mē). The excision of a nerve or of a part of it.

neuritis (nūr-ī'tis). Inflammation of or in a nerve.

neurofibroma (nūr-ō-fīb-rōm'a). A tumor of nerves and/or nerve sheaths.

neurologist (nūr-ol'ō-jist). A physician who specializes in neurology.

neurology (nūr-ol'ō-jē). *See* introductory paragraphs.

neurolysis (nūr-ō-lī'sis). LYS=destroy. The operative freeing of perineural adhesions; also, degeneration of nerve tissue.

neuroma (nūr-ōm'a). A tumor or scarification growing from a nerve, particularly from a damaged one.

neuron (nūr'on). The basic cell of the nervous system. It consists of dendrites, a cell body, and an axon. (Fig. 11, below)

axon (aks'on). The efferent branch of the neuron by which impulses leave the cell body. It may communicate with dendrites of the next neuron in the chain. *See* **synapse.** (Fig. 11, below)

cell body. The coordinating center of the neuron which changes afferent impulses which are received from dendrites into efferent impulses which leave by the axon. (Fig. 11, below)

dendrite (den'drīt). One of several afferent nerve-cell branches which receive impulses and convey them to the cell body for coordination and conduction by the efferent axon. (Fig. 11, below)

synapse (sin'aps). The "relay station" which conveys efferent impulses from an axon to the dendrites of the next neuron in the impulse chain. The transmitter substances are **catecholamines.** (Fig. 11, below)

neurosurgeon (nūr-ō-surj'on). A specialist in neurosurgery.

neurosurgery (nūr-ō-surj'er-ē). *See* introductory paragraphs.

obturator nerve (ob'tūr-ā-tor). An important spinal nerve innervating several muscles of the thigh region.

oculomotor nerve (ok-yūl-ō-mōt'or). The third cranial nerve (paired) innervating muscles which move the eye and eyelid. It is also involved in regulating the size of the pupil.

olfactory nerve (ol-fak'tō-rē). The first cranial nerve (paired) involved in the sense of smell.

optic chiasm (kī'azm)—**optic chiasma** (kī-az'ma). OP=eye. The x-shaped body located behind and between the eyes which is formed by the crossed and uncrossed fibers of the **optic nerve.**

optic nerve. The second cranial nerve (paired) involved with the sense of sight.

otorrhea (ō-tō-rē'a). OT=ear. Fluid discharge from the ear. Free escape

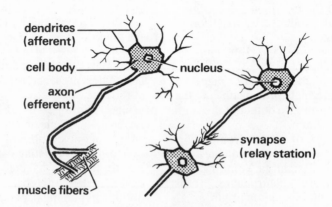

dendrites (afferent)

cell body

nucleus

axon (efferent)

synapse (relay station)

muscle fibers

FIG. 11. Neurons

of spinal fluid from the ear indicates a basal skull fracture.

pachymeningitis (pak-i-men-in-jī'tis). Inflammation involving only the dura mater layer of the **meninges,** producing symptoms similar to those of meningitis proper.

paresthesia (pair-es-thē'zha). ESTH= feeling. A sensation of prickling, tingling, or of "pins and needles" (as though asleep). It may be the first evidence of **neuritis.**

parkinsonism (park'in-son-izm). A progressive syndrome of middle or late life associated with several characteristic features. (Also called **paralysis agitans** or **Parkinson's disease.**)

past pointing. A manifestation of disturbance of coordination.

phrenic nerve (fren'ik). PHREN=diaphragm. The spinal nerve supplying innervation to the diaphragm.

phrenicotomy (fren-i-kot'ō-mē). Surgical interruption of the phrenic nerve.

pia mater (pē'a mā'tr). The innermost of the three layers comprising the meninges, generally referred to simply as "the pia."

pituitary gland (pit-ū'i-tair-ē). A twolobed glandular body connected with the base of the brain. It is of great importance in the endocrine system and is generally referred to as "the pituitary."

plantar nerves (plan'tar). Two nerves (external and internal) supplying sensory and motor branches to the sole of each foot.

plexus (pleks'us). In neurology, one of the networks of nerve fibers or nerve centers found in various parts of the body. (*plural,* — plexuses — not plexi.) Prominent plexuses are *lumbosacral, pudendal, cervical, celiac (solar), mesenteric, lumbar, brachial,* and *Auerbach's.*

pons (pōnz). The part of the brain which connects the cerebrum, the cerebellum and the medulla.

presacral neurectomy (prē-sāk'ral nūrek'tō-mē). Surgical division of the anterior roots of the sacral nerves. It is occasionally used for the relief of intractible pelvic pain.

radiculitis (rad-ik-yū-lī'tis). Inflamation of the root of a spinal nerve.

reflex (rē'fleks). The involuntary response of a muscle or tendon when receiving a stimulus such as tapping, touching or stroking. A reflex demonstrates the continuity of the nerves and spinal cord involved in the action.

rhinorrhea (rīn-or-rē'a). RHIN=nose. In neurology, the escape of spinal fluid from the nose, sometimes following a fracture of the base of the skull.

rhizotomy (rīs-ot'ō-mē). Surgical division of the anterior and/or posterior roots of a spinal nerve, performed for the relief of intractable pain or muscle contracture.

sella turcica (sel'la tur'sik-a). The depression in the base of the skull in which the pituitary gland rests.

singultus (sing-gul'tus). A fancy name for hiccup.

Smithwick procedure. Sympathectomy of the lower thoracic nerves originally done for the relief of hypertension.

speech areas. The brain centers involved in the transferring of thoughts into spoken words.

spina bifida (spīn'a bif'i-da). A congenital failure of the spinal canal to close completely over the spinal cord.

spinal accessory nerve. The eleventh cranial nerve (paired) innervating some of the neck muscles.

subarachnoid hemorrhage (sub-ar-ak' noyd). Hemorrhage into the space within or below the arachnoid network.

subarachnoid space. The space between the arachnoid and the pia mater.

subdural hemorrhage (sub-dūr'al). Hemorrhage into the **subdural space.**

subdural space. The space between the dura mater and the arachnoid.

sympathectomy (simp-a-thek'tō-mē). Surgical interruption of some of the pathways of the sympathetic nervous system, to accomplish certain specific purposes.

sympathetic nervous system. See **autonomic nervous system.**

syringomyelia (sir-ing-gō-mī-ēl'ē-a). A chronic progressive disease of the spinal cord characterized by the gradual formation of cavities within it.

tabes dorsalis (tāb'ēz dor-sal'is). A disease which results in various changes in the nervous system. It is generally a third stage of **syphilis** although it may also be caused by congenital syphilis. (Also called **neurosyphilis** or **locomotor ataxia.**)

tentorium (ten-tōr'i-um). A portion of the covering of the brain which forms a partition between the cerebrum and the cerebellum.

thalamus (thal'a-mus). The brain center which relays sensory impulses to the cerebrum.

tic (tik). A spasmodic twitching, as of a part of the face.

tic douloureux (dūl'ū-rū). **Neuralgia** of the fifth cranial nerve.

tremor (trem'or). An involuntary trembling.

trephine (trē'fīn). In neurology, a cylindrical saw used for removing a disk of bone from the skull. (Also used as a verb.)

trigeminal nerve (trī-jem'i-nal). GEMIN=double. The fifth cranial nerve (paired). It has three branches which

supply sensory or motor innervation to various parts of the face.

trochlear nerve (trōk'lē-ar). The fourth cranial nerve (paired). It rolls the eyeball downward.

vagotomy (vā-got'ō-mē). The cutting or excision of the **vagus nerve** to interrupt the distal innervation.

vagus nerve (vāg'us). The tenth cranial nerve (paired). This nerve sends both motor and sensory branches to many structures in the neck, the thorax and the abdomen. (Also called the **pneumogastric nerve.**)

vasomotor (vāz-ō-mōt'or). *adj.* Referring to changes in blood vessel walls, such as expansion and contraction, which are under the control of the autonomic nervous system.

vegetative nervous system (vej-e-tāt'iv). See **autonomic nervous system.**

ventriculogram (ven-trik'yūl-ō-gram) — **ventriculography** (ven-trik'yūl-og'ra-fē). GRAM=record. Visualization of the ventricles of the brain by x-ray techniques.

von Recklinghausen's disease (von Rek'ling-houz-enz). A condition characterized by the appearance of multiple tumors along the course of nerves (particularly cutaneous nerves) and some associated abnormalities.

white matter. The conducting portion of the brain and spinal cord which is located beneath the cortex. It is differentiated from gray matter.

13 Obstetrics and Gynecology

UNTIL SPECIALIZATION became popular, obstetrics was the third part of the medical practice triad — medicine, surgery and obstetrics. Obstetrics and gynecology are generally practiced by the same doctor: *obstetrics* focuses upon childbirth, including the prenatal and postdelivery care of the mother, and *gynecology* focuses upon the care of medical and surgical conditions which are strictly female, many of which are related to childbearing.

Obstetrics is as old, of course, as the human race. Its lack of regular hours is compensated for by the fact that the obstetrics floor is the happiest in the hospital, and by the special regard which the mother has for her obstetrician. Gynecology, on the other hand, is a relatively new speciality which was limited in its development until the advent of modern surgery. Nonetheless, only about fifteen percent of gynecologists' patients are hospitalized for surgery; the remaining portion of patients require only advice and medical treatment. The influence of endocrinology has been a large factor in the increasing number of nonsurgical gynecological patients.

Today the obstetrician is frequently aided by the pediatrician. The discovery of prenatal factors which may affect the mother's pregnancy, her delivery, and the condition of her newborn infant has led to the increasing involvement of pediatricians with prenatal and postdelivery infant problems.

The American Board of Obstetrics and Gynecology requires the completion of three years of postgraduate residency training, followed by one and one-half years of practice, prior to application for certification.

CONSULTANTS

Theodore S. Stashak, M.D., F.A.C.S.
Diplomate, American Board of Obstetrics and Gynecology
Santa Rosa, California

William J. Dunn, M.D.
Diplomate, American Board of Obstetrics and Gynecology
Santa Rosa, California

Clarence E. Toshach, M.D., F.A.C.S.*
Diplomate, American Board of Obstetrics and Gynecology
Saginaw, Michigan

*deceased

ablatio placentae (ab-lā'shē-ō pla-sen' tē). Premature separation of the normally implanted placenta from the uterine wall. Sometimes called **abruptio placentae.**

abort (a-bort'). *verb.* To **miscarry** during the first trimester of pregnancy; also, to cause or bring about an **abortion.**

abortion (ab-ōr'shun). The spontaneous, or instrumental, termination of an early pregnancy. Types of abortions include criminal, habitual, imminent, induced, spontaneous, therapeutic, and threatened. *See* **miscarriage.**

accouchement forcé (a-kūsh-mon' fōr-sā'). Forced, rapid vaginal delivery of a child, carried out during a late stage of labor.

adnexa (ad-neks'sa). *plural.* A term indicating associated or connected parts of organs. In this specialty the organs of the female pelvis are generally implied.

adnexa uteri (yūt'er-ī). The ovaries and fallopian tubes.

allantois (al-an'tō-is). An embryonic structure through which the embryo is originally supplied with nourishment. (*adj.* — allanto'ic.)

amenorrhea (a-men-ōr-rē'a). MEN= menses. Absence or abnormal cessation of the **menses.** (*adj.* — amenorrhe' ic.)

amnion (am'nē-on). A membrane enclosing the fetus and amniotic fluid ("the bag of waters").

amniotic fluid (am-nē-ot'ik). The fluid surrounding the fetus and the umbilical cord, all of them contained by the amniotic sac (**amnion**).

anteflexion (an-tē-fleks'shun). FLEX= bend. A forward curvature (generally referring to that of the uterus) upon itself.

antepartum (an-tē-part'um). *adj.* PART=labor. Referring to the period shortly before delivery.

anteversion (an-tē-verzh'un). VERS= turn. A tipping forward of the whole uterus which differs slightly from **anteflexion.**

areola (ar-ē'ō-la). The dark area of skin surrounding the nipple of the female breast. (*adj.* — are'olar; *plural,* — are' olae.)

axis-traction forceps (aks'is-trak'shun for'seps). TRAC=draw. A type of delivery forceps which is sometimes used for more difficult births.

ballottement (bah-lot'mon *or* bal-lot' ment). A diagnostic procedure used in detecting pregnancy. The fetus is palpated with the hands through the abdominal wall.

Bartholin's glands (Bar'tō-linz). Paired mucus secreting glands at the lateral edges of the vaginal orifice.

bicornate uterus (bī-korn'āt) — **bicornuate uterus** (bi-korn'ū-āt). CORNU= horn. A congenital condition in which there is a pseudo partition thru the midline of the uterine cavity. Sometimes this develops to a stage where the fundus of the uterus resembles two points or "horns."

broad ligament. The paired peritoneal fold connecting the side of the uterus with the pelvic wall.

"B.S.O." (bilateral salpingo-oophorectomy) (sal-ping-gō-ūf-ōr-ek'tō-mē). Medical jargon referring to the surgical removal of both ovaries and both fallopian tubes.

castrate (kas'trāt). *verb.* To destroy the function of the gonads (ovaries, in this case) by surgical removal or by irradiation; also *noun,* the person castrated.

"caudal" (kawd'al). CAUD=tail. A type of anesthesia frequently used during delivery.

cervix uteri (serv'iks yūt'er-ī). The lower part, or neck, of the uterus which projects into the vagina. (Fig. 12, p. 119)

cesarean section (sē-zair'ē-an) — **caesarean section.** Delivery of a fetus by way of an abdominal incision ("CS" or "a Caesarean").

choriocarcinoma (kōr-ē-ō-kars-in-ōm'a). An occasionally seen uterine tumor, derived from both the uterus and from portions of the placenta. It is also called a **chorionepithelioma** (chorionepitheliom'a) and is very malignant.

chorionepithelioma (kōr-ē-on-epi-i-thēl-ē-ōm'a). A malignant tumor of the uterus originating from **chorionic** tissue. *See* **choriocarcinoma.**

choriogonadotropic hormone (kōr-ē-ō-gōn-ad-ō-trōp'ik) — **choriogonadotrophic hormone** (– trof'ik). A gonad-stimulating hormone evolved from placental tissue.

chorion (kōr'ē-on). The outermost of the coverings of the fertilized ovum (*Adj.* – chorion'ic.)

circumcision (ser-kum-sizh'un). CIS= cut. Surgical removal of the penile foreskin.

climacteric (klīm-ak-ter'ik). The phase of life associated with the cessation of reproduction. *See* **menopause.**

clitoris (klit'or-is). A female sexual organ, the homologue of the male penis.

coitus (kō'it-us). Sexual intercourse.

colostrum (kōl-ost'rum). A thin secretion from the breasts associated with childbirth, preceding the onset of lactation.

colpitis (kolp-ī'tis). COLP=vagina. Inflammation of the lining of the vagina. *See* **vaginitis.**

colpocleisis (kolp-ō-klī'sis). The partial or complete surgical closure of the vaginal canal.

colpoplasty (kolp-ō-plast'ē). Any plastic surgery, usually anterior or posterior, performed on the vaginal walls.

colporrhaphy (kolp-or'ra-fē). Surgical repair of the vaginal walls, subsequent to childbirth injury.

conception (kon-sep'shun). Fertilization of the **ovum.**

condyloma latum (kon-di-lōm'a lāt'um). A secondary **syphilitic** lesion sometimes seen in the genito-anal region. (*plural* – condylo'mata lat'a.)

conization (kōn-i-zā'shun). Surgical reshaping of the cervix uteri; also a method of obtaining a biopsy from the cervix.

contraception (kon-tra-sep'shun). The prevention of pregnancy.

contracted pelvis (pel'vis). A pelvic canal too small to allow vaginal delivery of a full-term fetus.

corpus (korp'us). CORP=body. The main body of an organ; in this specialty, generally referring to the uterus. (*plural* – cor'pora.)

corpus luteum (lūt'ē-um). The yellow mass which develops in the ovary at the site of the discharged egg. (*plural* – corpora lut'ea.)

curet (kyūr-et') — **curette.** A surgical instrument for scraping the lining of a cavity, particularly the uterine cavity.

curettage (kyūr-e-tahzh'). The surgical procedure of scraping the lining of the uterine cavity. Also called **curettement.**

cystocele (sist'ō-sēl). CYST=bladder. A bulging of the prolapsed bladder into the anterior vaginal wall.

"D&C" (**dilation and curettage**). Dilation of the cervical canal and scraping of the lining of the uterus.

decidua (dē-sid'jū-a). The lining of the uterine cavity during pregnancy.

delivery. The spontaneous expulsion or the manual extraction of a child at birth.

douche (dūsh). The cleansing or washing out of a cavity, generally with solution; also the equipment or solution used.

dysmenorrhea (dis-men-ōr-rē′a). Painful menstruation. Also called **menorrhagia.**

dyspareunia (dis-par-rūn′e-a). Painful intercourse.

dystocia (dis-tō′sē-a *or* dis-tō′sha.) Difficult labor.

eclampsia (ē-klamp′sē-a). A severe toxemia of pregnancy, sometimes accompanied by convulsions. Generally there is also associated hypertension.

ectopic pregnancy (ek-top′ik). TOP= position. Pregnancy occurring outside the uterus, generally within a fallopian tube.

embryo (em′brē-ō). An early developmental stage of the fertilized **ovum.** (*adj.* — embryon′al.)

emmenagogue (em-men′a-gog). An agent which stimulates **menstruation.**

endometriosis (end-ō-mē-trē-ō′sis). METR=uterus. Misplaced **endometrium,** generally found in a femal pelvis or in other parts of the abdominal cavity.

endometritis (end-ō-mē-trī′tis). Inflammation of the lining of the uterus.

endometrium (end-ō-mē′trē-um). The lining of the uterus. (*adj.* — endomet′-rial.)

enterocele (ent′er-ō-sēl). ENTER= bowel. Hernial protrusion of the bowel into the weakened posterior wall of the vagina.

episiotomy (e-pēz-ē-ot′ō-mē). A perineal incision sometimes made to facilitate vaginal delivery of the baby′s head. Types of episiotomy are med′-ian and mediolat′eral.

estrogen (es′trō-jen). An ovarian hormone, commonly called the "female hormone." (*adj.* — estrogenic.)

extrauterine (eks-tra-yut′er-in). *adj.* Outside the uterus.

fallopian tubes (fal-lōp′ē-an). Paired tubes, attached to and entering the uterus, which convey the **ova** from the ovaries to the uterus. (Fig. 12, p. 119)

fecundation (fē-kun-dā′shun). Impregnation or fertilization of the **ovum.**

fertile (fert′il). *adj.* Having the ability to conceive.

fertilization (fert-il-i-zā′shun). The fusion of an **ovum** with a **spermatozoon.**

fetus (fēt′us). What the embryo becomes at the third month of pregnancy. (*adj.* — fet′al.)

"fibroid" (fīb′royd). A common, *rarely malignant,* tumor of the uterine wall.

fimbria (fim′brē-a). The outer, fringe-like end of each **fallopian tube.** (*Plural* — fim′briae.)

follicle (fol′li-kl). *See* **graafian follicle.** (*adj.* — follic′ular.)

forceps (for′seps). An instrument sometimes used in deliveries.

fornix (for′niks). The space between the cervix and the vaginal walls (anterior, posterior and lateral). (*plural* — forn′ices.)

fundus (fun′dus). The dome or top of the uterus. (Fig. 12, p. 119)

funiculus (fūn-ik′yūl-us). The scientific name for the umbilical cord. (*adj.* — funic′ular.)

Gelpy retractor (Gel′pē). An instrument used to spread or expose tissues for carrying out surgical procedures. It is frequently used in **episiotomy** repairs.

gestation (jest-ā′shun). The total period of pregnancy.

gonad (gōn′ad). GONAD=sex The principal sex gland (male or female). (*adj.* — gonad′al *or* gon′adal.)

gonadotropic (gon-ad-o-trop′ik) — **gonadotrophic,** *adj.* Possessing the character of being stimulating to gonadal activity.

graafian follicle (graf′ē-an). The thin membraneous structure surrounding

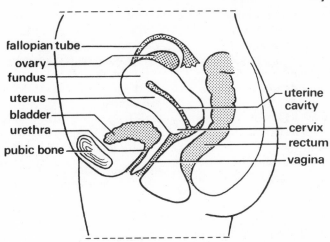

FIG. 12. Female Reproductive System

and including each **ovum** before its escape from the ovary.

gravid (grav'id). *adj.* GRAV=pregnancy. Referring to the condition of being pregnant.

Gravindex (Grav-in'deks). A test for detecting pregnancy.

"gyne" (gīn'ē). GYNE=woman. Medical jargon for **gynecology.**

gynecologist (jin-e-kol'ō-jist *or* gīn-e-kol'ōjist). A doctor who specializes in **gynecology.**

gynecology (jin-e-kol'ō-jē *or* gīn-e-kol'ō-jē). *See* introductory paragraphs.

hematocolpos (hem-a-tō-kol'pos). HEM =blood. An accumulation of blood in the vaginal cavity.

hematometra (hēm-a-tō-mēt'ra). An accumulation of blood in the uterine cavity.

hematoperitoneum (hēm-a-tō-per-i-tōn-ē'um). An accumulation of blood in the **peritoneal** cavity.

hematosalpinx (hēm-a-tō-sal'pinks). SALPING=fallopian tube. An accumulation of blood in a fallopian tube.

hermaphrodism (herm-af'rō-dizm) — **hermaphroditism** (herm-af'rō-dit-izm). HERMA=double. A congenital state in which both male and female sex organs are present, in greater or less degree, in the same individual.

hydatid mole (hī-dat'id). A type of benign uterine tumor arising from placental tissue. (*adj.* — hydatid'iform.)

hydramnios (hī-dram'nē-os). HYDR= water. An excessive quantity of **amniotic fluid** surrounding the fetus. (also called **polyhydram'nios.**)

hydrosalpinx (hī-drō-sal'pinks). A type of inflammation of the **fallopian tube,** usually subacute or chronic, resulting in an accumulation of fluid in the **lumen** of the tube.

hymen (hī'men). The membrane which partially covers the external surface of the vagina; the virginal membrane.

hyperemesis gravidarum (hī-per-em'ē-sis grav-i-dair'um). "Morning sickness" of pregnancy which is present in an abnormal degree.

hypermenorrhea (hī-per-men-or-rē'a). Excessive menstrual flow (**menorrhagia**).

hypomenorrhea (hī-pō-men-or-rē'a). Scanty menstrual flow.

hysterectomy (hist-er-ek'tō-mē). HYSTER=womb. The surgical removal of the uterus. Types of hysterectomy include abdom'inal, rad'ical (Wertheim), subto'tal, to'tal ("T.H."), and vag'inal.

hysterotomy (hist-er-ot′ō-mē). The surgical procedure of making an incision through the uterine wall.

infertile (in-fert′tl). *adj.* Relatively unable to conceive, or to be impregnated. (**Sterility** denotes absolute infertility.)

infundibulopelvic ligament (in-fun-dib yūl-ō-pel′vik). The ligamentous structure supporting the ovary and carrying its major blood supply.

introitus (in-trō′i-tus). The entrance to any body cavity, generally meaning the vagina.

involution (in-vōl-lū′shun). The normal shrinking of the uterus following childbirth. (*adj.* — involu′tional.)

isthmus (is′mus). In this specialty, the narrowed midportion of the **fallopian tube.**

kraurosis vulvae (kraw-rōs′is vūlv′ē). Dryness and shriveling of the female external genitalia, generally of elderly women.

labia (lāb′ē-a). *plural.* The folds of the female external genitalia. (*Singular*—lab′ium.)

   labia, majora (ma-jōr′a). *plural.* The outer folds.

   labia, minora (min-ōr′a). *plural.* The inner folds.

labor. The function (work) of childbirth.

lactation (lak-tā′shun). LAC=milk. The secretion of milk.

leiomyoma (lī-ō-mī-ōm′a). LEIO= smooth muscle. The well-known "fibroid tumor" of the uterus.

leucorrhea (lūk-or-rē′a) — leukorrhea. LEUC=white. A vaginal discharge, especially a whitish discharge. It is generally pathological.

lochia (lōk′ē-a). The vaginal discharge following childbirth.

lutein (lūt′ē-in). A hormone secreted by the **corpus luteum** of the ovary. Also called **progesterone.**

maceration (mac-er-ā′shun). The condition of the skin following prolonged or repeated wetting. In obstetrics, refers to the tissue changes occurring in an unborn dead fetus.

Mackenrodt's ligament (Mahk′en-rōts). The main paired ligament supporting the uterus. It contains the uterine artery, and is also called the cardinal ligament.

mastitis (mast-ī′tis). MAST=female breast. Inflammation of or in a mammary gland.

meconium (mē-kōn′ē-um). A new baby's first fecal discharge, generally black.

menarche (men-ark′ē). MEN=month. The beginning of **menses.**

menopause (men′ō-paws). The period when menstruation ceases; often called the **climacter′ic.**

menorrhagia (men-or-rāj′ē-a). Excessive menstrual flow. Also called **hypermenorrhea.**

menorrhalgia (men-or-ral′jē-a). ALG= pain. Pain during menstruation. Also called **dysmenorrhea.**

menorrhea (men-or-rē′a). A synonym for menses but sometimes referring to unusually profuse menstruation (**menorrhagia**).

menses (men′sēz). Another term meaning **menstruation** or menorrhea.

menstruation (men-strū-ā′shun). The cyclic, monthly uterine bleeding. (*adj.* — men′strual.) Synonyms are **menses** and **menorrhea.**

mesosalpinx (mē-zō-sal′pinks). The paired **peritoneal** fold by which each **fallopian tube** is suspended.

mesovarium (mē-zō-vair′ē-um). The paired fold of **peritoneum** by which the ovary is suspended.

metritis (mē-trī′tis). Inflammation of or in the body of the uterus.

metrorrhagia (met-ror-rāj′ē-a). Uterine bleeding occurring between the regular menstrual periods. It is considered pathological except when occurring with ovulation.

miscarriage. A common name for a spontaneous abortion.

Monilia (Mōn-il′ē-a). A type of yeast growth (Candida albicans) sometimes found in vaginal secretions.

"morning sickness." The morning nausea which sometimes accompanies pregnancy during the early months.

müllerian ducts (mil-lāir′ē-an). Embryological forerunners of certain female organs.

multigravida (mul-ti-grav′i-da). A woman who has had two or more pregnancies. The term has no reference to whether or not she delivered the fetus as a viable offspring.

multipara (mul-tip′a-ra). PARA=birth. A woman who has had two or more pregnancies which she has completed.

myometrium (mī-ō-mēt′rē-um). The muscular body of the uterus.

nabothian glands (na-bōth′ē-an). Glands found in the cervix uteri which may become **cystic**.

"OB" Medical jargon for **obstetrics.** Also "OBS."

obstetrician (ob-ste-trish′un). A doctor who specializes in obstetrics.

obstetrics (ob-stet′riks). *See* introductory paragraphs.

oligomenorrhea (ol-i-gō-men-or-rē′a). OLIGO=few. Infrequently occurring, or scanty, menstrual periods.

oophorectomy (ūf-ō-rek′tō-mē). The surgical removal of an ovary (unilateral or bilateral).

oophoritis (ūf-ō-rīt′is). Inflammation of an ovary.

ovarian cycle (ō-vair′ē-an sī′kl). OVA= egg. The rhythmic changes associated with ovarian function. Menses are one end result.

ovariectomy (ō-vair-ē-ek′tō-mē). **Oophorectomy.**

ovary (ō′ver-ē). The paired female reproductive gonad. (Fig. 12, p. 119)

ovulation (ov-yūl-ā′shun). Release of the egg from the ovary ("laying the egg").

ovum (ō′vum). The female reproductive cell (or egg). (*Plural*—o′va.)

panhysterectomy (pan-hist-er-ek′tō-mē). The surgical removal of the entire uterus, including the cervix. Also called *total hysterectomy.*

parametritis (par-a-mē-trī′tis). Inflammation of the **parametrium.**

parametrium (par-a-mēt′rē-um). The tissue adjacent to the lower segment of the uterus (sometimes called the **"cardinal" ligament** or **Mackenrodt's ligament**).

parturition (par-tūr-ish′un *or* par-tyūr-ish′un). The process of "having a baby." (*adj.*—parturient.)

perineorrhaphy (pair-in-ē-or′ra-fē). An operation frequently performed to repair **perineal** damage from childbirth.

perineum (pair-in-nē′um). The area between the anus and the genitalia. (*adj.*—perine′al.)

pessary (pes′a-rē). An appliance placed in the vagina to maintain or influence uterine position.

placenta (pla-sent′a). The structure providing intrauterine fetal nourishment (it becomes the "afterbirth").

polymenorrhea (pol-i-men-or-rē′a). Too frequent menstrual periods.

postpartum (pōst-part′um). *adj.* Occurring after delivery. Also adverb, meaning after delivery.

preeclampsia (prē-ē-klamp′sē-a). A less severe phase of **eclampsia**—eclampsia prior to convulsions.

pregnancy (preg′nan-sē). Everybody knows this one!

"pregnancy tests." Laboratory tests used to confirm the presence of a pregnancy. Although animal tests were exclusively used in the past, biochemical tests have been developed and are now generally used. Types of tests include Aschheim-Zondek (mouse), Friedman (rabbit), Rana (frog), Gravindex, Pregnosticon, and "H.C.G." tests.

premature (prē-ma-tūr′). *adj.* Born before full term, technically between the 28th and 36th week of pregnancy. Also noun, a child born prematurely — a "premie."

prenatal (prē-nāt′al). *adj.* NAT=birth. Before birth.

presentation (prē-zen-tā′shun). The portion of the fetus emerging first during birth. Types of presentation are cephal′ic (occiput, vertex, sinciput, face, chin), shoulder, and breech (frank, footling).

primigravida (prīm-i-grav′i-da). A woman who is pregnant for the first time.

primipara (prīm-ip′pa-ra). A woman who has had her first child.

primordial follicle (prīm-ord′ē-al). The original (ovarian) site of the ovum.

procidentia uteri (prōs-i-den′shē-a yūt′er-ī). Extreme prolapse of the uterus, the cervix protruding through the vulva.

progesterone (prō-jes′ter-ōn). A hormone produced by the corpus luteum of the ovary. *See* **lutein.**

progestin (prō-jes′tin). A name for a group of hormones of which **progesterone** is one.

pruritus vulvae (prūr-ī′tus vul′vē). PRUR=itch. Itching of the female external genitalia.

pseudohermaphrodism (sū-dō-herm-af′rō-dizm) — **pseudohermaphroditism** (sū-dō-herm-af′rō-dit-izm). A congenital abnormality causing doubt regarding the true sex.

pseudopregnancy (sū-dō-preg′nan-sē). A condition in which there are signs and symptoms suggesting a pregnancy which is not actually present. Also called "false pregnancy."

puerpera (pū-er′per-a). PUER=child. A woman who has just given birth. (*adj.* — puer′peral.)

puerperium (pūr-per′ē-um). The period following the birth of the child.

pyosalpingitis (pī-ō-sal-pin-jī′tis). SALPING=fallopian tube. Inflammation, with pus formation, of a fallopian tube. *See* **hydrosalpinx.**

pyosalpinx (pī-ō-sal′pinks). **Pyosalpingitis.**

rectocele (rek′tō-sēl). Bulging of the rectum through the weakened posterior vaginal wall. *See* **enterocele.**

round ligament (lig′a-ment). A paired ligament connecting the top of the uterus with the **inguinal** canal.

salpingectomy (sal-pin-jek′tō-mē). The surgical removal of a **fallopian tube.**

salpingitis (sal-pin-jī′tis). The term covering any general type of inflammation of a **fallopian tube.**

salpingo-oophorectomy (sal-pin-gō-ūf-or-ek′tō-mē). The surgical removal of an ovary and its fallopian tube.

salpinx (sal′pinks). Another name for a **fallopian tube.** (*plural* — salpin′ges.)

secundines (sek-un′dēnz). *plural.* The intrauterine tissues associated with pregnancy; a nicer name for "the afterbirth."

septate vagina (sep′tāt vaj-ī′na). A congenital defect resulting in a dividing partition within the vagina.

souffle (sūf′fl). An abdominal sound produced by the placental or uterine blood vessels, sometimes audible during late pregnancy.

sterility (ster-il′i-tē). The inability to reproduce, or to have children. (*adj.* — ster′ile.)

stress incontinence (in-kon′ti-nens). The inability to hold one's urine on coughing, sneezing, or straining.

suspension (sus-pen′shun). The surgical correcting of an abnormal position of the uterus. Types include Baldy-Webster, Gilliam, and others.

tampon (tamp′on). A plug of cotton or gauze used to absorb secretions, particularly vaginal secretions.

Trendelenburg position (Tren-del′en-berg). A specific position of the patient on the examining or operating table, the head being lower than the hips.

Trichomonas vaginalis (Trik-ō-mōn′as vaj-i-nal′is). A **protozoan** organism which sometimes causes vaginal infection (**vaginitis**).

trimester (trī′mes-ter). A term designating each third of the total gestation period (first, second, or third trimester).

umbilical cord (um-bil′i-kl). The connecting structure through which the fetus obtains nourishment from the mother. *See* **funiculus.**

umbilicus (um-bil′i-kus *or* um-bil-ī′kus). The navel. (*adj.* — umbil′ical.)

urachus (yūr-āk′us). An embryonic excretory structure which later persists as a ligament.

urethrocele (yūr-ēth′rō-sēl). Herniation of the urethra into the vagina.

uterosacral ligament (yūt-er-ō-sāk′ral). An important ligament supporting the uterus posteriorly.

uterus (yūt′er-us). The womb. (*adj.* — ut′erine.) (Fig. 12, p. 119)

vagina (vaj-ī′na). The part of the female genital system which extends from the uterine cervix to the vulva. (*adj.* — vag′inal.) (Fig. 12, p. 119)

vaginismus (vaj-in-is′mus). Painful vaginal spasm.

vaginitis (vaj-in-ī′tis). Inflammation of the lining of the vagina. *See* **colpitis.**

version (verzh′un). VERS=turn. A maneuver sometimes used in delivering a child. Types are podal′ic and Braxton-Hicks.

viable (vī′a-bl). *adj.* VI=life. Denoting the ability of a newly born infant to live and sustain life.

vulva (vulv′a). The external genitalia of the female.

Wertheim operation (Vert′īm). A surgical procedure used in certain cases of uterine malignancy, especially that of the cervix uteri.

14 Ophthalmology

VISION IS OF great concern to individuals and, unlike the patients of other specialists, many patients with eye problems come to the "eye doctor" directly without first being seen by another physician. Newspaper feature writers enjoy writing about advances in the handling of eye problems, and the ophthalmologist figures heavily in bridge table conversation.

The ophthalmologist not only treats the eye. Examinations of the interior of the eye may reveal hidden arteriosclerosis, diabetes, blood dyscrasias, thyroid disease or brain tumors. Advances in ophthalmologic technique, including contact lenses, cataract removal improvements, corneal transplants, and reattachment of detached retinas, among others, are well-known.

An **ophthalmologist** was formerly called an **oculist.** When you receive a prescription from an ophthalmologist for glasses, the prescription is filled by an **optician.** An optician is not a doctor but a technician trained to grind lenses according to the ophthalmologist's prescription. An optician never examines the patient. An **optometrist,** on the other hand, has a degree in optometry and a license from the State Board of Optometry. He is allowed to examine patients for refractive errors, and to prescribe glasses or contact lenses to overcome them but he is not allowed to dilate the pupil of the eye nor to prescribe drugs. Optometrists generally refer patients with other than refractive difficulties to ophthalmologists.

The American Board of Ophthalmology requires three years of an approved residency, plus one year of active practice, before examining applicants for certification.

CONSULTANTS

Samuel D. Aiken, M. D.
Diplomate, American Board of Ophthalmology; Former Assistant Clinical Professor, Ophthalmology, University of California Medical Center, San Francisco
Santa Rosa, California

A. Paul Keller, Jr., M. D.
Diplomate, American Board of Ophthalmology; Diplomate, American Board of Otolaryngology
Athens, Georgia

abducens muscle (ab-dūs′ens). Another name for the external **rectus muscle** which rotates the eye outwardly.

abduction (ab-duk′shun). In ophthalmology, the act of rotating the eye outwardly.

accommodation (ak-kom-ō-dā′shun). The ability of the lens to change its shape in adjusting to near and far vision.

achromatopsia (a-krōm-a-top′sē-a). CHROM=color; OP=see. Total color blindness. (*adj.*—achromatop′sic.)

achromatosis (a-krōm-a-tō′sis). Lack of normal pigmentation in the iris.

acuity (a-kyū′i-tē). The capacity of the eye to discriminate fine details of objects.

albinism (al′bin-izm *or* al′bīn-izm). In ophthalmology, absence of normal pigment in the eye. Albinism is, fortunately, rare.

amaurosis (am-aw-rō′sis). Complete loss or lack of vision, occurring without an apparent lesion of the eye structures.

amblyopia (am-blē-ōp′ē-a). Impairment of vision, with no detectable organic lesion.

ametropia (am-e-trōp′ē-a). Inability of the eye to focus an image exactly upon the retina. *See myopia, hyperopia, astigmatism.*

angioid streaks (anj′ē-oyd). Pigmented lines sometimes seen in the fundus, simulating a blood vessel pattern. It is associated with several systemic illnesses.

aniseikonia (an-i-sī-kōn′ē-a). ANISO= unequal. A condition in which the size or shape of an object as seen by one eye differs from the image seen by the other eye.

anisocoria (an-i-sō-kōr′ē-a). Inequality in the diameter of the two pupils.

anisometropia (an-i-sō-me-trō′pē-a). Inequality of the refractive power of the two eyes.

anophthalmia (an-off-thal′mē-a) — **anophthalmos** (an-off-thal′mos). OPHTHAL=eye. The absence of an eye (congenital, or following its removal).

anterior chamber. The space between the cornea and the iris. (Fig. 13. p. 127)

aphakia (a-fāk′ē-a). Absence of the lens of an eye, as following an operation for **cataract.**

aqueous humor (ā′kwē-us hew′mer). AQUA=water. The watery fluid filling the space between the cornea and the lens.

arcus senilis (ark′us sen′il-is). A gray or whitish ring in the periphery of the cornea sometimes seen in older people.

Argyll Robertson pupil. A pupil which has lost the ability to accommodate to different degrees of light, but which does accommodate to different distances.

asthenopia (as-thēn-ōp′ē-a). ASTHEN=weakness. Any symptoms or distress resulting from, or accompanying, the use of an eye ("eye strain").

astigmatism (a-stig′ma-tizm). A vision defect usually caused by unevenness in the curvature of the cornea. (*adj.*,—astigmat′ic.)

atropine (at′rō-pēn). A drug used in ophthalmology, principally for dilating the pupil. When used to allow better examination of the retina with the ophthalmoscope, it may be referred to as "drops." It is also used as a **cycloplegic** (to paralyze the focusing power of the eye) during examination.

bifocal (bī-fōk′al). A common name of an artificial lens which is made in two parts with different focuses to improve both near and far vision. Also used as an adjective.

binocular vision (bīn-ok′yū-lar). The ability of the brain to fuse and correlate the separate images produced on the two retinas.

blepharitis (blef-a-rī′tis). BLEPH=eyelid. Inflammation of the margins of the eyelids.

blepharoptosis (blef-er-op-tō′sis). The involuntary drooping down of an eyelid, generally due to a nervous system defect.

blepharospasm (blef′a-rō-spazm). Inability to separate the eyelids, resulting from muscular spasm.

blind spot. A spot in the **retina,** where the **optic nerve** enters, which is not sensitive to light.

bulbar (bul′bar). *adj.* In ophthalmology, referring to the eyeball.

canaliculus (kan-al-ik′yūl-us). One of the canals in the upper and lower eyelids which carries the tears from the eyes to the tear sacs. (*plural—* canalic′uli.) (Fig. 14, p. 129)

canthus (kan′thus). The angle formed by the eyelids at either end of the eye.

capsulotomy (kap-sul-lot′ō-mē). An incision made surgically into the capsule of the lens.

caruncle lacrimalis (kar′ung-kl lak-rim-al′is). The pinkish mound at the inner **canthus** of the eye.

cataract (kat′ar-akt). A condition in which the lens of the eye becomes opaque. Types of cataract are cap′-sular, congen′ital, cor′tical, hypermature′, incip′ient, mature′, nuc′-lear, se′nile, tox′ic, and traumat′ic.

chalazion (ka-lā′zē-on). A cyst like enlargement of a **meibomian gland** of an upper eyelid.

chemosis (kēm-ō′sis). **Edema** limited to the part of the **conjunctiva** covering the eyeball.

choked disk. A name given to swelling of the optic nerve where it enters the eye posteriorly. Also called **papilledema.**

chorioretinitis (kōr-ē-ō-ret-in-īt′is). Inflammation of the **choroid** as well as of the **retinal** layer of the eye.

choroid (kōr′oyd). The middle one of the three coats of the eye. It carries blood vessels to the other parts of the eye. (Fig. 13, p. 127)

choroiditis (kōr-oyd-ī′tis). Inflammation of the **choroid** coat of the eye.

cilia (sil′ē-a). *plural.* The eyelashes. The singular, cil′ium, is seldom used.

ciliary body (sil′ē-air-ē). That part of the vascular coat of the eye which contains the ciliary muscles. The ciliary muscles control the ability of the lens to change its shape, as required for **accommodation.** (Fig. 13, p. 127)

color vision. The faculty of distinguishing different colors.

cones (retinal) (kōnz). Specialized visual cells in the retina which are responsible for sharpness of vision and for color vision.

conjunctiva (kon-junk-tīv′a). The delicate membrane that lines the eyelids (**palpebral** portion) and covers the exposed surface of the eyeball (**bulbar** portion).

conjunctival sac (kon-junk′tiv-al). The space between the eyelids and the eyeball which is lined by **conjunctiva.**

conjunctivitis (kon-junk-tiv-ī′tis). Inflammation of the **conjunctiva,** generally only the **palpebral** portion.

contact lens. A corrective lens made of transparent plastic, molded to cover part or all of the surface of the cornea, eliminating the need for conventional eyeglasses.

convergence (kon-verj′ens). VERG= turn. The turning in of the two lines of sight when focusing on a nearby point.

cornea (korn'ē-a). The transparent structure forming the anterior part of the external layer of the eyeball. It is the principal refracting medium of the eye. (Fig. 13, below)

corneal reflex (korn'ē-al re'fleks). Blinking or winking in response to approaching, touching, or irritating the cornea.

cyclitis (sī-klī'tis). Inflammation of the **ciliary body.**

cyclodialysis (sī-klō-dī-al'i-sis). CYCLO=ciliary muscle. A surgical procedure used to reduce intraocular pressure in certain types of **glaucoma.**

cycloplegia (sī-klō-plēj'ē-a). Loss or lack of accommodation power of the lens due to paralysis of the **ciliary** muscle. *See* **atropine.**

dacryoadenectomy (dāk-rē-ō-ad-en-ek'-tō-mē). Surgical removal of the **lacrimal gland.**

dacryoadenitis (dāk-rē-ō-ad-en-ī'tis). DACRYO=tears; ADEN=gland. Inflammation of the **lacrimal gland** which is located above the upper eyelid.

dacryocystitis (dāk-rē-ō-sist-ī'tis). CYST=sac. Inflammation of the conducting portion of the **lacrimal apparatus.**

dacryocystorhinostomy (dāk-rē-ō-sist-ō-rīn-ost'ō-mē). RHIN=nose. The surgical procedure of forming a communication between the **lacrimal sac** and the interior surface of the nose.

Descemet's membrane (Des-e-maz'). A thin internal membrane between the substantia propria and the endothelial layer of the cornea.

detachment of retina. A condition in which the inner layers of the retina become separated from the pigment layer.

dilator pupillae (pyū'pil-lē). The radiating elastic fibers of the iris which dilate the pupil.

diopter (dī-op'ter). A unit used in designating the refractive power of a lens.

diplopia (dip-lōp'ē-a). **Double vision.**

divergence (dī-verj'ens). Deviation of the lines of sight of the two eyes, causing faulty vision.

double vision. A weakness or disturbance of nerve function resulting in the seeing of an object as double or as two objects.

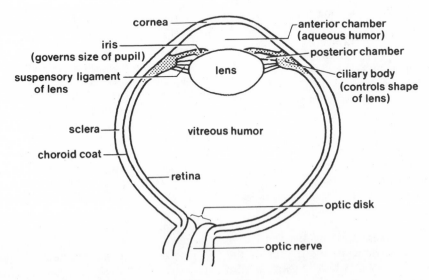

FIG. 13. Eye

ectropion (ek-trōp'ē-on). The **eversion** (turning out) of the edge of an eyelid.

emmetropia (em-e-trōp'ē-a). The normal condition of the eye with respect to **refraction.**

endophthalmitis (end-off-thal-mī'tis). Inflammation of the internal tissues of the eye.

enophthalmos (en-off-thal'mos). Abnormally deep recession of the eyeball into the socket.

entropion (en-trōp'ē-on). The **inversion** (turning in) of the edge of an eyelid.

enucleation (ē-nūk-lē-ā'shun). In ophthalmology, the surgical removal of an eye.

epicanthus (ep-i-kan'thus). A congenital skin fold alongside the nose which conceals the "inner corner" of the eye.

epiphora (ē-pif'ōr-a). An abnormal overflow of tears over the cheek, generally due to some affection of the tear-conducting apparatus.

episcleritis (ep-i-skler-ī'tis). Inflammation of the outer coat of the **sclera** and of the tissues overlying the sclera.

esophoria (es-ō-fōr'ē-a). A tendency of the eyes to turn inward with relation to each other.

esotropia (es-ō-trōp'ē-a). Manifest turning inward of one eye ("crossed eyes").

exophoria (eks-ō-fōr'ē-a). A tendency of the eyes to turn outward with relation to each other.

exophthalmos (eks-off-thal' mos). Abnormal forward protrusion of the eyeball.

exotropia (eks-ō-trōp'ē-a). Manifest turning outward of one eye.

fluorescein (flūr-es'sin). A stain sometimes used to demonstrate ulceration or laceration of the cornea. It turns the damaged portion of the cornea green.

fovea centralis (fōv'ē-a cen-tral'is). A depressed area in the center of the **macula lutea,** where vision is the most distinct.

fundus (fun'dus). In ophthalmology, the concave interior of the eye which is visible through an **ophthalmoscope** ("eyeground").

fusion (fyū'zhun). The normal, unconscious blending of the separate images in the two eyes of the same object into one mental image.

glaucoma (glaouw-kōm'a). A condition in which the intraocular pressure is abnormally high. Types of glaucoma are absolute, acute, chron'ic, congen'ital, closed angle, and open angle.

gonioscope (gōn'ē-ō-skōp). The instrument used in examining the anterior chamber of the eye.

gonioscopy (gōn-ē-os'kō-pē). The examination, using a **gonioscope,** of the angle between the iris and the cornea.

goniotomy (gōn-ē-ot'ō-mē). A surgical procedure used in the treatment of congenital **glaucoma.**

Graefe's sign (Grā'fēz). Slowness of the upper lid to follow the movement of the eyeball on looking downward. It sometimes indicates thyroid trouble.

hemianopsia (hem-ē-an-op'sē-a). Blindness in one-half of the field of vision of one or both eyes.

heterochromia (het-er-ō-krōm'ē-a). A difference in the coloration of the iris of the two eyes.

heterophoria (het-er-ō-fōr'ē-a). Any tendency to deviation from normal muscle balance.

heterotropia (het-er-ō-trōp'ē-a). An obvious deviation of the visual axis of one eye from that of the other **(strabismus).**

hordeolum (hor-dē'ō-lum). A big name for a **sty.** (Also spelled stye.)

humor (hew'mer). A term used to designate the fluids in the eye (**vitreous** or **aqueous**).

hyperopia (hī-per-ōp'ē-a). "Farsightedness"; a condition in which light rays converge behind the retina, generally the result of a smaller-than-normal eyeball.

hypertropia (hī-per-trōp'ē-a). Elevation of one of the visual axes.

hyphema (hī-fēm'a). Hemorrhage into the anterior chamber of the eye.

hypopyon (hī-pōp'ē-on). PYO=pus. An accumulation of pus in the anterior chamber of the eye.

hypotony (hī-pot'ō-nē). TON=tension. A condition in which the intraocular tension is too low. (*adj.* – hypoton'-ic.)

image (im-āg'). In ophthalmology, the mental representation produced by an object "seen" by the eye.

injection (injek'shun). A term sometimes used to refer to redness of the **conjunctiva.**

instillation (in-stil-lā'shun). In ophthalmology, a term referring to the introduction of liquid into the **conjunctival sac,** usually by drops.

interstitial keratitis (in-ter-stish'al ker-a-tī'tis). A particular inflammation of the cornea, generally due to congenital **syphilis.**

intraocular (in-tra-ok'yūl-ar). *adj.* Within the eye.

iridectomy (ir-i-dek'tō-mē). IRI=iris. The surgical removal of a portion of the iris.

iridocyclitis (ir-i-dō-sī-klī'tis). Simultaneous inflammation of both the iris and the ciliary body.

iridodialysis (ir-i-dō-dī-al'i-sis). A separation or tearing away of the iris from its attachment.

iridotomy (ir-i-dot'ō-mē). Any surgical incision made into the iris.

iris (ī'ris). The colored, circular, perforated membrane surrounding the pupil, which regulates the amount of light entering the eye by shaping the size of the pupil. (*plural* – ir'ides or i'rises.) (Fig. 13, p. 127)

iritis (ī-rīt'is). Inflammation of the iris.

Ishihara's color plates (Ish-i-har'az). A set of colored patterns used in determining color blindness.

Jaeger's test types (yāg'erz). Lines of mixed type for testing near vision.

keratitis (ker-a-tī'tis). Inflammation of the cornea which is sometimes characterized by loss of transparency.

lacrima (lak'rim-a). LACRI=tear. A tear. (*adj.* – lacrimal; *plural* – lac'-rimae.)

lacrimal canaliculus (lak'rimal kan-al-ik'yūl-us). One of four short tubes (one in each eyelid) through which tears are conveyed from the **puncta** to the **lacrimal sac.** (Fig. 14, below)

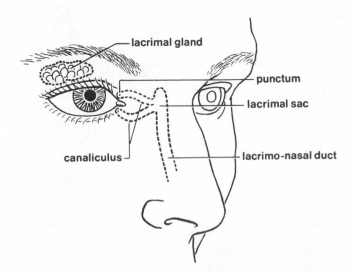

FIG. 14. Lacrimal System

lacrimal duct. The paired duct which conveys the tears from the lacrimal sac to the inner surface of the nose. Also called the **nasolacrimal duct.** (Fig. 14, p. 129)

lacrimal gland. The gland which secretes the tears, located in the upper and outer part of each orbit. (Fig. 14, p. 129)

lacrimal punctum (punk'tum). The opening, near the medial border of each lid, by which tears enter the **canaliculus.** (*plural*—punc'ta.) (Fig. 14, p. 129)

lacrimal sac. The dilated portion of each lacrimal duct into which the canaliculi drain. (Fig. 14, p. 129)

lacrimation (lak-rim-ā'shun). The production and shedding of tears.

lagophthalmos (lag-off-thal'mos). A condition in which the upper lid, when lowered, does not completely cover the eye.

lens (lenz). The transparent body within the eye which converges light rays on their way toward the retina. (*adj.*—lentic'ular.) (Fig. 13, p. 127)

leukoma (lūk-ōm'a). A dense white opacity of the cornea.

levator palpebrae (lēv-ā'tor pal-pēb'rē). A muscle which raises the upper eyelid.

limbus (lim'bus). The circular edge of the **cornea,** where it joins the **sclera.**

loupe (loop). A convex lens for examining the exterior tissues of the eye or for concentrating light upon them. Some loupes are binocular.

luxation (luks-ā'shun). Dislocation; in ophthalmology, referring to dislocation of the lens.

macula lutea (mak'yūl-a lū-tē'a). A small circular area in the retina where vision is the most acute, and the most responsive to color vision.

meibomian glands (mī-bōm'ē-an). Certain sebaceous glands located in the eyelids.

metamorphopsia (met-a-mor-fop'sē-a). MORPH=shape. The technical name for an eye condition in which objects appear distorted.

microphthalmia (mī-krof-thal'mē-a). A developmental condition resulting in abnormally small eyeballs.

miosis (mī-ō'sis). An abnormally small, contracted pupil seen in certain conditions. (*adj.*—miot'ic.)

monocular (mōn-ok'yūl-ar). *adj.* Pertaining to, or having only one eye.

mydriasis (mid-rī'a-sis). Extreme **dilatation** of the pupil.

mydriatic (mid-rē-at'ik). A drug used for **dilating** the pupil.

myopia (mī-ōp'ē-a). An eye condition in which light rays coverge in front of the retina, generally the result of a larger-than-normal eyeball ("nearsightedness").

naso-lacrimal duct (nā-zō-lak'rim-al). The duct conveying tears from the lacrimal sac to the interior of the nose.

nearsightedness. A common name for **myopia.**

nyctalopia (nik-tal-ōp'ē-a). "Night blindness."

nystagmus (nis-tag'mus). A repeating, involuntary movement of the eyeball, generally in one plane. It is slow, with a fast return.

ocular (ok'yūl-ar). *adj.* Pertaining to the eye.

oculist (ok'yūl-ist). A physician specializing in diagnosis and treatment of diseases of the eye. More recently he is referred to as an **opthalmologist.**

oculomotor (ok-yūl-ō-mōt'or). The third cranial nerve. Also used as an adjective, relating to eye movements.

opaque (ō-pāk'). *adj.* Partially or completely impervious to light rays. (*noun*—opac'ity.)

ophthalmia (of-thal'mē-a). **Conjunctivitis;** also, infection of the eye itself.

ophthalmia neonatorum (nē-ō-nā-tōr'um). Gonorrheal **conjunctivitis** of the newborn.

ophthalmodynamometer (of-thal-mō-dīn-a-mom'e-ter). MET=measure.

An instrument sometimes used for measuring the blood pressure in the retinal vessels.

ophthalmologist (of-thal-mol′ō-jist). A specialist in ophthalmology.

ophthalmology (of-thal-mol′ō-jē). *See* introductory paragraphs.

ophthalmoplegia (of-thal-mō-plēj′ē-a). Paralysis of some of the eye muscles.

ophthalmoscope (of-thal′mō-skōp). SCOPE=look, see. An instrument used for inspecting the interior of the eye. It employs a light source and a perforated mirror.

ophthalmoscopy (of-thal-mos′kō-pē). Examination of the interior of the eye with the **ophthalmoscope.**

optic (op′tik). *adj.* OP=sight, eye. Pertaining to sight, or to the eye.

optic atrophy (at′rō-fē). Degeneration of the optic nerve fibers, usually accompanied by loss of vision.

optic chiasm (kī′azm)—**optic chiasma** (kī-az′ma). An arrangement of the optic nerves, allowing the crossing of some fibers to the opposite side of the brain.

optic disk. A round, yellowish, disklike area seen in the **fundus.** It represents the spreading out of the optic nerve fibers connecting with the **retina.** Also called the **optic papilla.**

optic nerve. The second cranial nerve which carries visual images from the retina to the brain. (Fig. 13, p. 127)

optic papilla (pa-pil′a). Another name for the **optic disk.**

optician (op-tish′un). A technician who makes eyeglasses or optical instruments in accordance with a prescribed formula.

optics (op′tiks). The science dealing with light and vision.

optometrist (op-tom′e-trist). One trained in measuring and overcoming mechanical visual defects. His license generally does not allow the use of any drugs.

optometry (op-tom′e-trē). Nonmedical visual care.

ora serrata (ō′ra ser-rā′ta). The outer edge of the retina where it attaches to the underlying **choroid** coat.

orbicularis oculi (orb-ik-yūl-ar′is ok′-yūl-ē). A circular eyelid muscle which closes the eyelids.

orbit (orb′it). The bony eye socket.

orthophoria (or-thō-fōr′ē-a). The condition of normal eye muscle balance (straight eyes).

orthoptics (or-thop′tiks). The teaching and training process aimed at improving or eliminating **strabismus.**

palpebra (pal-pē′bra). The eyelid, any one of four. (*plural*—palpe′brae.)

palpebral fissure (pal-pē′bral). The space between the two eyelids.

pannus (pan′us). An abnormal condition in which blood vessels invade the normally transparent cornea. (*plural*—pan′ni.)

panophthalmitis (pan-of-thal-mī′tis). An inflammatory process involving all the structures of the eyeball.

papilledema (pap-il-e-dēm′a). Noninflammatory swelling of the optic disk, as seen in advanced **nephritis** or in increased intracranial pressure.

papillitis (pap-il-lī′tis). Inflammation of the **optic disk.**

perimeter (per-im′e-ter). An instrument used to determine the extent of the field of vision.

peripheral vision (per-if′er-al). What one is able to perceive outside the direct line of vision.

phlyctenula (flik-ten′yūl-a). An ulcerated nodule occurring on the conjunctiva (**phlyctenular conjunctivitis**) or on the cornea (**phlyctenular keratitis**).

photopsia (fō-top′sē-a). The perception of sparks or flashes of light caused by retinal disease.

phthisis bulbi (thī′sis bul′bē). Shrinkage, wasting, and atrophy of the eye.

pilocarpine (pī-lō-karp′ēn). A drug sometimes used in the treatment of **glaucoma.**

pinguecula (pin-gwek′yūl-a). A benign yellowish spot on the **bulbar conjunctiva.**

"pink eye". The name of a common type of **conjunctivitis** (applied by the public to almost every red eye).

plica semilunaris (plēk′a sem-ē-lūn-ar′-is). The fold of **conjunctiva** in the medial corner of the eye.

posterior chamber. The space between the back of the iris and the front of the lens. (Fig. 13, p. 127)

presbyopia (pres-bē-ōp′ē-a). The usual impairment of vision associated with advancing years or old age ("the far-sightedness of the forties"). It results from weakening of the power of the eye to focus or accommodate.

prism (prizm). In ophthalmology, the transparent component of any optical system which is used to bend light rays.

prosthesis (pros-thē′sis). In ophthalmology, generally refers to an artificial eye ("glass eye"). (*plural* — prosthe′-ses.)

pseudo-isochromatic charts (sūd-ō-ī-sō-krōm-at′ik). A set of colored charts used in testing color vision.

pterygium (ter-ij′ē-um). A triangular membrane growing from the conjunctival border toward the center of the cornea.

ptosis (tōs′is). A paralytic drooping of the upper eyelid. (*plural* — pto′ses.)

pupil (pyū′pil). The opening at the center of the iris through which light rays pass. Its size changes as the iris contracts or relaxes in accordance with the brightness of the light, or in the process of **accommodation.**

pupillary reflex (pyū′pil-ler-ē). The involuntary constriction of the pupil which occurs when bright light strikes the eye, or when the eye **accommodates** (focuses).

rectus muscle (rek′tus). One of the muscles attached to the eyeball to accomplish eye movement.

refraction (rē-frak′shun). The deviation given to light rays when they pass from one transparent medium to another of a different density. Also, the diagnostic process of determining the refractive errors of the eye, and their correction by glasses.

refractive error (rē-frac′tiv). An eye defect which prevents light rays from focusing exactly on the retina.

retina (ret′in-a). The image-receiving, inner coat of the eye. The light-sensitive **rods** and **cones** are located in the retina. (Fig. 13, p. 127)

retinal detachment (ret′in-al). An abnormal separating of the retina from the next underlying tissues.

retinitis (ret-in-ī′tis). Inflammation of the retina.

retinopathy (ret-in-op′a-thē). PATH= disease. A diseased condition of the retina due to various causes. Types include diabet′ic and hyperten′sive.

retinoscope (ret′in-ō-skōp). An instrument for determining the refractive state of the eye. The examination procedure is called **retinoscopy** or **skias′copy.**

retrolental fibroplasia (ret-rō-len′tal fīb-rō-plāz′ē-a). A retinal disease seen in some premature babies.

rods (retinal). Specialized visual cells in the retina which respond to low levels of illumination and give black and white responses.

Schlemm's canal (Schlemz). The circular canal draining the anterior chamber of the eye, located at the junction of the sclera and the cornea.

sclera (skler′a). The "white" or thick outer covering of the eyeball. (*plural* — scler′ae.) (Fig. 13, p. 127)

sclerectomy (skler-ek′tō-mē). Surgical excision of part of the **sclera.**

scleritis (skler-ī′tis). Inflammation of the **sclera.**

sclerokeratitis (skler-ō-ker-a-tī′tis). Simultaneous inflammation of the **sclera** and the **cornea.**

sclerotomy (skler-ot′ō-mē). A surgical incision made into the **sclera.**

scotoma (skō-tōm′a). A "blind spot" in the visual field. (*plural* — scotom′ata.)

"second sight." A condition which sometimes occurs in older people, resulting in their being able to discard their reading glasses for a time. It is generally a symptom of **cataract** formation.

slit lamp. A particular kind of instrument (**biomicroscope**) used in examining the anterior chamber of the eye.

Snellen's chart (Snel'enz). A set of lines and letters used in testing distant vision.

squint (skwint). A common name for **heterophoria, heterotropia,** or **strabismus.**

Stellwag's sign (Stel'wagz). Diminution of the ability to wink.

stereoscopic vision (stēr-ē-ō-skop'ik). The perception of the visual field in three dimensions, accomplished through a mixture of images from the two eyes.

strabismus (stra-biz'mus). Uncontrollable deviation of one eye from the desired line of vision.

sty (stī). Inflammation of one or more of the sebaceous glands at the edge of the eyelids. Also called **hordeolum.**

substantia propria (sub-stan'shē-a prōp'rē-a). In ophthalmology, the parenchyma, or connective tissue, of the cornea.

supraorbital (sūp-ra-orb'i-tal). *adj.* Situated above the eye socket.

symblepharon (sim-blef'a-ron). An adhesion between the eyeball and one of the eyelids.

sympathetic ophthalmia (of-thal'mē-a). Inflammation of one eye following inflammation in the other eye.

synechia (sin-ek'ē-a). An adhesion of the iris to either the cornea *(anterior synechia)* or to the lens *(posterior synechia).*

tarsus (tar'sus). The thin framework of firm tissue which gives shape to the eyelids.

Tenon's capsule (Ten'onz). The fibrous sheath that envelops the eyeball.

tonometer (tōn-om'e-ter). An instrument for measuring the intra-ocular pressure.

trachoma (tra-kōm'a). A chronic, contagious infection of the **conjunctiva** and the **cornea.**

trichiasis (trik-ī'a-sis). TRICH=hair. The condition of "ingrown hairs" sometimes occurring with eyelashes ("ingrown eyelashes").

uvea (yūv'ē-a). A term referring to the entire pigmented vascular coat of the eyeball.

uveitis (yūv-ē-ī'tis). Inflammation of all the coats of the eye.

vergence (verj'ens). A comprehensive term for a particular group of eye movements—convergence, divergence, etc.

visual axis. The line of gaze.

visual field. The area visible to an eye in a given position.

vitreous humor (vit'rē-us). The transparent gelatinous mass that fills the part of the eyeball between the lens and the retina, giving the eye its shape. Also called "the vitreous." (Fig. 13, p. 127)

xanthelasma (zan-thel-az'ma). XANTH=yellow. The presence of small benign yellow tumors in the skin of the eyelids, sometimes seen in elderly people.

xerophthalmia (zēr-of-thal'mē-a). XERO=dry. A type of **conjunctivitis** which produces no liquid discharge. The end result is a dry **atrophic** eyeball.

15 Orthopedics

THE TERM **orthopedics** originally implied the study and treatment of diseases and deformities of the locomotor system. This concept has now been expanded to include those structures *associated with* the functions and articulations of the skeletal system.

Orthopedic surgery is one of the oldest specialties; old surgical records refer to the correction of the effects of deformities, injuries, and amputations. In fact, the term **orthopedics** originates from root words which mean "straight child."

Although happily such disabling diseases as poliomyelitis and tuberculosis of the bone are now disappearing from the orthopedic scene, improvements and refinements of technique (as well as advances in x-ray and anesthesiology procedures) are continually allowing more and more extensive and rewarding restorative operative procedures. The surgical procedure in which both components of the ball-and-socket joint of the hip are replaced with metal and plastic prostheses (the socket half of the joint is anchored in permanent plastic) may well expand to include other joints crippled by disease. Many other equally surprising procedures are being considered and developed.

The American Board of Orthopedic Surgery requires that a candidate complete four years of an approved residency before he may be examined by the board. It also requires one year of orthopedic practice and the submission of complete authentic hospital case records demonstrating the candidate's competence.

CONSULTANTS

T. Wesley Hunter, M.D., F.A.C.S.
Diplomate, American Board of Orthopedic Surgery; Assistant Clinical Professor, Orthopedics, University of California Medical Center
Santa Rosa, California

Douglas D. Toffelmier, M.D.
F.A.C.S.
Diplomate, American Board of Orthopedic Surgery
Oakland, California

abduction (ab-duk'shun). The moving or withdrawing of an arm or a leg *away from* the midline of the body; also, the resulting position.

acetabulum (as-e-tab'yūl-um). The socket of the ball-and-socket joint of the hip. (Fig. 16, p. 143)

Achilles tendon (A-kil'lēz). The **tendon** attaching the calf muscles to the heel bone.

acromioclavicular joint (ak-rō-mē-ō-klav-ik'yūl-ar). The slightly movable joint between the shoulder blade and the collar bone.

acromion (a-krōm'ē-on). The outermost tip of the shoulder; part of the shoulder blade.

adduction (ad-duk'shun). The moving or drawing of an arm of a leg *toward* the midline of the body; also, the resulting position.

Albee (Awl'bē). A name well-known in orthopedics, associated with many procedures, instruments, and pieces of equipment, Albee saw, Albee table, etc.

ankylosis (ang-kil-ō'sis). The loss or absence of mobility of a joint.

apophysis (a-pof'e-sis). An additional growth center not located in the ends of the long bones.

arthralgia (arth-ral'jē-a). ARTH=joint; ALG=pain. Pain in a joint.

arthritis (arth-rīt'is). Inflammation of one or more joints. Types include atroph'ic, degen'erative, gout'y, hy-pertroph'ic, rheum'atoid, and sup'-purative.

arthrocentesis (arth-rō-sen-tē'sis). Puncture of a joint cavity for withdrawal of fluid or for injection of medication.

arthrodesis (arth-rō-dē'sis). The surgical "fusing" or fixation of two or more adjacent joint surfaces.

arthropathy (arth-rop'a-thē). PATH= disease. A general comprehensive term which includes any disease of a joint.

articulation (art-ik-yūl-ā'shun). The natural joining or connecting of two adjacent bones, allowing varying degrees of mobility. Types include acromioclavic'ular, astragalocalcan'eal, costovert'ebral, intervert'ebral, metacarpophalan'geal, metatarsophalang'eal, sternoclavic'ular, substrag'aloid, and others.

astragalus (as-trag'a-lus). One of the very important bones comprising the ankle joint; the **talus**. (Fig. 4, p. 50)

Bradford frame. An orthopedic bed sometimes used in caring for immobilized patients.

bunion (bun'yon). A thickening of the skin and bursa overlying the medial surface of the great toe, forcing it against the other toes.

bursa (burs'a). A fluid-filled sac-like cavity found at frequent points where pressure or friction occurs, as between a muscle or a tendon and an underlying bone. Examples are: Achilles, glu'teal, olec'ranon, poplit'-al, prepatel'lar, and subdel'toid. (*adj.* — bur'sal; *plural* — bur'sae.)

bursitis (burs-ī'tis). Inflammation of or in a bursa.

calcaneus (kal-kān'ē-us). The heel bone.

calcareous (kal-kair'ē-us). *adj.* CALC= lime, stone. Consisting of, or characterized by, the presence of lime or calcium.

calcification (kal-sif-i-kā'shun). Hardening of body tissues by their infiltration with calcium.

callus (kal'lus). In orthopedics, a term referring to new bone formed at the site of a fracture.

cancellous (kan'sel-lus). *adj.* Referring to spongy or soft bone. (Fig. 15, p. 138)

capitellum (kap-i-tel'um). A name given to the lateral condyle of the humerus.

carpus (karp'us). CARP=wrist. A composite name for the wrist region and its parts, particularly the bones. (*adj.*—carpal.) (Fig. 3, p. 41)

cartilage (kart'i-lej). The elastic substance covering joint surfaces of bones. It also makes up some parts of the skeleton. It is sometimes called "gristle." (*adj.*—cartilag'inous.)

cast (kast). A stiff form-fitting support made of bandage impregnated with plaster of paris or other hardening material. It is used for immobilizing sprains, fractures or dislocations. (Also used as a *verb,* to apply a cast.)

Charcot's joint (Shar'kōz). A swollen, painless joint, formerly considered indicative of third stage syphilis, but now more commonly associated with corticosteroid injections.

"Charley horse." A common name for a muscle injury sometimes sustained when a contracted muscle receives a blow.

chondral (kond'ral). *adj.* CHONDR= cartilage. Referring to, or consisting of, cartilage.

chondromalacia (kond-rō-mal-ā'cē-a *or* —sha). MALAC=soft. Softening of a cartilage.

clavicle (klav'i-kl). The technical name for the collar bone. (*adj.*—clavic' ular.)

clubfoot. A common name for a congenital foot deformity. *See* talipes.

coccygodynia (kok-sē-gō-din'ē-a)—coccydynia (kok-sē-din'ē-a). A fancy name for pain in or around the coccyx.

coccyx (kok'siks). The tip of the spine ("tail bone"). (*adj.*—coccyg'eal.)

collateral ligaments (ko-lat'er-al). Strong longitudinal ligaments which help to support the knee, elbow and wrist joints.

condyle (kond'īl). A rounded projection of a bone, usually at its end, allowing articulation with an adjacent bone. (*adj.*—cond'ylar.)

contraction (kon-trak'shun). TRAC= draw. The temporary shortening of a muscle when it is activated and exerts force.

contracture (kon-trak'tchur). A sometimes temporary, but frequently permanent, shortening or distortion of muscles or of tendons.

coracoid process (kōr'a-koyd). A bony projection originating from the outer end of the scapula.

coronoid process (kōr'o-noyd). A bony projection from the upper end of the ulna.

cortex (kort'eks). In orthopedics, the outer shell of the many hard bones. (*adj.*—cort'ical.) (Fig. 15, p. 138)

costal (kost'al). *adj.* Referring to a rib or ribs.

crepitus (krep'i-tus). In orthopedics, the crackling heard or felt when fractured bony surfaces rub together. *See* crepitant.

cruciate ligaments (krūsh'ē-āt). Important knee-joint ligaments (two in each knee).

cuboid (kyūb'oyd). One of the seven ankle bones.

cuneiform (kyūn-ē'i-form). A name applied to three of the ankle bones and to one of the wrist bones.

diaphysis (dī-af'i-sis). The shaft of a long bone. See epiphysis and metaphysis.

"disk" (formerly "disc"). Medical jargon for a ruptured intervertebral disk which is giving rise to symptoms.

dislocation. The displacement of a bone or bones, generally traumatic, and always involving a joint.

dorsum (dors'um). The back portion of a body structure. (*adj.*—dors'al.)

Dupuytren's contracture (Dūp'ē-tronz). A deformity of the hand and fingers, mostly involving the medial half of

dysplasia

the hand. It produces varying degrees of **flexion** of the last three fingers, and wrinkling of the palm.

dysplasia (dis-plā'zha *or* – zē-a). A congenital abnormality which involves the interruption or cessation of the growth process in a part of the body, notably the bones.

epiphyseal line (ē-pif-e-sē'al). The cartilaginous line present near the ends of long bones during early life. It separates the **epiphysis** and **diaphysis** (shaft) and is the region where bone growth occurs. (Fig. 15, p. 138)

epiphysis (ē-pif'a-sis). The flared out portion of the long bones where most of their growth occurs and **ossification** begins. *See* **diaphysis** and **metaphysis.**

equinovarus (ē-kwīn-ō-vair'us). EQUI= horse. The technical name for a "clubfoot" deformity.

equinus (ē-kwīn'us). The composite name of several foot deformities in which the toes point downward, suggesting the hoof of a horse (hence the name).

erector spinae (ē-rek'tor spīn'ē). The group of back muscles which straightens the spinal column.

Ewing's tumor (yū'ingz). A malignant tumor occurring in the shafts of long bones. It is generally seen in young people.

exostosis (eks-os-tō'sis). OS=bone. A localized benign overgrowth on the surface of a bone.

extension. The straightening of a part of the body, or the moving of it toward a straightened position. Opposite of **flexion.**)

fabella (fa-bel'la). A **sesamoid** bone which is located behind the knee joint and is frequently involved in athletic injuries.

fascia (fash'a *or* fash'ē-a). The sheet of fibrous tissue enveloping, supporting, or separating muscles and organs.

femur (fēm'ur). The large thigh bone. (*adj.* – fem'oral.) (Fig. 4, p. 50; Fig. 16, p. 143)

fibula (fib'yūl-a). The outer and smaller of the two bones of the lower leg. It does not support weight. (Fig. 4, p. 50)

"flatfoot." A vernacular name for the condition of abnormal flattening of the sole of the foot (**pes planus**).

flexion (fleks'shun). FLEX=bend. The bending of a part of the body, or the moving of it toward a more angulated position. (Opposite of **extension.**)

fracture (frak'tchur). The accidental (or intentional) sudden breaking of a bone or tendon; also, the resulting condition. Types include Bennett's, Col'les, comminuted, compound, compression, depressed, epiphyse'al, greenstick, impacted, intercon'dylar, intracap'sular, lin'ear, oblique, patholog'ic, Pott's, spiral, stellate, and transverse.

fusion (fyūzh'un). The growing together of two or more adjacent, separate bones following their surgical joining. Also, the surgical procedure employed.

ganglion cyst (gang'glē-on). A subcutaneous cystic tumor, generally originating from a tendon sheath on the back of the wrist.

genu valgum (jē'nū val'gum). GENU= knee. The condition of "knock-knees."

genu varum (jē'nū vair'um). The condition of "bow legs."

glenohumeral subluxation (glen-ō-hūm'-er-al sub-luks-ā'shun). A very common type of shoulder dislocation.

glenoid cavity (glen'oyd). The socket of the ball-and-socket joint of the shoulder.

glenoid fossa (fos'sa). The socket in the temporal bone with which the lower jaw **articulates.**

hallux (hal'luks). The big toe.

hallux valgus (val'gus). A deformity characterized by the turning of the great toe toward the other toes. It is often associated with **bunion** formation.

hamate (ham'āt). One of the eight **carpal** (wrist) bones.

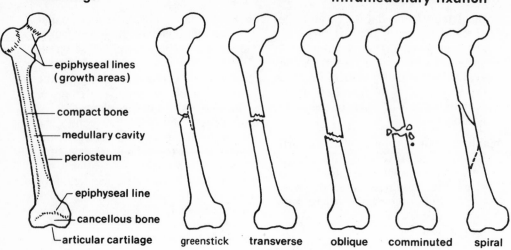

epiphyseal lines
(growth areas)

compact bone

medullary cavity

periosteum

epiphyseal line

cancellous bone

articular cartilage

greenstick   transverse   oblique   comminuted   spiral

FIG. 15. Structure and Formation of Bone and Types of Fractures

hamstrings. The tendons of the posterior thigh muscles, which flex the leg at the knee.

haversian canals (hav-ers′ē-an). The interlaced system of canals in compact bone. It contains the blood vessels carrying nourishment to the bone.

hemarthrosis (hēm-arth-rō′sis). A collection of blood within a joint cavity.

"hip nailing." Fixation of the fragments of a fractured hip by using internal fixation (pins, etc.).

"hip spica" (spīk′a). A term commonly given to a type of cast sometimes used in treating fracture of the **femur.**

humerus (hūm′er-us). The large bone of the upper arm.

hydrarthrosis (hī-drarth-rō′sis). A collection of nonbloody fluid in a joint cavity.

hyperostosis (hī-per-os-tō′sis). A large abnormal projection on the surface of a bone (a large **exostosis**).

iliac crest (il′ē-ak). The upper, lateral free edge of the **ilium.** (Fig. 16, p. 143)

ilium (il′ē-um). The uppermost of the three fused bones (paired) forming the bony pelvis. (Fig. 16, p. 143)

insertion. The attachment of a muscle or its tendon to the part of the skeleton which the muscle moves when it contracts. *See* **origin.**

internal fixation. A method of fracture treatment in which stabilizing material is inserted into the interior of the fractured bone.

interspinous ligament (in-ter-spīn′us). The ligament joining the spinous projection of each vertebra to that of its adjacent neighbor.

intertrochanteric (in-ter-trō-kan-ter′ik). *adj.* Referring to the location between the major and minor **trochanters** of the **femur.** It is a frequent fracture site.

intervertebral disk (in-ter-ver-tēb′ral). One of the several flat cartilaginous pads which occur between adjacent vertebral bodies. Disks are frequently fractured, allowing herniation of the **nucleus pulposus,** which may cause nerve symptoms.

intramedullary fixation (in-tra-med′yūl-lair-ē). The introduction of foreign materials into the marrow cavity of long bones to assist in their alignment and immoblization following fracture.

ischium (isk'ē-um). The lowermost of the three fused bones (paired) forming the bony pelvis. We sit on it. (Fig. 16, p. 143)

Kirschner wire (Kersh'ner). A rigid wire which is drilled through a bone to facilitate the use of traction in treating a fracture.

kyphosis (kīf-ō'sis). An abnormal backward bowing of a part of the spinal column (concavity facing forward—"hunchback"). *See* **lordosis.**

lamina (lam'in-a). One of the two flattened sides of the arch of a vertebra. (*plural*—lam'inae.)

laminectomy (lam-in-ek'tō-mē). The surgical removal of a spinal **lamina** to allow approach to the intervertebral space.

lateral condyle (kon'dīl). The lateral enlargement of the lower end of the **femur.**

ligamentum flavum (lig-a-ment'um flāv'-um). One of the several short pairs of ligaments which connect each two adjacent vertebral arches. (*plural*—ligament'a flav'a.)

lordosis (lord-ō'sis). An abnormal forward bowing of a part of the spinal column, the concavity facing backward. It is commonly referred to as "swayback." *See* **kyphosis.**

lumbar (lum'bar). *adj.* LUMB=loin. Referring to the loins or lower back.

lumbosacral joint (lum-bō-sāk'ral). The semisolid junction of the **sacrum** with the fifth **lumbar vertebra.**

lunate (lūn'āt). One of the eight carpal (wrist) bones.

luxation (lux-ā'shun). A dislocation.

malar bone (māl'ar). The cheek bone, generally called the zygoma.

malleolus (mal-lē'ō-lus). Either of the two bony prominences of each ankle. (*plural*—malle'oli.)

mandible (man'di-bl). The lower jaw. (Fig. 18, p. 148)

manubrium sterni (man-ūb're-um stern'ē). The upper segment of the breastbone. (Fig. 4, p. 50)

medial condyle (mēd'ē-al kon'dīle). The medial enlargement of the lower end of the **femur.**

meniscus (men-isk'us). One of the two crescent-shaped joint cartilages found in each knee joint. (*plural*—menis'ci.)

metacarpals (met-a-kar'plz). The five bones positioned between the wrist and the fingers in each hand. (Fig. 3, p. 41)

metaphysis (met-af'i-sis). The flaring-out portion of the diaphysis (shaft) of the long bones, where it joins with the epiphysis. *See* **epiphysis** and **diaphysis.**

metatarsals (met-a-tar'slz). The five bones in each foot corresponding to the **metacarpals** in each hand.

myelitis (mī-el-ī'tis). *See* **osteomyelitis.**

myeloma (mī'el-ō-ma). MYEL=marrow; OMA=tumor. A slowly growing tumor of the bone marrow, or of the bone marrow cavity wall.

navicular (nav-ik'yul-ar). One of the tarsal (ankle) bones; also, one of the carpal (wrist) bones.

nucleus pulposus (nūk'lē-us pul-pōs'us). The semisolid inner portion of each intervertebral disk. When the rim of the disk allows it to herniate, nerve pressure may be produced. (*plural*—nuclei pulposi.)

nutrient artery (nut'rē-ent). An artery found in some of the long bones. It supplies the bone with its nourishment and is an important factor in the healing of fractures.

olecranon (ō-lek'ra-non). The tip of the elbow.

origin. In orthopedics, the fixed attachment or anchor of a muscle. It allows the muscle to exert power when it contracts. *See* **insertion.**

orthopedics (orth-ō-pēd'iks). *See* introductory paragraphs.

orthopedist (orth-ō-pēd'ist). A doctor who specializes in orthopedics.

Osgood-Schlatter's disease (Os'good Shlat'erz). Traumatic separation of the tibial **tubercle** from the **tibia** by sudden strain thrown upon it through the knee cap ligament.

ossification (os-if-i-kā′shun). The normal process of the hardening or forming of bone through the deposition of calcium. *See* **ossification centers.**

ossification centers. The specific points, usually located in the **epiphyses** of bones, from which **ossification** spreads.

osteitis (os-te-ī′tis). Inflammation of a bone, generally also involving the marrow cavity of the bone. (Also called **osteomyeli′tis.**

osteitis deformans (dē-form′anz). **Paget's disease.**

osteoarthritis (os-tē-ō-arth-rī′tis). A noninfectious, chronic, degenerative disease which may involve many joints and which generally occurs in later life.

osteoarthropathy (os-tē-ō-arth-rop′a-thē). A broad term covering any disease of bones and joints.

osteochondritis (os-tē-ō-kon-drī′tis). CHONDR=cartilage. Disease or inflammation of the joint cartilage covering the end of a bone.

osteochondritis dissecans (dis′ē-kanz). An unexplained disease causing nutritional changes (and detachment of cartilage) in the joint of a long bone, generally the femur or the humerus.

osteochondrosis (os-tē-ō-kon-drō′sis). An abnormal change in the growth of **ossification** pattern, sometimes affecting children.

osteoclast (os′tē-ō-klast). A surgical instrument used for breaking a bone to improve its alignment or function.

osteomalacia (os-tē-ō-mal-ā′sha). Softening of a bone due to disease.

osteomyelitis (os-tē-ō-mī-el-ī′tis). Inflammation in the marrow cavity of a bone. It is sometimes called **myelitis.**

osteoporosis (os-tē-ō-pōr-ō′sis). A condition resulting in increased porousness, or loss of density, of a bone.

osteotomy (os-tē-ot′ō-mē). The surgical procedure of cutting through or into a bone to improve its alignment. Two types are subtrochanter′ic and supracon′dylar.

Paget's disease (Paj′ets). A deforming bone disease characterized by loss of calcium and sometimes causing increased thickening of bones.

patella (pa-tel′la). The kneecap. (Fig. 4, p. 50)

pedicle (ped′i-kl). In orthopedics, a name applied to a specific (paired) portion of each vertebra.

pelvic girdle. A composite term applied to the fused pelvic bones which form the firm connecting link between the vertebral column and the two femurs.

periosteum (per-ē-os′tē-um). The tightly adherent membrane covering the bones. (*adj.*—perios′teal.) (Fig. 15, p. 138)

periostitis (pair-ē-os-tī′tis). Inflammation of the **periosteum.**

Perthes′ disease (Per′thēz). A juvenile type of **osteochondrosis** in which the **epiphysis** of the head of the femur is affected. (Also called **Legg-Calvé-Perthes disease.**)

pes planus (pess plan′us). PES=foot. The medical name for "flat foot."

pes valgus (pess val′gus). One type of clubfoot in which the sole of the foot turns outward.

pes varus (pess vair′us). Another type of clubfoot in which the sole of the foot turns inward.

phalanx (fāl′anks). Any one of the 56 bones of the fingers or toes. (*plural*—phalan′ges) (Fig. 3, p. 41)

pisiform (pīs′i-form). The smallest of the eight **carpal** bones, located on the **ulnar** side of the wrist.

pollex (pol′eks). The thumb. (*plural*—poll′ices.)

polydactylism (pol-ē-dak′til-izm). A deformity characterized by the presence of additional fingers or toes.

Pott's disease. Tuberculous disease of the body of a vertebra. It may also involve vertebrae which are adjacent to the diseased vertebra.

Pott's fracture spondylitis **141**

Pott's fracture. A particular kind of fracture which involves both bones of the lower leg near the ankle.

prepatellar bursa (prē-pa-tel′lar bursa.) A bursa lying over the front of the patella (knee cap). It may become inflamed from constant or repeated pressure against the patella, and is then called "housemaid's knee." **(prepatellar bursitis).**

pronation (prōn-ā′shun). The act of rotating the hand palm-backward or palm-downward; or of turning the foot arch-downward at the ankle joint. Also, the resulting position.

pseudarthrosis — pseudoarthrosis (sūd-arth-rō′sis) (sūd-ō-arth-rō′sis). A "false joint" caused by callus growth between the poorly united bony fragments separated by a previous fracture.

pubis (pyūb′is). The most anterior of the three fused (paired) bones forming the pelvic girdle. (*adj.* — pub′ic.) (Fig. 4, p. 50; Fig. 16, p. 143)

pyarthrosis (pī-arth-rō′sis). PY=pus. The presence of pus within a joint cavity.

rachitic (rā-kit′ik). *adj.* Referring to or originating from **rickets.**

radiocarpal (rād-ē-ō-kar′pl). *adj.* Referring to a part or a function of the region comprising the wrist and the lower end of the radius.

radius (rād′ē-us). The smaller, outer bone of the forearm. Its use allows rotation of the forearm and hand. (Fig. 3, p. 41; Fig. 4, p. 50)

reduction. The "setting" or repositioning of the bony fragments produced and displaced by a fracture. Reductions may be closed (manipulated through the intact skin) or open (through a surgical incision).

rheumatoid arthritis (rūm′a-toyd). An inflammatory type of arthritis, generally severe and often involving several joints simultaneously.

sacrococcygeal (sāk-rō-kok-sij′ē-al). *adj.* Relating to the region of the lower spine, comprising the **sacrum** and the **coccyx.**

sacroiliac (sāk′rō-il′ē-ak). *adj.* Referring to the slightly movable **articulation** between the **ilium** and the **sacrum,** on each side. (Fig. 16, p. 143)

sacrospinalis (sāk-rō-spīn-al′is). A long paired muscle attached to the **sacrum.** It is part of the erector spinae group which straighten and support the spinal column.

sacrum (sāk′rum). The portion of the lower spine made up of the five (fused) sacral vertebrae.

scaphoid (skaf′oyd). A small bone in each wrist and each ankle. (Also called the **navic′ular.**)

scapula (skap′yūl-a). The shoulder blade.

scoliosis (skōl-ē-ō′sis). Curvature of the spine in a lateral direction.

sequestrum (sē-ques′trum). A piece of dead bone which has been completely separated from its parent bone and is without blood supply. This sometimes occurs following fractures.

sesamoid (ses′a-moyd). Any one of several small oval-shaped bones which develop in tendons at pressure sites. Their development is most frequent in the hand or foot.

Smith-Petersen nail. A supporting, flanged, immobilizing "nail" sometimes driven lengthwise through the neck of the **femur** following its fracture.

spinous process (spīn′us). The posterior, midline, downward-pointing extension of each vertebral body.

splint. An appliance used to support, immobilize, or rest an injured part of the body, generally a fractured bone. Common types of splints are aeroplane, banjo, coapta′tion, cock-up, Kanav′el, Roger Anderson, Sta′der, Thomas, and others.

spondylitis (spon-dil-ī′tis). Inflammation in one or more vertebrae, generally referring to **tuberculous** inflammation or to **rheumatoid arthritis.**

spondylolisthesis (spon-dil-ō-lis-thē'sis). Abnormal slipping forward of one vertebra upon the body of the next lower one. It generally occurs in the lower lumbar region.

spondylolysis (spon-dil-ō-lī'sis). A disease or defect of a vertebral body which allows spondylolisthesis to occur.

sprain (sprān). Wrenching of a joint with injury to its attachments but without fracture or dislocation.

Steinmann's pin (Stīn'manz). A steel pin sometimes driven crossways through a bone to assist in reducing or holding a fracture in correct position for healing.

sternum (stern'um). The breast bone.

styloid process (stīl'oyd). A slender projection extending outwardly from the main body of a bone, particularly the radius, the ulna, and the temporal bone.

subcoracoid dislocation (sub-kōr'a-koyd). A common type of shoulder dislocation in which the head of the humerus slips beneath the coracoid process of the scapula.

subluxation (sub-luks-ā'shun). An incomplete dislocation.

supination (sūp-īn-ā'shun). The act of rotating the palm-forward or palm-upward; also, the resulting position. *See* pronation.

sustentaculum tali (sus-ten-tak'yūl-um tāl'ē). A projection originating from the medial surface of the calcaneus (heel bone). The talus articulates with it.

symphysis pubis (sim'fis-is pyūb'is). The midline junction of the two pubic bones, forming the pubic prominence.

synovial fluid (sin-ōv'ē-al) A lubricating fluid contained in the capsules of movable joints and in bursae.

synovial membrane (sin-ōv'ē-al). A connective tissue membrane which lines joint cavities and bursae.

synovium (sin-ōv'ē-um). A term designating the entire (synovial) membrane lining a joint cavity.

talipes (tal'i-pēz). A broad term designating any congenital foot deformity resulting in its being twisted out of shape ("clubfoot").

talus (tāl'us). The uppermost and largest of the seven tarsal bones, and a vital part of the ankle joint. It is also called the astrag'alus.

tarsus (tar'sus). TARS=ankle. A compound term referring to the seven tarsal (ankle) bones. (*adj.*—tar'sal.)

tendon (ten'don). The fibrous inelastic band which attaches some muscles to the bones so that they move when the muscles contract.

tenotomy (ten-ot'ō-mē). The dividing or refashioning of a tendon, frequently for the purpose of lengthening it.

thoracolumbar (thōr-a-kol-um'bar). *adj.* Referring to the region of the lower thoracic and the upper lumbar vertebrae.

tibia (tib'ē-a). The large (weight bearing) bone of the lower leg (shin bone). (*adj.*—tib'ial.) (Fig. 4, p. 50)

traction. The application or exerting of pull on bones (and/or muscles) in order to relieve displacement, overriding, or pressure.

transverse process (of a vertebral body). A large lateral bony projection from each side of a vertebra. It is attached to several muscles and may articulate with other bones.

trapezium (trap-ē'zē-um). One of the eight carpal bones. It is located on the thumb side of the wrist.

trauma (trawm'a). TRAUM=wound. A wound or injury or the force producing it. (*adj.*—traumat'ic.)

triquetrum (trī-kwet'rum). One of the eight wrist bones (carpals).

trochanter (trō-kant'er). One of the two prominences (major and minor) of the upper femur, located just below the neck of the femur. It is a frequent fracture site. (Fig. 16, p. 143)

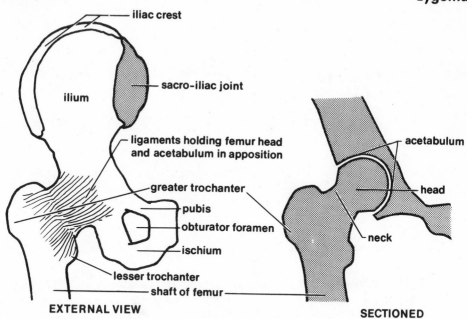

FIG. 16. Region of the Hip Joint

tubercle (tūb′er-kl). A jutting prominence on the surface of a bone. It generally serves as the attaching point for a muscle or a tendon.

ulna (ul′na). The medial (larger) bone of the forearm. (Fig. 3, p. 41; Fig. 4, p. 50)

vertebra (vert′ē-bra). Any one of the 33 bones of the spinal column, of which some are fused. Types of vertebra are: cerv′ical, C 1-7; sac′ral, S 1-5; thorac′ic, T 1-12; coccyg′eal, C 1-4; and lum′bar, L 1-5. (*plural* — vert′ebrae.)

Vitallium (Vit-al′ē-um). The proprietary name of an alloy frequently used in making orthopedic appliances.

xiphoid process (zī′foyd) — **xyphoid process.** The lower end of the breastbone (**sternum**). (Fig. 4, p. 50)

zygoma (zī-gōm′a). The cheek bone. (*adj.* — zygomat′ic.)

16 Otolaryngology

THE TERM **otolaryngology** designates the diagnosis and treatment of diseases of the ear, nose and throat. Originally the specialty was more inclusive and the present "E.N.T. man" was the "E.E.N.T. man," as his province also included the care of eye conditions. That segment of practice has since developed into a specialty of its own called **ophthalmology.**

Although the OPHTHALMO– (eye) root was dropped from the original OPHTHALMO-RHINO-OTO-LARYNGOLOGY for logical reasons, the root RHINO– (nose) was apparently deleted merely to accomplish easier pronunciation, as the specialty still covers the care of nasal conditions. Probably PHARYNGO– (throat) was omitted because there just wasn't enough room in the title. OTOLOGY (ear), has recently shown signs of splitting off into its own separate specialty with the advent of microsurgery of the ear and the development of audioelectric equipment.

With the passing years, the requirements for certification in the specialty have been increased and now four years of special training are stipulated for a candidate. Interest in otolaryngology temporarily declined with the advent of chemotherapeutic and antibiotic agents, but interest has revived because of exciting medical and surgical advances in this field during the past quarter of a century.

CONSULTANTS

A. Paul Keller, Jr., M.D.
*Diplomate, American Board of
Otolaryngology; Diplomate, American
Board of Ophthalmology
Athens, Georgia*

Bruce G. Whitaker, Ph.D., M.D.
*Diplomate, American Board of Otolaryngology; Assistant Clinical Professor,
Otolaryngology, University of California Medical Center
Santa Rosa, California*

Joseph J. Littell, M.D., F.A.C.S.*
*Diplomate, American Board of Otolaryngology; Former Assistant Professor,
Otolaryngology, University of Indiana
College of Medicine, Indianapolis
Santa Rosa, California*

*deceased

acoustic (a-kūs'tik). *adj.* ACOU=hear. Relating to sound or hearing.

adenoidectomy (ad-en-oyd-ek'tō-mē). ADEN=gland. The surgical removal of the adenoids.

adenoids (ad'-en-oyds). *plural.* Lymphoid tissue normally found in the nasopharynx of children.

allergen (al'er-jen). A substance capable of producing an allergic reaction. It frequently results in **rhinitis.**

antrum of Highmore (an'trum of Hī'-mōr). The technical name for the paranasal sinus (paired) located in the maxillary bone. It is generally called the **antrum,** or the **maxillary sinus.**

anulus tympanicus (an'yūl-us tim-pan'i-kus). That portion of the temporal bone which surrounds the ear drum (**tympanic membrane**).

aphonia (ā-fōn'ē-a). PHON=sound. The condition of being unable to speak.

aphtha (af'tha). A characteristic mouth lesion for which there are several causes. They are commonly called "canker sores." (*plural*—aph'thae.)

arytenoid (a-rit'e-noyd). A part of the larynx.

atrophic rhinitis (a-trōf'ik rīn-ī'tis). RHIN=nose; ITIS=inflammation. A chronic nasal condition resulting in thinning of the nasal lining. *See* **ozena.**

audiogram (awd'ē-ō-gram). AUD=hearing; GRAM=record. A curve transcribed by a technician recording the patient's ability to hear sounds of different pitch.

audiometer (awd-ē-om'e-ter). MET=measure. An instrument used to measure the ability to hear.

aural (awr'al). *adj.* Pertaining to the ear. Differentiate **oral.**

aural vertigo (vert'i-go). VERT=turn. Dizziness due to conditions within the ear.

auricle (awr'i-kl). The projecting portion of the ear. (Fig. 17, p. 146)

branchial (brang'kē-al). *adj.* Relating to the fish-like gill clefts. They are embryonic structures, but they occasionally persist.

buccal (buk'kl). *adj.* Referring to the cheek.

cancrum oris (kang'krum ō'ris). OR=mouth. A **gangrenous** mouth condition.

"catarrh" (ka-tahr'). A commonly used name for a postnasal discharge resulting from a variety of causes.

catarrhal deafness (ka-tahr'al). A type of deafness often caused by inflammatory swelling around the nasal opening of the **eustachian tube.**

"cauliflower ear." The well-known "boxers' ear."

cerumen (ser-ū'men). CER=wax. Ear wax.

cholesteatoma (kōl-es-tē-a-tōm'a). OMA=tumor. A particular kind of tumor of the middle ear.

circumoral (ser-kum-ōr'al). *adj.* Referring to the area around the mouth.

cochlea (kok'lē-a *or* kōk'lē-a) The spiral part of the inner ear in which the auditory nerve endings are located. (Fig. 17, p. 146)

concha (kong'ka). The shell like, sound catching portion of the external ear.

coryza (kōr-ī′za). A more dignified name for a "head cold."

cricoid cartilage (krī′koyd kar′til-ij). A ring shaped cartilage making up the lower part of the larynx.

croup (krūp). An acute disease sometimes causing **edema** of the vocal cords and noisy, difficult breathing.

deaf-mutism (def-myūt′izm). The absence of ability to hear or speak.

deafness. The partial or complete loss, or lack, of the sense of hearing. Types include central, conduction, functional, inner ear, nerve.

decibel (des′i-bl). The unit used in measuring sound intensity when testing hearing ability. (*abbr.*–db.)

deglutition (deg-lū-tish′un). The act of swallowing.

deviated nasal septum (dē′vē-ā-ted nāz′al sep′tum). A deformed or crooked "partition" between the two nasal cavities, often the cause of difficult breathing or of obstructed sinus drainage.

dysphagia (dis-fāj′ē-a *or* –fāj′a). DYS= difficult; PHAG=eat, swallow. Pain or difficulty when swallowing.

epistaxis (ep-is-taks′is). Nosebleed.

epulis (ep′yūl-is). A tumor of the gums. It is usually attached to the jaw bone.

ethmoid sinus (eth′moyd sīn′us). The paranasal sinus (paired and multiple) located medial to the eye ("the ethmoids").

eustachian catheter (yūs-tāk′ē-an kath′e-ter). A hollow instrument which can be inserted into the nasal end of the **eustachian tube.**

eustachian tube (yūs-tāk′ē-an). The paired tube connecting the nasopharynx with the middle ear. Fig. 17, below)

external ear. The projecting part of the ear. (Fig. 17, below)

fauces (faw′sēz). *plural.* The passage from the mouth to the pharynx.

fenestration operation (fen-es-trā′shun). A surgical procedure used to relieve a certain type of deafness, usually that due to **otosclerosis.**

follicular tonsillitis (fol-lik′yūlar ton-sil-lī′tis). One of the many kinds of tonsillar infections.

frontal sinus (front′al). The paranasal sinus (paired) located in the frontal bone above the eye socket ("the frontals").

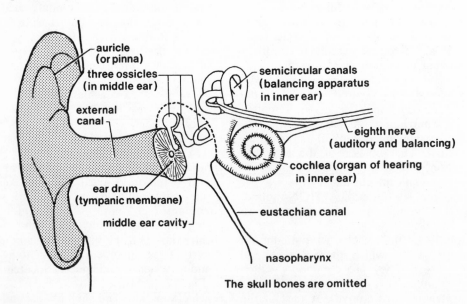

The skull bones are omitted

FIG. 17. Human Ear

gingiva (jin'jiv-a). The gum. (*plural* — gin'givae.).

gingivitis (jin-jiv-ī'tis). Inflammation of the gums.

globus hystericus (glōb'us his-ter'i-kus). A hysterical reaction involving the throat ("Doc, I've got a ball in my throat").

glossitis (glos-sī'tis). GLOSS=tongue. Inflammation of the tongue.

glossopharyngeal nerve (glos-sō-fair-in'jē-al). The ninth cranial nerve (paired). It supplies sensation to the back part of the mouth and taste to the posterior third of the tongue.

glossopharyngeal neuralgia (nūr-al'jē-a). NEUR=nerve; ALG=pain. One type of "sore throat."

harelip (hair'lip). A congenital deformity of the upper lip which resembles a hare's split upper lip.

hay fever. An allergic sensitivity resulting in the well-known "hay fever" symptoms. Although originally considered seasonal and related to pollens, the term now also includes these symptoms when caused by perennially contacted allergens.

hyoid (hī'oyd). A U-shaped bone at the base of the tongue to which several muscles are attached.

incus (ing'kus). One of the three **ossicles** of the middle ear (the **anvil**).

intubation (in-tūb-ā'shun). The procedure of placing a tube (generally into the trachea) for purposes of treatment, drainage, or relief of respiratory obstruction.

labia (lāb'e-a). *plural.* The lips. (*Sing.* — lab'ium; *adj.* — lab'ial)

labyrinth (lab-i-rinth). The part of the inner ear concerned with equilibrium.

laryngectomy (lair-in-jek'tō-mē). The surgical removal of the larynx.

laryngismus stridulus (lair-in-jis'mus strid'yūl-us). A sudden spasm of the larynx which sometimes occurs in cases of laryngeal inflammation, causing a crowing type of inspiration.

laryngitis (lair-in-jī'tis). Inflammation of the larynx, often causing hoarseness.

laryngoscope (lair-ing'gō-skōp). SCOPE=look, see. An instrument used in examining the larynx.

laryngoscopy (lair-ing-gos'kō-pē). Visual inspection of the larynx. Types are **indirect** (by means of an angle mirror held in the throat) and **direct** (by means of a speculum or laryngoscope).

laryngotracheitis (lar-ing-gō-trāk-ē-ī'tis). Simultaneous inflammation of the larynx and the trachea.

larynx (lair'inks — *not* lar'niks). The anatomical name for the "voice box."

lingua (ling'gwa). The tongue. This term is used in connection with several conditions affecting the tongue.

lobe (lōb). The soft, fleshy appendage at the bottom of the ear.

Ludwig's angina (Lūd'vigs anj-ī'na). A specific type of inflammation of the floor of the mouth.

macroglossia (māk-rō-glos'sē-a). GLOSS=tongue. A congenital enlargement of the tongue.

malleus (mal'ē-us). One of the middle ear **ossicles** (the **hammer**).

mandible (man'i-bl). The technical name for the lower jaw. (Fig. 4, p. 50; p. 148)

mastoid process (mas'toyd). The part of the temporal bone which contains the **mastoid cells,** spaces in the mastoid bone which sometimes become infected (**mastoiditis**).

mastoidectomy (mas-toyd-ek'tō-mē). The surgical removal of the mastoid cells or of diseased mastoid bone.

maxilla (maks-il'la). The upper jaw. It is not movable. (*plural* — maxil'ae.) (Fig. 18, p. 148)

maxillary sinus (maks'il-lair-ē). The paranasal sinus (paired) located in the maxillary bone. *See* **antrum of Highmore.**

Meniere's syndrome (Men-ē-airz' sin'drōm). A specific inner ear condition often associated with dizziness, nausea, vomiting, tinnitus, and hearing loss.

moniliasis (mōn-il-ī'a-sis). A disease which may affect the lining of the mouth. It is due to a specific infection and is generally called **"thrush."**

myringotomy (mīr-ing-got'ō-mē). The surgical procedure of incising the ear drum (generally for draining the middle ear cavity).

nares (nair'ēz). *plural.* The paired external openings into the divided nasal cavities. The term generally refers to the anterior nares or nostrils. (*Sing.* – nar'is.)

nasal polyp (nāz'al pol'ip). A small-based benign tumor which sometimes occurs in the nasal passages.

nasolacrimal ducts (nāz-ō-lak'rim-al). NASO=nose; LACRIM=tears. The tear ducts (one from each eye). They discharge upon the inner surface of the nose often causing "sniffles."

nasopharyngitis (nāz-ō-fair-in-jī'tis). PHARYN=throat. Inflammation of the nose and throat.

nasopharyngoscope (nāz-ō-fair-ing'gō-skōp). An instrument used in examining the nasopharynx.

nasopharynx (nas-ō-fair'inks). The space above the roof of the mouth. It extends from the posterior end of the nasal septum to about the level of the soft palate. (Fig. 18, below)

oral (ōr'al). *adj.* OR=mouth. Pertaining to the mouth. *See* **aural.**

ossicle (os'i-kl). OS=bone. Any small bone. It generally refers to one of the three small bones of the middle ear (**incus, malleus, stapes**). (Fig. 17, p. 146)

otitis media (ōt-ī'tis mēd'ē-a). OT, OTO=ear; MED=middle. Inflammation of or in the middle ear.

otolaryngologist (ō-tō-lair-in-gol'ō-jist). A physician who specializes in otolaryngology.

otolaryngology (ō-tō-lair-in-gol'ō-jē). *See* introductory paragraphs.

otologist (ōt-ol'ō-jist). A specialist in diseases of the ear. *See* Introduction.

otology (ōt-ol'ō-jē). OLOGY=science. *See* introductory paragraphs.

otomicroscope (ōt-ō-mīk'rō-skōp). A light-bearing microscope used for visualizing and magnifying the interior of the ear during certain operations.

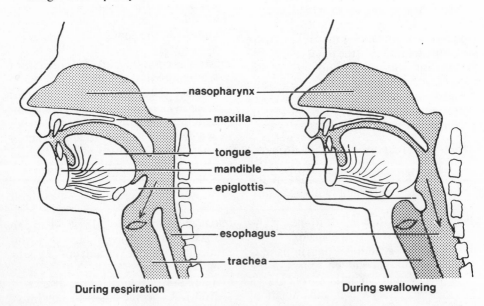

FIG. 18. Epiglottis and Nasopharynx

otorhinolaryngology (ōt-ō-rīn-ō-lair-ing-gol'ō-jē). *See* introductory paragraphs.

otorrhea (ōt-or-rē'a). A discharge from the ear.

otosclerosis (ōt-ō-skler-ō'sis). SCLER= hard. A condition causing conduction deafness associated with fixation of the **stapes.**

otoscope (ōt'ō-skōp). An instrument used in examining the ear canal and the ear drum.

ozena (ōz-ēn'a). A very offensive odor originating in the nasal passages. It is associated with **atrophic rhinitis.**

palate (pal'et). The roof of the mouth, also called the hard palate. (adj.— pal'atal *or* pal'atine.) *See* **soft palate.**

papilla (pa-pil'a). Any one of the tiny projections on the tongue which give it its granular appearance. (*plural.*— papil'lae.)

paranasal sinuses (pair-a-nāz'al). The four groups of nasal sinuses, all of which drain into the nose. The names are ethmoid, frontal, maxillary (antrum of Highmore), and sphe'noid.

paratonsillar abscess (pair-a-ton'sil-lar) — peritonsillar abscess (per-ē-ton'sil-lar). An abscess in the tissues adjacent to the tonsil ("quinsy").

parotid gland (par-ot'id). A paired saliva-producing gland located near the ear.

parotitis (pair-ō-ti'tis). Inflammation of the **parotid gland.** If you've ever had **mumps,** then you've had parotitis.

perceptive deafness. A specific type of nerve deafness.

petrous (pēt'rus *or* pet'rus). *adj.* Referring to a certain portion of the temporal bone.

pharyngitis (fair-in-jī'tis). Inflammation of the pharynx ("sore throat").

pharynx (fair'inks — *not* far'niks). The throat. (*adj.*—pharyng'eal; *plural.*— pharyn'ges.)

pinna (pin'na). The outer projecting part of the ear. (Also called the **aur'icle.**) (Fig. 17, p. 146)

"Politzer" (Pol'itz-er). Medical jargon for a treatment consisting of inflation of the middle ear with air via the eustachian tube.

"Proetz" (Pretz). Medical jargon for a type of treatment which uses suction applied to the nasal sinuses.

"quinsy" (quin'zy). Medical jargon for a **peritonsillar abscess.**

ranula (ran'yūl-a). A particular type of cyst which is located beneath the tongue.

rhinitis (rīn-ī'tis). Irritation of the lining of the nose, due to any one of several causes.

rhinophyma (rīn-ō-fīm'a). A particular **bulbous** type of nasal deformity.

rhinoplasty (rīn-ō-plast'ē). Surgical reshaping of the nose.

rhinorrhea (rīn-or-rē'a). A nicer name for a "runny nose." (Very occasionally, cerebrospinal fluid will escape from the nose, indicating a certain kind of skull fracture.)

sacculus (sak'yūl-us). In otolaryngology, a part of the inner ear. (*plural.*— sac'culi.)

saliva (sal-īv'a). The secretion produced by the salivary glands. (*adj.*— sal'ivary.)

semicircular canals. *plural.* Parts of the inner ear involved with balancing and equilibrium.

Shrapnell's membrane (Shrap'nelz). The upper portion of the tympanium **(tympanic membrane).**

sialadenitis (sī-al-ad-eni'tis). Inflammation in one of the salivary glands.

snare (snair). A surgical instrument sometimes used in removing tonsils or nasal polyps.

soft palate (pal'et). The horseshoe-shaped muscle forming the top and sides of the opening of the mouth into the throat. The **uvula** hangs down from the middle of the oval structure.

sphenoid sinus (sfē'noyd). The paranasal sinus (paired) located in the anterior portion of the sphenoid bone. The sphenoid sinuses are generally referred to as "the sphenoids."

stapedectomy (stāp-e-dek'tō-mē). The surgical removal of the **stapes**.

stapes (stāp'ēz). The third **ossicle** of the middle ear (the **stirrup**).

Stensen's duct (Sten'senz). The paired tube carrying saliva from the **parotid gland** to the mouth.

stomatitis (stōm-a-tī'-tis). STOM= mouth. Inflammation of the lining of the mouth. Types are aph'thous, herpet'ic, mercur'ial, and Vin'cent's.

stridor (strīd'or). A characteristic high-pitched respiratory sound.

sublingual (sub-ling'gwal). *adj.* Positioned beneath the tongue.

submucous resection (sub-myūk'us). The surgical correction of a deformed nasal septum.

tegmen tympani (teg'men tim'pan-ē). The roof of the middle ear.

tensor tympani (ten'sor tim'pan-ē). A muscle which keeps the ear drum tight through action on the **malleus**.

"thrush." A vernacular name for **moniliasis.**

thyroglossal cyst (thī-rō-glos'sl). A persisting (embryonic) structure in the neck (a persistent thyroid duct).

tinnitus (tin-nī'tus *or* tin'ni-tus). A buzzing sensation in the ears.

tonsillectomy (ton-sil-lek'to-mē). The surgical removal of one or both tonsils.

tonsillitis (ton-sil-lī'tis). Inflammation of one or both tonsils.

trachea (trāk'ē-a). The tube extending down from the larynx which divides into the two bronchial tubes. (The "windpipe.") (Fig. 18, p. 148; Fig. 24, p. 232)

tracheostomy (trāk-ē-ost'ō-mē) — *or* **tracheotomy** (trāk-ē-ot'ō-mē). An opening made into the trachea from the front portion of the neck for the insertion of a tube to facilitate breathing.

tragus (trāg'us). A part of the external ear. (*plural.* — trag'i.)

transillumination (trans-il-lūm-in-ā'shun). The technique of shining a light through a cyst or cavity for diagnostic purposes.

"trench mouth." Medical jargon for **Vincent's angina.**

trigeminal nerve (trī-jem'i-nl). The fifth cranial nerve (paired).

turbinate bodies (tur'bin-āt). *plural.* Three specific ridges (one above the other) on the lateral wall of each nasal cavity beneath or between which the ducts of the paranasal sinuses, as well as the lacrimal duct, empty.

tympanoplasty (tim-pan'ō-plast'ē). A surgical procedure involving the tympanic membrane, middle ear, and mastoid, often done for eradication of ear disease and in an attempt to restore hearing.

"U.R.I." Medical jargon for upper respiratory tract infection.

utriculus (yū-trik'yūl-us). A part of the inner ear.

uvula (yūv'yūl-a). The terminal, dependent "tongue" of tissue hanging down from the soft palate.

vasomotor rhinitis (vāz-ō-mō'tor rīn-ī'tis). A nice name for the "runny nose" of hay fever.

vertigo (vert'i-gō). A type of dizziness associated with the sensation of whirling, sometimes originating from disturbances of the semicircular canals.

vestibule (vest'i-byūl). A part of the inner ear.

Vincent's agina (Vin'sents anj-ī'na). A specific disease of the gums, mouth, or tonsils. (Often called "trench mouth".)

vocal cords — vocal chords. *plural.* The two membranous bands in the larynx with which voice sounds are produced.

vomer (vōm'er). A small bone which forms part of the nasal septum.

17 Pathology

PATHOLOGY IS DEFINED as the study of disease. It is one of the two medical specialties — Public Health is the other — which do not include the actual direct care of patients. Few specialties, however, require the making of decisions which so profoundly affect the lives of patients and their families.

A pathologist must supervise and be responsible for the functioning of tissue laboratories. Generally he also directs and supervises clinical laboratories and blood banks. In a *tissue laboratory* a pathologist investigates the detectable changes in body tissues by which many diseases manifest themselves; for example, he investigates the nature of a tumor so that appropriate treatment can be prescribed. A *clinical laboratory* investigates changes in the body fluids of the patient; their correct interpretation may determine or change the physician's method of treatment. A *blood bank* stores and checks the compatibility and suitability of all blood and other fluids used in transfusions.

The performing of autopsies, which is another of the pathologist's numerous duties, has provided valuable information on which much of medical knowledge is based. In addition, a pathologist's findings in determining the cause of death are often very influential with juries or in settling insurance claims, in cases of possible suicide or of a traffic accident in which the driver may have died at the wheel from natural causes and not from the impact of collision.

Certification by the American Board of Pathology requires a four-year residency (which may include internship) before the applicant can be examined by the Board.

CONSULTANTS

Robert L. Dennis, M. D.
Diplomate, American Board of Pathology; Director, Pathology, San Jose Hospitals and Health Center
San Jose, California

Marvin A. Brownstein, M. D.
Diplomate, American Board of Pathology
Oakland, California

achalasia (ak-a-lā′zha *or* −zē-a). CHALASIA=failure to relax. A constriction of a tube due to failure of the smooth muscle fibers to relax. It is most frequently seen at the lower end of the esophagus where it is also given the name of **cardiospasm.**

achondroplasia (a-kon-drō-plā′zha *or* −zē-a). CHRONDR=cartilage. A congenital disturbance of cartilage growth at the ends of the long bones, resulting in one type of dwarfism.

acromegaly (ak-rō-meg′a-lē). MEG=large. A disorder of bony development due to overproduction of a growth hormone produced by the pituitary gland. The usual result is a characteristic enlargement of hands, feet, face, and thorax.

adenitis (ad-en-ī′tis). ADEN=gland; ITIS=inflammation. Inflammation of a gland.

adenocarcinoma (ad-en-ō-kars-i-nōm′a). OMA=tumor. A malignant tumor composed of glandular cells or of cells derived from glands.

adenocystoma (ad-en-ō-sist-ōm′a). CYST=hollow space. A cystic benign tumor with dilated gland spaces which form cysts.

adenofibroma (ad-en-ō-fīb-rōm′a). FIBR=hard. A benign tumor consisting of combined glandular and fibrous elements.

adenoma (ad-en-ōm′a). A benign tumor of glandular origin.

aneurysm (an′yūr-izm)−aneurism. A localized dilatation of a blood vessel, generally an artery, due to weakening

of the vessel wall (a potential "blow out").

angioma (anj-ē-ōm′a). ANG=vessel. A benign tumor consisting of blood vessels (**hemangioma**) or of lymph vessels (**lymphangioma**).

angiosarcoma (anj-ē-ō-sark-ōm′a). SARC=flesh. A malignant tumor composed of multiple blood or lymph vessels, or of cells derived from such vessels.

anomaly (an-om′a-lē). An anatomical alteration which differs markedly from the normal.

aortitis (ā-or-tī′tis). An inflammation of the wall of the aorta, frequently resulting in **aneurysm** at the site (often of **syphilitic** origin).

arcus senilis (ark′us sen-il′is). ARC=bow; SENIL=old. A gray or whitish ring in the periphery of the cornea which is sometimes seen in older people.

atelectasis (at-el-ek′ta-sis). ECTASIS=expansion. Collapse or incomplete expansion of a lung or of part of it. There are two types: primary, an infant lung that has never been inflated; secondary, a lung (or a portion of it) which has collapsed, for any reason, and contains no air.

atheroma (ath-er-ōm′a). A plaque-like lesion in the inner lining of an artery which probably begins as a fatty deposition. In smaller arteries this may cause obstruction.

autopsy (aw′top-sē). A post mortem examination done to study disease processes and to determine the cause of death.

blastomycosis (blas-tō-mīk-ō′sis). MYCO=yeast; OSIS=condition. An inflammatory disease caused by yeast-like fungi known as **blastomycetes.** It is generally confined to the skin, but may involve other organs.

bleb. A superficial blister or vesicle filled with fluid.

Boeck's sarcoid (Beks sark′oyd). A disease which is generally symptomless in early stages and is characterized by granulomatous lesions. (Also called **sarcoido′sis**.)

Brodie's abscess (Brōd′ez ab′ses). A chronic bone abscess usually following **osteomyelitis** which is generally seen at the ends of long bones, particularly the **tibia**.

bronchiectasis (brong-kē-ek′ta-sis). Chronic dilatation of the large or small bronchi of a lung.

Buerger's disease (Berg′erz). Another name for **thromboangiitis obliterans**.

cadaver (ka-dav′er). A dead human body. (*adj.* — cadav′eric.)

cancer (kan′ser). A malignant cellular tumor which pursues a fatal course unless removed, or treated radiologically or chemically.

carcinoma (kar-sin-ōm′a). CARC=cancer; OMA=tumor. A malignant tumor consisting mostly of epithelial cells which sometimes have a tendency to invade the lymph spaces of the neighboring tissue. Some types are: ba′sal cell, epider′moid, in′filtrating, med′ullary, metastat′ic, pap′illary, scir′rhous, and squa′mous cell.

chancre (shang′ker). The firm, localized, primary lesion of syphilis. A chancre may also be the lesion of a few other seldom-seen diseases.

chancroid (shang′kroyd). A wart-like venereal genital infection which resembles syphilis, but is not syphilitic.

Charcot's joint (Shar′kōz joint). A painless destructive type of joint disease generally associated with the third stage of **syphilis**.

chondroma (kon-drōm′a). CHONDR=cartilage. A benign, firm, generally encapsulated tumor consisting of cartilage.

chondrosarcoma (kon-drō-sark-ōm′a). SARC=connective tissue. A malignant tumor which is generally derived from cartilaginous elements.

choriocarcinoma (kor-ē-ō-kar-sin-ōm′a). CHORIO=fetal membrane. A malignant uterine tumor derived from portions of the placenta. It usually

responds well to treatment with **methotrexate** (a chemical agent). (Also called **chorionepitheliom′a**.)

cicatrix (sik′a-triks). A scar; the end stage of a healed wound. (*plural* — cicat′rices.)

contrecoup injury (kon-tra-kū′). A bruising injury sustained by the brain or skull on the side opposite to that side of the head receiving the blow.

contusion (kon-tūzh′un). A bruising injury sustained by tissue without the presence of an overlying break in the skin.

cyst (sist). A lesion consisting of a wall or membrane surrounding a space which usually contains fluid or other material. It is usually round or ovoid. Some types are: der′moid, echinococ′cus, endomet′rial, follic′ular, hydat′id, ovarian, reten′tion, seba′ceous, subdur′al, and thyroglos′sal.

cystadenoma (sist-ad-en-ō′ma). CYST + ADEN + OMA. A generally benign tumor consisting of localized areas of epithelial growth enclosed in a cyst. (**Cystadenocarcinoma** is a malignant variant.)

diverticulum (dī-vert-ik′yūl-um). VERT =turn aside. An abnormal sac-like pouch projecting from a defect in the wall of a tube or cavity. (*adj.* — divertic′ulous; *plural* — divertic′ula.)

elephantiasis (el-e-fan-tī′a-sis). Extreme enlargement of an anatomical part, usually the legs or the scrotum, due to obstruction of the lymphatic drainage channels.

embolism (em′bōl-izm). The blocking or plugging of an artery or a vein by an **embolus**.

embolus (em′bōl-us). A mass of detached matter, usually air, fat, or a blood clot, which is loose in the circulating blood stream.

emphysema (em-fīs-ēm′a). The abnormal distention of connective tissue with air, generally referring to the enlargement of the alveolar air spaces of the lungs.

empyema (em-pī-ēm′a). PY=pus. A collection of pus in a closed cavity, most frequently the chest cavity.

endometriosis (end-ō-mē-trē-ō′sis). A condition in which tissue resembling the uterine lining appears in abnormal locations, generally in the female pelvis or in other parts of the abdominal cavity.

endometritis (end-ō-mē-tri′tis). Inflammation of the **endometrium** (lining of the uterus).

Ewing's tumor (yū′ings). A highly malignant tumor which occurs in the bone marrow in the shafts of long bones. It is generally seen in young people.

excoriation (eks-kōr-i-ā′shun). COR=skin. The loss of a portion of the superficial layer of the skin.

exhumation (eks-hyūm-ā′shun). The removal of a dead body from a grave.

exostosis (ek-os-tō′sis). OS=bone. A localized benign overgrowth of the surface of a bone.

exudate (eks′yūd-āt *or* eks′ū-dāt). Material secreted by tissues either normally, or as a response (generally reparative) in conditions of disease or injury.

fibroma (fi-brō′ma). A benign tumor consisting of fibrous tissue.

fibromyoma (fīb-rō-mī-ōm′a). MYO=muscle. A benign muscular tumor of the uterus commonly called a "fibroid."

fibrosarcoma (fī-brō-sark-ō′ma). FIBR+SARC+OMA. A malignant tumor consisting of tissue derived from fibrous elements.

fistula (fist′yūl-a). An abnormal tube-like canal or tract extending from one organ to another, or from an organ to the surface of the body.

formaldehyde (form-al′de-hīd). A solution generally used for preserving dead bodies or tissues removed for laboratory examination.

fragilitas ossium (fraj-il′i-tas os′ē-um). FRAG=break; OS=bone. A bone disease in which the bones become fragile and are easily broken.

gangrene (gang-grēn′). Death of tissue (generally from lack of blood supply) sometimes accompanied by bacterial growth.

glioma (glī-ōm′a). A tumor arising from the supporting tissues of the brain and spinal cord. Its effects are mostly those caused by pressure.

granuloma (gran-yūl-ōm′a). A broad term for a lesion consisting of certain cellular elements packed together in a specific way.

Grawitz's tumor (Gra′wits-ez). A name applied to a malignant kidney tumor, ordinarily called a **hypernephroma,** or a renal cell carcinoma.

hemangioma (hēm-anj-ē-ōm′a). HEM=blood + ANG + OMA. A tumor consisting of an abnormal growth of blood vessels.

hematoma (hēm-a-tōm′a). A collection of escaped blood in the tissues.

hemorrhage (hem′or-ij). Bleeding from the vascular system.

hydrocele (hī′drō-sēl). HYDR=water; CELE=hollow tumor. A collection of serous fluid within the scrotum, generally within the cavity of the **tunica vaginalis.**

hydronephrosis (hī-drō-nef-rō′sis). NEPH=kidney. An advanced stage of dilatation of the pelvis of the kidney, secondary to obstruction farther down the urinary tract. Infection may or may not be involved.

hyperemia (hī-per-ēm′ē-a). HYPER=increased. Excessive amounts of blood in an area or region of the body, secondary to increased inflow, obstructed outflow, or (occasionally) to inflammation.

hyperplasia (hī-per-plā′zha *or* −zē-a) Enlargement, by virtue of increased numbers of individual cells. *See* **hypertrophy.**

hypertrophy (hī-per′trof-ē). Enlargement, by virtue of enlarged individual parts or cells. *See* **hyperplasia.**

icterus (ik'ter-us). Jaundice (a yellowish condition of the skin and **conjunctivae**) caused by an increase of bilirubin in the circulation. (*adj.* –icter'ic.)

infarct (in'farkt). Local death of tissue due to interference with its blood supply. (**Infarction** is a common but improper term.)

inflammation (in-flam-mā'shun). A type of tissue response with cellular infiltrates, redness and swelling. It is generally associated with infection or injury.

involucrum (in-vol-ūk'rum). A covering of new bone which generally forms around a fragment of separated, dead bone.

keloid (kē'loyd). An idiopathic overgrowth of scar tissue.

leiomyoma (lī-ō-mī-ōm'a). LEI=smooth. A benign tumor consisting of smooth muscle. The most common example is the well-known "fibroid" of the uterus.

leiomyosarcoma (lī-ō-mī-ō-sar-kōm'a). A malignant tumor arising from smooth muscle tissue.

lipoma (līp-ōm'a *or* lip-pōm'a). LIP= fat. A benign tumor consisting of normal fatty tissue, generally divided into irregular lobules.

liposarcoma (līp-ō-sark-ōm'a). LIP + SARC + OMA. A malignant tumor arising from fatty tissue.

lymphangioma (limf-anj-ē-ōm'a). A tumor consisting of lymphatic vessels.

lymphoma (limf-ōm'a). A malignant tumor consisting of lymphoid and related cells.

lymphosarcoma (limf-ō-sark-ōm'a). A malignant tumor consisting of malignant lymphocytic cells.

Meckel's diverticulum (Mek'elz). A persistent, congenital outpouching of the wall of the terminal **ileum,** which in embryonic life connected the umbilical cord to the ileum.

melanocyte (mel'an-ō-sīt). A cell capable of developing into pigmented tissue. (*adj.* – melanocyt'ic.)

melanoma (mel-a-nōm'a). MELA= black. A neoplasm composed of **melanocytic** cells arising generally in skin. They are malignant and must be differentiated from benign **nevi** (nevuses).

meningioma (men-inj-ē-ōm'a). A tumor arising from the meningeal brain covering, usually the dura mater.

meningocele (men-ing'gō-sel *or* men-inj' ō-sel). A congenital defect of the skull or lower spine through which the coverings of the brain or spinal cord (meninges) may protrude.

meningomyelocele (men-in-jō-mī'e-lō-sēl). A meningocele containing a protruding part of the spinal cord as well as cerebrospinal fluid.

mole (mōl). A common name for a congenital, generally raised, benign skin tumor.

morgue (morg). The room where dead bodies are kept. Autopsies may he performed in morgues.

multiple myeloma (mī-el-ōm'a). MYEL=marrow + OMA. A malignant bone marrow tumor most frequently seen as multiple lesions in the ribs, skull, and other bones.

myelitis (mī-el-ī'tis). Inflammation of the spinal cord. *See* **poliomyelitis.**

myelocele (mī'e-lō-sēl). A protrusion of parts of the spinal cord through a defect in the spinal canal.

myeloma (mī-el-ōm'a). A slow-growing (often multiple) tumor of the bone marrow or of the bone marrow cavity. *See* **multiple myeloma.**

myxoma (miks-ōm'a). MYX=mucus. A rare benign connective tissue tumor which is jelly-like in consistency.

nabothian follicle (nā-bōth'ē-an fol'li-kl). A spherical cystic collection of fluid sometimes found in the lower end of the cervix uteri.

necropsy (nek'rop-sē). NECRO=death. Another name for an **autopsy.**

necrosis (ne-krō'sis). The death of a group of contiguous cells or of a cellular structure. (*adj.* –necrot'ic.)

neoplasm (nē'ō-plazm). Any new or abnormal growth, such as a tumor.

neuroma (nūr-ōm'a). NEUR=nerve. A benign tumor consisting of and occurring along the course of nerve fibers.

neurosarcoma (nūr-ō-sark-ōm'a). NEUR + SARC + OMA. A malignant tumor arising from the neural elements. There are several types of neurosarcomas.

nevus (nēv'us). A benign congenital tumor of the skin, generally discolored. (*plural,* – nev'i.)

occlusion (ok-klū'zhun). The process of closing or being closed, particularly referring to a blood vessel.

oophoritis (ūf-or-ī'tis). OOPH=ovary. Inflammation of an ovary.

orchitis (ork-ī'tis). ORCH=testicle. Inflammation of a testicle.

osteitis deformans (ost-ē-ī'tis dē-form' anz). OS + ITIS. A deforming bone disease characterized by loss of calcium and sometimes by increased thickening of bones, and by other features. It is sometimes called **Paget's disease.**

osteitis fibrosa (fīb-rōs'a). A bone disease characterized by degeneration and absorption of bone, and by other features.

osteochondritis (ost-ē ō-kon-drī'tis). OS + CHONDR + ITIS. An inflamed condition of unknown cause which involves cartilage and adjacent bone.

osteochondroma (ost-ē-ō-kon-drōm'a). OS + CHONDR + OMA. A benign tumor made up of both bony and cartilaginous elements.

osteoma (ost-ē-ōm'a). A benign tumor made up of bony elements.

osteomyelitis (ost-ē-ō-mī-el-ī'tis). Inflammation of a bone and its medullary (marrow) cavity.

otitis media (ō-tī'tis mēd'i-a). OT=ear. Inflammation of the middle ear.

Paget's disease (Paj'ets). *See* **osteitis deformans.** There is also a Paget's disease of the breast which is a variety of breast carcinoma.

papilloma (pap-il-lōm'a). A benign tumor of epithelial origin originating from the skin or mucous membrane and projecting above the surrounding tissue.

parametritis (par-a-mē-trī'tis) METR= uterus. Inflammation of the **parametrium.** *See Obstetrics and Gynecology.*

pathologist (path-ol'ō-jist). A doctor who specializes in pathology.

pathology (path-ol'ō-jē). *See* introductory paragraphs.

periostitis (per-ē-ost-ī'tis). Inflammation of the membrane covering a bone.

peritonitis (per-i-ton-ī'tis). Inflammation of the lining of the abdominal cavity.

phagocytosis (fag-ō-sīt-ō'sis). PHAG= eat. The engulfing by certain body cells (**phagocytes**) of bacteria, foreign bodies, and other cells.

phimosis (fīm-o'sis). A narrowing of the end of the foreskin of the penis.

phlebolith (fleb'ō-lith). PHLEB=vein; LITH=stone. A **calculus** formed in a vein.

pilonidal cyst (pīl-ō-nīd'al). A congenital cyst in skin and subcutaneous tissue overlying the coccyx. It generally contains hair and may become abscessed.

polycystic kidney (pol-ē-sist'ik). A congenital condition in which kidney tissue is gradually replaced by cysts.

polyp (pol'ip). A benign tumor characterized by a fingerlike protrusion generally emanating from a smaller base. (*plural,* – pol'ypi.)

polyposis (pol-i-pōs'is). A condition in which there are multiple **polypi** in an area or organ.

postmortem (pōst-mort'em). *adj.* MORT=death. After death; often used as a noun to denote an autopsy.

Pott's disease (Pots). **Tuberculous** disease of the body of a vertebra.

prostatitis

prostatitis (prost-a-tī'tis). Inflammation of the prostate gland.

putrefaction (pyūt-rē-fak'shun). Decomposition of tissue, particularly protein tissue, generally with resultant disagreeable odor. It is frequently initiated by infection and/or by infarct.

pyelonephritis (pī-el-ō-nef-rī'tis). PYELO=kidney pelvis; NEPH= kidney. Inflammation of both the pelvis and the cortex of the kidney.

pyosalpinx (pī-ō-sal'pinks). PYO=pus; SALPINX=fallopian tube. A collection of pus due to an infection within a fallopian tube.

Raynaud's disease (Rā-nōz'). A condition involving the terminal arteries of the extremities which sometimes results in degenerative changes. These may include **gangrene** which is due to obstruction of the blood supply.

Recklinghausen's disease (Rek'ling-how-zenz). A disease of one or more cutaneous nerves, frequently producing multiple nerve tumors. Also, a bone condition associated with parathyroid overactivity. Also called **von Recklinghausen's disease.**

rhabdomyoma (rab-dō-mī-ōm'a). A benign tumor consisting of voluntary, striated muscle. **Rhapdomyosarcoma** is a malignant form.)

rhabdomyosarcoma (rab-dō-mī-ō-sark-ōm'a). A malignant tumor arising from striated muscle tissue.

rickets (rik'ets). A disease of early life characterized by bone softening and Vitamin D deficiency.

rigor mortis (rig'or mort'is). RIG=stiff; MORT=dead. The stiffening of muscles which begins shortly after death.

salpingitis (sal-ping-jī'tis). SALPING + ITIS. Any type of inflammation of the fallopian tube.

sarcoidosis (sar-koyd-ō'sis). A disease characterized by **noncaseous** granulomas which may occur in numerous tissues.

sarcoma (sark-ōm'a). SARC + OMA. A malignant tumor arising from connective tissue. Types are: alve'olar, fibrosarcom'a, giant cell, Hodg'kins, leiomyosarcom'a, liposarcom'a, melanot'ic, metastat'ic, my'eloid, osteogen'ic, retroperitone'al, and rhabdomyosarcom'a.

Schimmelbusch's disease (Shim'mel-būsh-ez). A disease characterized by the presence of multiple cysts in the breasts.

seminoma (sem-i-nōm'a). SEM=seed. A malignant tumor of testicular tissue arising from the cells of the semen-producing tubules.

septicemia (sep-ti-sēm'ē-a). SEPT= poison. A condition characterized by the presence of bacteria and their associated toxins in the blood.

spermatocele (sperm'a-tō-sēl). SPERM=seed. A cyst in the **epididymis** which contains spermatozoa.

splenomegaly (splen-ō-meg'a-lē). Enlargement of the spleen, often chronic, due to a number of causes.

spondylitis deformans (spon-dil-ī'tis). Rigid, deforming inflammation of the spinal column. Also called **Marie-Strumpell spondylitis.**

sporotrichosis (spōr-ō-trik-ō'sis). A chronic, rare infection produced by a particular fungus.

synovitis (sīn-ō-vī-'tis). SYNOV=joint lining. Inflammation of the **synovial membrane** lining a joint.

telangiectasis — telangiectasia (tel-anj-ē-ek'ta-sis) (tel-anj-ē-ek-tāz'ē-a). A group of dilated capillary blood vessels. (*plural,* — telangiec'tases.)

tenosynovitis (ten-ō-sīn-ō-vī'tis). TENO=tendon. Inflammation of a tendon and its sheath.

teratocarcinoma (ter-a-tō-kar-sin-ōm'a). A **teratoma** with a malignant epithelial component.

teratoma (ter-a-tōm'a). A compound tumor composed of tissues exhibiting more than one type of embryonic element. Teratomas may contain teeth, hair, nails, etc.

thromboangiitis obliterans (throm-bō-anj-ē-ī'tis ob-lit'er-anz). THROMB= clot. A chronic disease of the terminal arteries, veins and nerves of the lower extremities. It predisposes to **gangrene** because of circulatory interference. Also called **Buerger's disease.**

thrombophlebitis (thromb-ō-flēb-ī'tis). THROMB + PHLEB + ITIS. Inflammation in the wall of a vein, accompanied by clot formation at the site.

thrombosis (thromb-ō'sis). THROMB + OSIS. The presence or formation of a **thrombus.**

thrombus (thromb'us). A blood clot which remains at the site of its formation in the circulatory system. When it becomes detached it becomes an **embolus.** (*adj.* — thrombot'ic.)

trichinosis (trik-in-ō'sis). A condition, occasionally fatal, caused by eating undercooked pork infected with pork worms (Trichinella spiralis).

tubercle (tūb-er'kl). The characteristic lesion of tuberculosis. It is generally a small, rounded nodule containing characteristically arranged cells and tubercle bacilli.

tuberculosis (tū-berk-yūl-ō'sis). Infection with the tubercle bacillus ("T.B.") Types are: bronchogen'ic, os'seous, fibrocas'eous, menin'geal, mil'iary, pul'monary, ren'al, and ul'-cerative.

tubo-ovarian abscess (tū-bō-ōv-air'ē-an). An abscess involving a fallopian tube and its ovary.

tumor (tūm'or). A generic term designating any swelling or enlargement, particularly an abnormal overgrowth of tissue, benign or malignant.

urachus (yūr-āk'us). A congenital remnent of the embryonic urinary bladder; it extends from the under surface of the umbilicus to the summit of the bladder, and is usually nonfunctional.

urethritis (yūr-ē-thrī'tis). Inflammation of the urethra.

varix (vair'iks). A dilated and tortuous vein, most commonly seen in the legs. (*plural,* — var'ices.) Also called **varicose vein.**

xanthelasma (zan-the-las'ma). XANTH=yellow. A condition characterized by soft yellowish spots on the eyelids.

xanthoma (zan-thōm'a). XANTH + OMA. A yellowish skin nodule which contains a type of fat.

Pathology – Clinical Laboratory

CONSULTANTS

Robert L. Dennis, M.D.
Diplomate, American Board of Pathology; Director, Pathology, San Jose Hospitals and Health Center
San Jose, California

Marvin A. Brownstein, M.D.
Diplomate, American Board of Pathology
Oakland, California

Frank L. Prior, M.S.
Director, Empire Medical Laboratory
Santa Rosa, California

acetone (as'e-tōn). A substance sometimes found in the urine when a hyperacid condition exists in the body, as in **diabetes** or in extreme dehydration.

acid-fast. A staining characteristic which differentiates a few kinds of bacteria, notably tubercle bacilli.

aerobacter (air-ō-bak'ter). An important species of pathogenic bacteria now called **enterobacter.**

A/G ratio. A quantitative relationship between the amounts of **albumin** and **globulin** present in the blood or in the urine.

agglutination (ag-glū-tin-ā'shun). GLUT=clump. Clumping of blood cells which can be caused by mixing incompatible types of blood; also, the precipitation or clumping of certain bacteria on their being exposed to the action of appropriate **agglutinins** (agglut'inants).

agglutinin (ag-glūt'in-in) – **agglutinant** (ag-glūt'in-ant). An antibody which causes **agglutination.**

albumin (al-byūm'in). A protein found in most body tissues and body fluids. Abnormal amounts in the urine indicate kidney malfunction.

amorphous (a-morf'us). *adj.* MORPH= shape. Without constant form or shape (not crystalline), relating particularly to some constituents of urinary sediments.

amylase (am'el-lās). A digestive enzyme which converts starch into sugar.

anaerobe (an'er-ōb). A microorganism which grows in situations or locations where oxygen is not present.

anemia (a-nēm'ē-a). An abnormal diminution in the quality or quantity of the red blood corpuscles, with a decreased amount of hemoglobin in the blood.

anisocytosis (an-i-sō-sīt'ō-sis). ANISO =unequal; CYT=cell. Variations in the size of blood corpuscles.

Ascaris lumbricoides (Ask'ar-is lumbra-koyd'ēz). A parasite ("round worm") sometimes found in the human bowel. It may be recovered from the feces. *See* **ascariasis.**

Ascaris vermicularis (Ask'ar-is vermik-yūl-air'is). The technical name for "pinworm", also called **Enterobius vermicularis.** *See* **enterobiasis.**

bacillus (ba-sil'us). A large class of bacteria, the form of which is relatively elongated, differentiating them from cocci which are round. (*plural*—bacil'li; *adj.*—bacil'liform.)

bacteriophage (bak-tēr'ē-ō-fāj). A virus-like organism which, when brought into contact with bacteria, causes a breakdown of the bacterial structure.

basophil (bās'ō-fil). A **leukocyte,** the granules of which characteristically absorb basic (generally blue) dyes. In increased numbers they may have clinical significance.

Bence Jones protein. A specific protein which sometimes appears in the urine in cases of myeloma and in some other diseases.

bilirubin (bil-ē-rūb'in). A yellowish-red bile pigment measured because of its diagnostic connection with liver function.

blood groups. The groups into which human blood is divided. The classifications are O, A, B, and AB.

blood smear. A thinly spread layer of blood on a glass slide, prepared and stained for microscopic examination.

blood typing. The classifying into specific groups of blood from potential donors or recipients for blood transfusion in order to determine probable compatibility or incompatibility of the cells.

buffer. Something added to a solution to preserve its balance of acidity or alkalinity.

carbolfuchsin (kar-bol-fūk'sin). An intensely red stain commonly used in clinical laboratory practice.

casts. *plural.* Moulds of renal tubules which may be found in urine sediments. Their presence generally indicates some type of kidney malfunction. Types are: hyaline, granular, blood, waxy, epithelial, fatty, false (elements resembling casts).

cell fragility (fraj-il'i-tē). This term refers to the point at which cells break down into fragments; if red blood corpuscles are abnormally fragile, they rupture spontaneously, causing **anemia** and **jaundice.**

centrifuge (sent'ri-fūj). FUGE=to fly away from. A piece of laboratory equipment which by spinning (centrifugation) separates, precipitates, or concentrates the formed elements present in liquids being examined.

cholesterol (kōl-est'er-ol). A fatty constituent of normal blood. Excessively high levels are reputedly contributory to **arteriosclerosis** and **hypertension.**

coagulation time (Lee-White). A test used to determine the clotting ability of blood. It is often used preceding surgery

coccus (kok'us). A large class of bacteria, the form of which is round or relatively round. (*plural*—coc'ci.)

color index. An old term indicating the amount of hemoglobin present in the blood in proportion to the number of red blood corpuscles present. It thus discloses the amount of hemoglobin in each red corpuscle, and may be helpful in detecting abnormalities.

creatinine (krē-at'in-in). A waste product found in the blood. Abnormally high levels indicate kidney disease.

crenated (krēn'āt-ed). *adj.* Referring to a shrunken, scalloped appearance which red blood corpuscles assume under certain conditions.

cross match. The ultimate test for determining whether the blood of a particular donor will be compatible or incompatible with the blood of a particular recipient. The determining factor is the resultant clumping or nonclumping of the blood corpuscles when the samples are combined.

culture. The placing of material into sterile substances (**media**) prior to incubation to determine if bacteria are present, and to identify them and study their growth characteristics. (Also used as a verb.)

culture media. *plural.* Various types and kinds of sterile material conducive to bacterial growth after inoculation and incubation.

cylindroids. *plural.* Cylindrical structures often consisting of mucus and sometimes found in urine sediments. Although resembling renal casts, cylindroids generally have no clinical significance.

cytoplasm (sīt'ō-plazm). The protoplasm of a cell, surrounding the nucleus. It may or may not contain granules.

differential count. The result of microscopic examination of a blood smear to determine and express the relative percentage of various types of leukocytes.

diplococcus (dip-lō-kok'us). A **coccus** which normally occurs in pairs.

E. coli (E kōl'ē)—**Escherichia coli** (Esker-ish'ē-a kōl'ē). A common type of bacillus normally found in the intestinal tract. It may cause infections in various parts of the body.

electrolyte balance (ē-lek'trō-līt). The state in which the vital body electrolytes are present within normal physiologic ranges.

eosinophil (ē-ō-sin'ō-fil) — **eosinophile**. A leukocyte, the granules of which characteristically absorb eosin stain (red). Abnormal numbers suggest certain disorders.

erythrocyte (ē-rith'rō-sīt). ERYTH= red. A red blood corpuscle.

flagella (flaj-el'a). *plural.* Small, hair like processes attached to one or both ends of certain protozoa or bacteria. (*Sing.* — flagel'lum.)

flagellate (flaj'el-lāt). FLAG=whip, hair. A one-celled parasitic organism which is equipped with **flagella** (see above).

glucose (glūk'ōs). One type of sugar.

glucose tolerance. A test used to determine the rate at which a person can utilize (burn) sugar and clear it from the blood.

glycosuria (glīk-ō-sūr'ē-a). GLY= sweet. The presence of sugar in the urine. When present in abnormal amounts, it is suggestive of diabetes.

gonococcus (gon-ō-kok'us). The specific organism which causes **gonorrheal** infections. (*plural* — gonococ'ci.).

gram-negative. *adj.* A term used to describe stained bacteria which have released their **Gram stain** under certain controlled conditions (decolorized) and have been stained a different color (counter stained).

gram-positive. *adj.* A term referring to stained bacteria which have retained the **Gram stain** under controlled conditions.

Gram stain. A blue stain which can be used to divide most bacteria into two groups: gram-positive and gram-negative.

granulocyte (gran'yūl-ō-sīt). A form of white blood cell containing **granules** in the cytoplasm.

hematocrit (hem-at'ō-krit). HEM= blood. A figure which indicates the percentage volume of the red blood corpuscles in a stated amount of blood.

hematocytometer (hēm-a-tō-sīt-om'e-ter). A counting chamber used for determining the number of blood cells per cubic centimeter of whole blood, by the use of a microscope. It is also called a **hemacytom'eter** or a **hemocytom'eter.**

hematology (hēm-a-tol'ō-jē). The study of blood and its components, and their relationship to health and disease.

hematoxylin and eosin (hēm-a-toks'il-in and ē'ō-sin). A combination stain (H &E) commonly used in preparing thin slices of tissue specimens for microscopic examination.

hemoglobin (hēm-ō-glōb'in). A pigment contained in the red blood corpuscles, which carries and delivers oxygen and carbon dioxide.

hemolysis (hēm-ol'i-sis). The lysis or dissolution of red blood corpuscles with escape of hemoglobin into the plasma. It may be caused by transfusion of mismatched blood.

hemolytic streptococcus (hēm-ō-lit'ik strep-tō-kok'us). An important type of streptococcus which causes **hemolysis** of red blood corpuscles.

hyperchlorhydria (hī-per-klōr-hid'rē-a). The condition in which there is excessive hydrochloric acid in the gastric juice.

hyperchromia (hī-per-krōm'ē-a). HYPER=increased; CHROM= color. An increased concentration of hemoglobin in the red blood corpuscles.

hypochromia (hī-pō-krōm'ē-a). HYPO=decreased. A decreased concentration of hemoglobin in the red blood corpuscles.

icterus index (ik'ter-us). A figure expressing the amount of bilirubin in the blood. It indicates degrees of liver function or of biliary tract obstruction.

incubate (in'kyūb-āt). *verb*. To keep an **inoculated** culture at a warm temperature (usually body temperature) to encourage bacteria multiplication.

inoculate (in-ok'yūl-āt). *verb*. To apply infected material to sterile culture media to induce the bacteria to multiply, for easier recognition and classification by the pathologist.

ketones (kē'tōnz). *plural*. Chemical substances found in the body when a hyperacid condition exists. There are a number of ketones, the most important of which is **acetone.**

17-ketosteroids (kē-tō-stēr'oyds). Substances sometimes found in urine which aid in the detection of endocrine disorders.

leukocyte (lūk'ō-sīt). LEUK=white. A broad term covering all the different types of white blood cells.

leukocytosis (lūk-ō-sīt-ō'sis). An increase in the number of white cells in the blood. Leukocytosis generally indicates infection.

leukopenia (lūk-ō-pēn'ē-a). PENIA= scarcity. A diminished number of white cells in the blood.

lymphocyte (lim'fō-sīt). A type of white blood cell having a round to ovoid, nonlobulated nucleus and sparse cytoplasm. Lymphocytes normally make up to 25% to 50% of the white cells in the blood (the percentage may be higher in children). (*adj.*— lymphocyt'ic.)

methylene blue (meth'il-ēn). A commonly used blue stain which aids in identifying bacteria.

microtome (mik'rō-tōm). An instrument used to cut very thin slices of tissue (biopsy specimens) for microscopic examination.

myeloblast (mī'el-ō-blast). An immature bone marrow cell; a blood cell precursor.

myelocyte (mī'el-ō-sīt). A more mature bone marrow cell.

nitrazene paper (nīt'ra-zēn). An impregnated paper strip with which the acidity or alkalinity of a fluid can be determined.

nucleated red cells (nūk'lē-āt-ed). Erythrocytes (red blood cells) which exhibit a nucleus (normally red blood corpuscles are nonnucleated). The presence of nucleated red blood cells is frequently suggestive of important blood disorders.

ova (ōv'a). *plural*. OV=egg. In laboratory practice, the eggs of parasites. They are frequently sought for and identified in feces or in certain body fluids. (*sing.*—ov'um.)

oxylate crystals (oks'sil-āt). The crystalized salts of oxalic acid. They occur in urine and are not significant unless present in very great numbers.

"Pap smear." A common name for a diagnostic examination (Papanicolau test) of secretions (particularly from the uterus and the lungs). It is done to detect abnormal cells suggestive of possible malignancy.

pH (pē-ātch'). A symbol used to express the acidity or alkalinity of substances. It actually expresses hydrogen ion concentration.

phosphate crystals (fos'fāt). Crystalline salts of phosphoric acid. They occur in urine and are not significant unless present in very great numbers.

platelets (plāt'lets). Small cell like structures found in the blood which are concerned with the mechanism of blood coagulation. They number 200,000 to 350,000 per cmm of blood in normal people.

polycythemia (pol-i-sī-thēm'ē-a). POLY=many. A disease state characterized by overactivity of **erythrocyte** production, resulting in an abnormally large number of red corpuscles in the blood.

"polys" (pol'ēz). Abbreviation for **polymorphonuclear leukocytes.** Excessive or diminished numbers suggest possible disease states. They normally make up 50% to 75% of the white cells of the blood.

postprandial. *adj.* Relating to the period after the taking of food.

protein-bound iodine (PBI). Iodine that is bound to a protein fraction of the blood plasma. Its amount is fairly constant in health; alterations from normal suggest certain disease states, particularly those concerned with thyroid function.

prothrombin (prō-throm′bin). THROMB=clot. A precursor of thrombin, which is necessary for blood coagulation. Normally prothrombin is in an inactive state. Prothrombin determinations are useful in evaluating blood coagulability.

protozoa (prō-tō-zō′a). *plural.* Primitive one-celled organisms which may be found in various parts of the body in certain specific diseases. (*sing.*—protozo′on *or* protozo′an; *adj.*—protozo′al.)

PSP. The abbreviation for the phenolsulphonphthalein test for kidney function.

reagent (rē-āj′ent). Any substance employed to produce a chemical reaction.

refractometer (rē-frak-tom′e-ter). MET =measure. The instrument used for determining the **specific gravity** of liquids. *See* **urinom′eter.**

reticulocyte (rē-tik′yū-lō-sīt). An immature or young red blood corpuscle, the presence of which indicates a stage of blood formation or regeneration occurring in the bone marrow.

Rh factor (R-ātch′). An important hereditary factor present in the red blood corpuscles of some people. It becomes very important in blood transfusions to expectant mothers.

Salmonella (Sal-mon-el′a). A genus of bacteria responsible for some types of **dysentery** as well as **typhoid fever.**

saprophyte (sap′rō-fīt). A bacterial organism which lives upon dead or decaying organic matter. It usually does not cause disease.

serology (sēr-ol′ō-jē). The study and testing of blood serum, particularly in connection with antigen-antibody reactions.

sickle cell (sik′el). A crescent shaped (sickle shaped) red blood corpuscle found in the blood in a specific kind of anemia **(sickle cell anemia).**

specific gravity (sg). GRAV=heavy. The weight of a liquid or a substance as compared with the weight of water. It is an important test in urinalysis.

spirochete (spīr′ō-kēt). A spiral shaped bacterium (of many types) which may be found in the blood or body secretions in certain diseases, notable among which are **syphilis, trench mouth,** and **yaws.**

Staphylococcus (Staf-il-ō-kok′kus). A type of bacteria which occurs characteristically as clumps or groups of **cocci.** (*plural*—staph′ylococci.)

steroids (stēr′oyds). *plural.* Compounds produced by the adrenal cortex which chemically resemble cholesterol. They may influence salt and water metabolism, glucose metabolism and androgenic activity. Many steroids are produced synthetically and are administered by doctors.

Streptococcus (Strep-tō-kok′kus). A type of bacteria which occurs characteristically as long or short chains of **cocci.** (*plural*—strep′tococci.)

Sulkowitch's test (Sulk′ō-witch-ez). A test used for detecting the excretion of excessive quantities of calcium in the urine.

titer (tīt′er). In laboratory practice, a term denoting degrees of dilution.

total serum protein. The quantity of protein in a stated volume of blood serum (usually expressed as grams per 100 cc of blood).

transaminase (trans-am′i-nāz). A blood enzyme measured because of its relationship to heart damage (SGOT) and liver damage (SGPT).

trichina (trik-ēn′a). TRICH=hair. The type of parasite responsible for trichinosis (pork worm disease). Also called **Trichinel′la spiralis.** *See* **trichinosis.**

Trichomonas (Trik-ō-mōn′as). A flagellated type of protozoa responsible for some important infections, notably **Trichomonas vaginalis.**

tubercle bacillus (tūb′er-kl ba-sil′us). A specific organism which causes **tuberculosis.** Its scientific name is Mycobacterium tuberculosis.

urea (yūr-ē′a). A waste product found in the blood and in the urine. Abnormal amounts in either signify the need for diagnostic study.

uric acid (yūr′ik). Another waste product found in the blood and in the urine. Abnormally high levels may indicate kidney malfunction or **gout.**

urinometer (yūr-i-nom′e-ter). An instrument used for determining the **specific gravity** of urine. *See* **refractom′eter.**

VDRL test. Abbreviation for a commonly used **agglutination** test for **syphilis.**

virus (vīr′us). An infectious agent too small to be visualized with an ordinary microscope.

xanthochromia (zan-thō-krōm′ē-a). In laboratory practice, a yellowish coloration (particularly of the spinal fluid) which may have diagnostic significance.

18 Pediatrics

ALTHOUGH THE TERM **pediatrics** usually implies care from birth through puberty, the interest of the pediatrician is actually much wider. It sometimes begins with conception, shares concern with the obstetrician through gestation, and provides post-delivery assistance to infants with blood dyscrasias and other congenital conditions.

Pediatric care includes attention to nutrition and growth (mental as well as physical), immunization against infectious diseases, and the management of acute and chronic illnesses. Pediatrics dictates no set age limits, and many pediatricians find interest in adolescent care with its many special problems. Although most young adults will have contacted other physicians by the age of eighteen, many continue to ask the pediatrician's advice because they value the rapport which has been established with the doctor who helped them and watched them develop during their formative years, dating back to the time when they were unable to communicate information.

Specialty certification by the American Board of Pediatrics requires, after graduation from medical school, three years of graduate pediatric training followed by two years of pediatric practice. The candidate is then required to pass appropriate written examinations and oral sessions with four or more examiners.

CONSULTANTS

Louis W. Menachof, M.D.
Diplomate, American Board of Pediatrics; Assistant Clinical Professor, Pediatrics, University of California Medical Center
Santa Rosa, California

Edward B. Shaw, M.D.
Diplomate, American Board of Pediatrics; Emeritus Professor and former Chief, Pediatrics, University of California Medical Center
San Francisco, California

acapnia (a-kap′nē-a). A condition of diminished carbon dioxide in the blood, sometimes responsible for nonbreathing in infants.

achalasia (ak-a-lā′zha *or* –zē-a). The lack of normal relaxation of any **sphincter,** particularly those of the gastrointestinal tract.

achondroplasia (ā-kon-drō-plā′zha *or* –zē-a). CHONDR=cartilage. A particular type of dwarfism generally characterized by short extremities resulting from imperfect cartilage development.

acne (ak′nē). An affliction of the sebaceous glands which is frequently seen in adolescents.

adenoids (ad′e-noydz). ADEN=gland. Glandular tissue normally found in the nasopharynx.

adolescence (ad-ō-les′ens). The period between childhood and adult life ("the teens"). (*adj.* – adoles′cent.)

adrenogenital syndrome (ad-rēn-ō-jen′i-tal sin′drōm). A group of changes suggestive of increased masculinity. It is due to abnormal functioning of the adrenal glands.

agranulocytosis (a-gran-yūl-ō-sīt-ō′sis). A disease characterized by too few white blood cells.

albino (al-bīn′ō). A person afflicted with **albinism** (lack of skin pigment).

amblyopia (am-blē-ōp′ē-a). AMBLY= dullness; OP=vision. Dimness of vision sometimes found in children in whom there is no demonstrable eye lesion.

amebiasis (am-ē-bī′a-sis). An infection with a particular type of intestinal parasite, an **ameba.** (*adj.* – ame′bic.)

anaphylaxis (an-a-fil-aks′is). An exaggerated patient reaction to a substance, generally a substance which he has received before. (*adj.* – anaphylac′tic.)

anoxia (a-noks′ē-a). A frequent cause of fetal or postnatal death due to insufficient delivery or utilization of oxygen.

antiemetic (an-tē-em-et′ik). A drug or substance given to prevent or stop vomiting.

anuria (a-nūr′ē-a). Absence or loss of urine production.

antihistaminic (an-tē-hist-a-min′ik). One of a group of drugs used to control or stop allergic reactions. Also used as an adjective.

apnea (ap′nē-a *or* ap-nē′a). Lack of breathing. In pediatrics it generally refers to the absence of the initial act of breathing in a newborn infant.

ascariasis (ask-a-rī′a-sis). A term referring to infestation of the intestinal tract with worms of the genus Ascaris. Types commonly seen are Ascaris lumbracoides ("round worms" localized in the small intestine) and Ascaris vermicularis ("pin worms" – also called Oxyuris vermicularis – limited to the colon and rectum).

ascorbic acid (as-korb′ik). A compound known as Vitamin C.

ataxia (a-taks′ē-a). TAX=order. Loss or lack of muscular coordination. (*adj.* – atax′ic.)

athetosis (ath-e-tōs′is). Constant, recurring movement of the extremities, generally because of a brain lesion. (*adj.* – ath′etoid.)

atresia (a-trē′zha). Absence of a normally present passageway or opening. (*adj.* – atrēs′ic *or* atret′ic.)

"BCG". A name given to a particular vaccine consisting of weakened tubercle bacilli.

bilirubin (bil-ē-rūb'in). One of the bile pigments produced by the breakdown of red blood cells. When present in excess in blood, it gives a yellow color to the skin.

bradycardia (brād-ē-kard'ē-a). CARD= heart. Slow heart rate.

bronchodilator (brong-kō-dī'lā-tor). An agent given to open the air passages to make breathing easier; therefore, used to treat asthma.

brucellosis (brū-sel-lō'sis). Undulant fever.

celiac disease (sēl'ē-ak). A disease of early childhood having many features, notably malabsorption of certain basic components of foods.

chalasia (ka-lā'zha *or* −zē-a). A continuous relaxation of the esophagus or of the gastric sphincter. It sometimes causes regurgitation of feedings in infants. *See* **achalasia.**

chickenpox. Almost everybody's had it! Also called **varicel'la.**

chorea (kōr-ē'a). A convulsive disease causing jerking movements **(St. Vitus dance).**

chromosome (krōm-ō-sōm). One of several specific particles in cell nuclei which appear at the time of cell division. They carry the **genes.**

cleft palate (kleft pal'et). A congenital fissure in the midline of the roof of the mouth.

colic (kol'ik). In pediatrics, generally refers to abdominal pain occurring in spasms.

congenital (kon-jen'i-tal). *adj.* Present at birth.

convulsion (kon-vul'shun). VULS= pull. Violent uncontrolled muscle contraction.

craniotabes (krān-ē-ō-tāb'ēz). CRAN= skull. Abnormally soft places in the skull of infants, usually unexplained, but occasionally associated with **rickets.**

cretinism (krēt'in-izm). A congenital condition due to diminished or absent thyroid secretion. It is generally accompanied by dwarfism and mental retardation.

croup (krūp). A severe inflammation of the laryngeal area, causing difficult and noisy ("croupy") breathing.

cystic fibrosis (sist'ik fĭb-rō'sis). A hereditary disease involving many organs of the body, including the pancreas, lungs, liver, and sweat glands.

deciduous teeth (dē-sid'yū-us). "Baby teeth."

dental caries (den'tal kār'ēz). Decay of the teeth; cavity formation.

dextrocardia (deks-trō-kard'ē-a). DEXTR=right. Displacement or rotation of the heart toward the right side of the chest.

diphtheria (dif-thēr'ē-a). A severe infectious disease, usually in the throat (now fortunately uncommon).

dwarf. An abnormally short person, sometimes because of glandular dysfunction.

eczema (ekz'e-ma). A skin disease which may exhibit one of many kinds of rashes. It is frequently due to allergies. (*adj.* − eczem'atous.)

emetic (em-et'ik). Something given or taken to induce vomiting.

enanthem (en-an'them). A rash appearing inside the mouth or on other mucous membranes.

encephalitis (en-sef-a-lī'tis). CEPH= head. Inflammation of the brain.

enterobiasis (en-ter-ō-bī'a-sis). Pinworm infestation. *See* **ascariasis.**

enuresis (en-yūr-ē'sis). Involuntary urination during sleep, usually at night (*nocturnal enuresis*).

epilepsy (ep-i-lep'sē). A nervous disorder generally characterized by convulsions. (*adj.* − epilep'tic.)

epileptic (ep-i-lep'tik). A person afflicted with **epilepsy.** (Also used as an adjective.)

erythroblastosis fetalis (ē-rith-rō-blas-tō'sis fēt-al'is *or* er-rēth-rō-blas-tō'sis). An abnormal blood condition sometimes seen in newborns. It is caused by conflicting blood types in mother and infant.

exanthem (eks-an'them). A fast appearing, generally extensive, skin eruption which is generally part of a systemic disease such as **measles.**

exanthem subitum (sūb'i-tum). An acute pediatric disease characterized by a rash which appears as the three-day unexplained temperature abruptly subsides; also called **roseola infantum.**

exchange transfusion (trans-fū'zhun). The substitution of a large quantity of donor blood; most frequently carried out in newborns.

folic acid (fōl'ik). One of the vitamins.

fontanelle (font-a-nel'). The "soft spot" in a baby's skull.

foramen ovale (for-ā'men ō-val'ē). A congenital opening in the wall between the two cardiac atria. It normally closes at birth with the advent of respiration.

gamma globulin (gam'a glob'yūl-in). A protein constituent of human blood, used for the prevention and treatment of some diseases.

gene (jēn). GEN=origin. The unit which transmits hereditary characteristics. The gene is generally attached to a particular **chromosome.** (*Plural*—genes.)

genetics (jen-et'iks). The study of heredity.

genu recurvatum (jē'nū rē-kurv-a'tum). GENU=knee. Backward curvature of the legs at the knee joints.

genu valgum (val'gum). "Knock knees."

genu varum (vair'um). "Bow legs."

German measles. "Three-day measles"; best called **rubella.**

Gomco clamp (Gom'ko). A surgical device sometimes used in performing circumcision on male infants.

gonadotrophin — gonadotropin (gon-ad-ō-trof'in) (gon-ad-ō-trōp'in). GONAD=sex. A naturally present hormonal substance which stimulates gonadal activity.

grand mal (grahn mahl). A severe convulsion with unconsciousness and twitching, resulting from one of several causes but most commonly associated with **epilepsy.**

hereditary (her-ed'i-te-re). *adj.* Inherited from one's parents or ancestors.

herpetic stomatitis (her-pet'ik stōm-a-tī'tis). STOM=mouth. A common disease of young children characterized by blisters in the mouth and by other symptoms; also called **aphthous stomatitis.**

hydrocephalus (hī-drō-sef'a-lus). HYDR=water; CEPH=head. A birth condition (large head, due to excessive fluid within the skull).

hydrops fetalis (hī'drops fēt-al'is). A retention of fluid in the tissues of a newborn infant. It is seen in cases of severe Rh factor conflict and is usually fatal.

hypoprothrombinemia (hī-pō-prō-throm-bin-ēm'ē-a). THROMB=clot. A deficiency of **prothrombin** (a clotting factor) in the blood, sometimes associated with insufficient Vitamin K.

hypoxia (hip-poks'ē-a). HYPO=diminished. Lack, want, or deficiency of oxygen—a frequent cause of fetal or postnatal death.

icterus neonatorum (ik'ter-us nē-ō-nāt-ōr'um). **Jaundice** in the newborn, generally due to **Rh factor** abnormality in the blood.

infectious mononucleosis (in-fek'shus mōn-ō-nūk-lē-ō'sis). A common disease of older children and adults which is characterized by fever and swelling of the lymph glands, particularly of the neck.

lactic acid (lak'tik). A constituent found in sour milk and in fermented foods.

laryngotracheobronchitis (lair-ing-gō-trāk-ē-ō-brong-kī'tis). Inflammation, right where the word indicates (one form of "croup").

leukemia (lūk-ēm'ē-a). LEUK=white. A usually fatal blood disease characterized by massive overproduction of white blood cells ("cancer of the blood").

marasmus (mar-az'mus). A progressive wasting away of the tissues, sometimes seen in infants. Frequently there is no obvious cause.

measles. Everybody's old acquaintance! "Hard measles" "two-week measles"). Also called **rubeola.**

Mendel's laws (men'delz). *Plural.* Some of the basic principles of heredity.

meningitis (men-in-jī'tis). An acute epidemic disease which was once frequently fatal but now, only rarely so.

meningocele (men-inj'jō-sēl *or* men-ing'gō-sēl). A congenital condition sometimes seen in babies. It consists of a hernial protrusion of the meninges through a defect in the skull or spinal column.

mongolism (mon'gō-lizm). A congenital condition accompanied by mental retardation (**Down's disease**).

myelocele (mī'el-ō-sēl). MYEL=nerve. A congenital defect in the posterior wall of the spinal canal.

myopia (mī-ōp'ē-a). Nearsightedness. (*adj.* — myop'ic.)

nasopharyngitis (nā-zō-fair-in-jī'tis). Inflammation of the nose and throat.

neonatal (nē-ō-nāt'al). *adj.* NAT=birth. Newborn; generally referring to the first four weeks of life.

oliguria (ol-i-gūr'ē-a). Scanty secretion of urine.

ossification (os-si-fi-kā'shun). OS= bone. The developmental process of hardening to bony consistency.

otitis externa (ōt-ī'tis eks-ter'na). OT= ear. Inflammation of the external ear canal.

otitis media (mēd'ē-a). Inflammation of the middle ear.

parotitis (pair-ot-ī'tis). Parotid gland inflammation; **mumps** is the commonest type.

pediatrician (pēd-ē-a-trish'un). A doctor who specializes in pediatrics.

pediatrics (pēd-ē-at'riks). *See* introductory paragraphs.

pediculosis (ped-ik-yūl-ō'sis). Infestation with lice.

pediculosis capitis (kap'i-tis). Infestation with head lice.

pediculosis corporis (kor'por-is). Infestation with body lice.

perianal (per-ē-ān'al). *adj.* Around or surrounding the anus.

perinatal (per-i-nāt'al). *adj.* A term indicating relationship to events or factors present at the approximate time of birth. It is generally supposed to include the period from the twenty-eighth week of pregnancy until the end of the first month after birth.

pertussis (per-tus'sis). A nicer name for whooping cough.

petit mal (pet'ē mahl *or* pet-ēt' mahl'. Momentary "black out" sometimes accompanied by dizziness and other sensations; it is considered by some to be a form of **epilepsy.**

pica (pīk'a). A perverted appetite, characterized by an abnormal craving for unusual or bizarre articles of food.

pinworm infestation. Infestation of the large bowel and rectum with typical "pinworms." *See* **enterobiasis.**

"PKU"—phenylketonuria (fēn-il-kē-tōn-ūr'ē-a). The presence of phenylketone in the urine, found in some cases of mental retardation.

pneumonitis (nūm-ō-nī'tis). PNEUM= lung. A form of lung inflammation frequently seen in children (**pneumonia**).

poliomyelitis (pōl-ē-ō-mī-el-ī'tis). A well-known disease, happily decreasing in incidence. Also called **infantile paralysis** or "**polio.**"

postmaturity (post-matūr'i-tē). The opposite of **prematurity**; the condition of being born later than the termination of the normal **gestation** period.

precocious (prē-kō'shus). *adj.* Advanced beyond one's years.

premature (prē-ma-tūr'). *adj.* Born too soon. (*noun* — prematur'ity.)

"premie" (prēm'ē). Medical jargon designating a prematurely born infant.

prepuce (prep'yūs *or* prēp'yūs). The fold of skin (**foreskin**) covering the end of the penis. (*adj.* — prepu'tial.)

puberty (pyūb′er-tē). The age of arrival at sexual maturity.

pyloric stenosis (pī-lor′ik sten-ō′sis). STEN=narrow. A congenital condition of overdevelopment of the **pyloric** musculature preventing normal emptying of the stomach.

respirator (res′pir-ā-tor). A machine used for artificial respiration.

Rh factor. A hereditary quality present in some patients' red blood cells. It is a frequent, very important cause of **jaundice** in the newborn.

rheumatic endocarditis (rūm-at′ik en-dō-kard-ī′tis). A type of heart disease associated with **rheumatic fever.**

rheumatic fever. An infectious disease of childhood, causing joint inflammation and sometimes **endocarditis.**

rhinitis (rīn-ī′tis). RHIN=nose. Inflammation of the lining of the nose, frequently seen in children as hay fever (**allergic rhinitis**).

riboflavin (rēb-ō-flāv′in). Vitamin B 12.

rickets (rik′ets). A deficiency disease of early childhood causing bone deformity. It is prevented by Vitamin D. (*adj.* — rachit′ic.)

roseola infantum (rōs-ē-ō′la in-fant′um). Another name for **exanthem subitum.**

rubella (rūb-el′la). RUB=red. **German measles.**

rubeola (rūb-ē-ō′la). "Hard measles"; "regular measles." The preferred term is **measles.**

scabies (skā′bēz). A parasitic skin infection sometimes called "the seven year itch."

scarlet fever. A contagious disease due to streptococci and most often seen during childhood or early adolescence.

seizure. A "polite" name for a convulsion.

splenomegaly (splen-ō-meg′a-lē). SPLEN=spleen. Abnormal enlargement of the spleen.

spondylitis (spon-dil-ī′tis). Inflammation of a vertebral body of the spine.

Stanford-Binet test (Bin-ā′). An intelligence test.

stridor (strīd′or). A harsh, high pitched respiratory sound, generally of **inspiration.**

"S.U.D." *or* **"S.I.D."** An abbreviation for "sudden unexpected death" or "sudden infant death."

tachycardia (tak-i-kard′ē-a). Excessively rapid heart action.

tachypnea (tak-ip-nē′a). Excessively rapid, shallow respiration which is a neurotic manifestation in some children.

tetanus (tet′a-nus). An acute infectious disease generally acquired through puncture wounds ("lockjaw").

tetany (tet′a-nē). A disorder marked by intermittent muscular contractions. It is sometimes caused by decreased blood calcium. (*adj.* — tetan′ic.)

thrush. A specific mouth infection due to a fungus and sometimes seen in very young infants.

thymus gland (thīm′us). A ductless gland in the neck which normally disappears during infancy or early childhood. It is important in producing cells essential for resistance to infection.

thyroglossal (thī-rō-glos′al). *adj.* GLOSS=tongue. Pertaining to both the thyroid and the tongue, and generally referring to the thyroglossal duct, a fetal passage from the thyroid to the base of the tongue.

tinea (tin′ē-a). A superficial skin infection caused by a fungus; in children it is sometimes seen as "ringworm."

torticollis (tort-i-kol′lis). TORT=twist; COLL=neck. A spastic condition of some of the neck muscles ("wryneck").

toxoplasmosis (toks-ō-plas-mō′sis). TOX=poison. A parasitic disease due to protozoa. It is seen in adults and is occasionally acquired from the mother by newborns.

tracheobronchitis (trāk-ē-ō-brong-kī′tis). An acute infection of the bronchial tubes and trachea which is frequently seen in young children.

tracheoesophageal fistula (trăk-ē-ō-ē-sof-a-jē′al fist′yūl-a). A congenital anomaly of the trachea in which there is a passage between the trachea and the esophagus.

tremor (trem′or *or* trēm′or). Continuous involuntary trembling.

urticaria (ert-i-kair′ē-a). An allergic skin reaction characterized by raised itching areas, generally called "hives."

vaccine (vak′sēn). Medication which consists of weakened or dead bacteria, or their products, and is used for immunization.

varicella (vair-i-sel′a). A Latin name for chickenpox.

variola (vair-ī′ō-la *or* vair-ē-ō′la). **Smallpox.**

vernix caseosa (ver′niks kās-e-ō′sa). CAS=milk. The white, waxy substance covering a newborn baby's body.

vestigial (ves-tij′ē-al). *adj.* In pediatrics, generally referring to a useless part or organ which is a "throwback" to a previous stage of evolutionary development.

vitamin (vīt′a-min). VIT=life. A substance needed by the body for proper growth and development.

19 Physical Medicine and Rehabilitation

PHYSICAL MEDICINE—more than any of the other medical specialties—makes primary use of physical measures (including the application of hot and cold, electric stimulation, massage, active and passive exercise) in treatment. Treatment may also include the use of chemical or pharmacological agents and psychotherapy; of late, the practice of physical medicine has shown a tendency to become oriented toward electrodiagnostic testing, particularly electromyography and nerve conduction studies.

In the United States this specialty is called *Physical Medicine and Rehabilitation.* The specialist in physical medicine is frequently referred to as a **physiatrist.** He diagnoses the patient's conditions and the needs, and prescribes the course of treatment. The treatments are generally given by a **physical therapist** who is working under the direction of the physiatrist. The physical therapist is a technician who has had special training in physical therapy and who is licensed by the State Board of Physical Therapy Examiners. In actual practice, physical therapists also give treatments under the direction of doctors other than physiatrists.

Rehabilitation—the restoration of a patient to his best attainable physical condition in the shortest amount of time—is the common goal of all personnel who work with disabled persons. Such disabilities may be the result of accidents, crippling diseases (strokes, polio, arthritis, etc.), amputations, congenital conditions, or just plain muscle weakness following surgery or long hospitalization.

The American Board of Physical Medicine and Rehabilitation requires a three-year residency program, and two years of actual practice, before the applicant can be examined for certification.

CONSULTANTS

Sedgwick Mead, M.D.
Diplomate, American Board of Physical Medicine & Rehabilitation; Chief, Neurology, Kaiser Rehabilitation Center
Vallejo, California

Robert A. Teckemeyer, R.P.T.
Washington, D.C.

abduction (ab-duk′shun). In physical medicine, the active or passive moving of a limb away from the midline of the body; also the resulting position. *See* **adduction.**

actinic (ak-tin′ik). *adj.* Pertaining to rays, solar or artificial, which lie beyond the violet end of the spectrum and cause chemical effects.

actinotherapy (ak-tin-ō-ther′a-py). Treatment by ultraviolet rays.

adduction (a-duk′shun). The moving or drawing of an arm or a leg toward the midline of the body; also, the resulting position. *See* **abduction.**

adhesion (ad-hē′zhun). The abnormal sticking together of tissues, resulting in pain or in limitation of motion.

adipose tissue (ad′i-pōs). ADIP=fat. Fatty tissue.

ambulation (am′byū-lā-shun). The ability to walk as opposed to enforced bed confinement.

ampere (am′pēr). The unit of measurement of the strength of electric current.

amputee (am-pyū-tē′). A person who has lost an arm or a leg by surgical or accidental amputation.

amyotonia (ā-mī-ō-tōn′ē-a). MYO= muscle. Diminished or absent muscle tone.

anion (an′ī-on). An ion carrying a negative charge, and thus attracted to the positive pole or **anode.**

ankylosis (ang-ki-lō′sis). The total loss of mobility of a joint.

anode (an′ōd). The positive electrode or pole of a source of electrical current.

antagonist (an-tag′ō-nist). In physical medicine, a muscle producing an effect which is opposite to that produced by a corresponding muscle (antagonist) acting on the same part, as in producing **flexion** and **extension** of a phalanx.

apraxia (a-prak′sē-a *or* a-prak′sha). The loss of a previously possessed ability to perform certain skilled acts. (*adj.* – apract′ic *or* aprax′ic)

Artane (ar′tān). A proprietary **anti-tremor** drug sometimes used in treating Parkinson's disease.

asynergia (a-sin-er′jē-a) – **asynergy.** Lack of coordination between parts normally acting together, usually the result of brain disease or brain damage.

athetosis (ath-ē-tō′sis). Constant, recurring movement of the extremities, generally related to a brain lesion. (*adj.* – ath′etoid)

atlas (at′las). A name given to the first cervical vertebra upon which the skull rests. (Named for Atlas, who carried the world on his shoulders.)

atonia (a-tōn′ē-a) *or* **atony** (at′ō-nē). Absence or loss of muscle tone. (*adj.* – aton′ic.)

Balkan frame (Bawl′kan). An overhead frame placed over a bed to allow the use of traction in the treatment of bone or joint conditions.

bunion (bun′yon). A swelling on the medial surface of the great toe causing it to turn toward the other toes.

calisthenics (kal-is-then′iks). Gymnastic exercises designed to improve the function and strength of muscles.

cathode (kath′ōd). The negative electrode or pole of a source of electrical current.

Charcot's joint (Shar′kōz). A swollen but painless joint, generally associated with third-stage *syphilis.*

"claw hand" (klaw hand). A claw like deformity of the fingers and hand, sometimes seen in **ulnar** nerve disease.

clonus (klō′nus). A type of spasm in which alternate relaxation and contractions follow each other rapidly. (*adj.* — clon′ic.)

coccygodynia (kok-sē-gō-din′ē-a) or **coccydynia.** Pain in the region of the **coccyx.**

conduction (kon-duk′shun). The process of transmitting or conveying energy from one place to another.

contracture (kon-trak′chur). Shortening or distortion of tissue, generally muscle tissue.

cryotherapy (krī-ō-ther′a-py). CRYO= cold. The therapeutic application of cold in any form.

debility (dē-bil′i-ty). Lack or loss of strength. (*adj.* — debil′itated.)

decalcification (dē-kal-si-fi-kā′shun). The physiological process in which lime salts are lost from the bones or the teeth. (*adj.* — decal′cified; also *noun*, the condition produced.)

decubitus ulcer. A skin ulceration caused by prolonged external pressure; "bedsores" are a common type.

deformity (dē-for′mi-ty). A disfiguring distortion or deviation from the normal contour or shape of a part of the body.

degeneration (dē-jen-er-ā′shun). Deterioration or retrogressive change of cells or tissue, generally resulting in progressive loss of function. (*adj.* — degen′erative.)

dehydration (dē-hī-drā′shun). The loss or removal of water; also, the condition resulting.

denervation (dē-ner-vā′shun). The interference or interruption of the function of a nerve by cutting, removing, or blocking it; also, the condition resulting.

diaphoresis (dī-a-for-rē′sis). Therapeutic production of excessive perspiration by one of many methods.

diathermy (dī′a-ther-my). THERM= heat. The use of high frequency current to generate or produce heat in the deeper tissues of the body; also, the apparatus used.

Dupuytren's contracture (Doo′pe-tronz). A deformity of the hand and fingers, mostly involving the medial half of the hand, producing varying degrees of flexion of the last three fingers, and wrinkling of the palm.

effleurage (ef-floo-razh′). A stroking movement used in massage.

electrode (ē-lek′trōd). In physical medicine, an instrument through the point of which current is discharged to a patient's body.

electromyograph (ē-lek-trō-mī′ō-graf). MYO=muscle; GRAPH=write. An apparatus for producing a record of the electrical response of muscles to either spontaneous or electrical stimulation.

electrotherapy (ē-lek-trō-ther′a-py). The use of electricity in the treatment of disease.

Erb's paralysis (Erbz). A paralysis of the muscles of the shoulder region and upper arm resulting from stretching of the fifth and sixth cervical nerve roots.

exercise (ek′ser-sīz). In physical medicine, a planned performance of a particular kind of physical exertion for the correction of deformities or of conditions resulting from injury, disease, or specific health problems. Types include: active, active assistive, active resistive, isometric, isotonic, passive, postural, and resistive.

farad (fair′ad). The unit of electrical capacity.

fibrositis (fī-brō-sī′tis). An inflammatory reaction, particularly of a muscle sheath, sometimes causing pain and immobility from adhesions.

flaccid (flak′sid). *adj.* Relaxed or weak, particularly relating to the condition of a muscle.

fomentation (fō-men-tā′shun). A hot, wet, external application for the relief of pain or inflammation ("hot packs").

gait (gāt). A manner of walking which is frequently diagnostic of a condition. Types are: atax'ix, e'quine, hemiple'gic, scis'sors, shuf'fling, spas'tic, tabet'ic, and wadd'ling.

gamma rays (gam'ma). A form of electromagnetic radiation used in treating certain tumors or conditions.

gastrocnemius (gas-trok-nē'mē-us). One of the two large calf muscles in the posterior portion of each leg.

goniometer (gō-nē-om'e-ter). MET= measure. A device for measuring the extent of movement of a joint.

heliotherapy (hēl-ē-ō-ther'a-pē). Exposure of the body to the sun's rays for therapeutic purposes.

hemiplegia (hem-i-plē'jē-a *or* –ja). HEMI=half: PLEG=paralysis. A one-sided paralysis involving the upper and the lower limb on the same side.

Hubbard tank. A large tank in which a person may be immersed for the performance of exercises under water.

hydrogymnastics (hī-drō-jim-nas'tiks). HYDRO=water. Underwater exercises.

hydrotherapy (hī-drō-ther'a-py). THERAP=treatment. The scientific use of water in the treatment of conditions or diseases. (*adj.*—hydrotherapeu'tic.)

hyperemia (hī-per-ē'mē-a). An excessive amount of blood in a part of the body. (*adj.*—hypere'mic.)

hyperesthesia (hī-per-es-thē'zē-a). ESTHE=feeling. Excessive sensitiveness, particularly of the skin. The antonym is **hyp'esthesia** or **hy'poesthesia.**

hyperhidrosis (hī-per-hid-rō'sis). Excessive sweating, sometimes artificially produced for therapeutic purposes.

hyperthermia (hī-per-ther'mē-a). Abnormally high body temperature.

hypothermia (hī-pō-therm'ē-a). Below normal temperature of all or of a part of the body, sometimes artificially produced.

incoordination (in-kō-or-di-nā'shun). Lack of muscle coordination.

infrared rays (in-fra-red'). The long, heat-producing rays of the spectrum, often used therapeutically.

intra-articular (in-tra-ar-tik'yū-lar). *adj.* Within the cavity of a joint.

irradiation (ir-rā-dē-ā'shun). Treatment by means of the application of various kinds of electromagnetic rays.

ischemia (is-kē'mē-a). A condition of localized diminished blood supply.

Kernigs' sign (ker'nigz). A particular muscle reflex, generally diagnostic of **meningitis.**

Kromayer's lamp (Krō'mī-erz). A well-known mechanical generator of ultraviolet rays.

lordosis (lor-dō'sis). The anteroposterior curvature (convexity forward) of the lumbar portion of the spinal column. "Swayback" is abnormal hyperlordosis.

lumbago (lum-bā'gō). LUMB=loin or back. An obsolete term still commonly used to designate pain in the lower back.

massage (ma-sazh'). The procedure of actively rubbing or kneading, generally performed to produce muscle relaxation.

metatarsalgia (met-a-tar-sal'jē-a). ALG=pain. Pain in the **metatarsal** region of the foot.

modality (mō-dal'i-ty). A method of applying or employing a therapeutic agent, particularly a physical one.

multiple sclerosis (sklē-rō'sis). A chronic, generally progressive, disease of the nervous system.

myalgia (mī-al'jē-a). Pain in or of muscles.

myasthenia gravis (mī-as-thē'nē-a gra'vis). STHEN=weakness. A chronic, generally progressive, weakness or paralysis of parts of the muscular system, without obvious **atrophy.**

myositis (mī-ō-sī'tis). Inflammation of or in a muscle, particularly a voluntary muscle.

myositis ossificans (os-sif'i-kanz). MYO=muscle; OS=bone. A disease of muscles characterized by their hardening, sometimes to bony consistency.

neuralgia (noo-ral'jē-a). NEUR=nerve. A general name for pain radiating along the course of a nerve.

neurasthenia (nūr-as-thēn'ē-a). A group of symptoms, generally on a psychogenic basis, resulting in extreme fatigue which is not necessarily related to exertion.

neuritis (nūr-ī'tis). Inflammation of a nerve resulting in various symptoms in the area supplied by that nerve.

nucleus pulposus (nūk'lē-us pul-pō'sus). The gelatinous mass in the center of each intervertebral disc. Its derangement, particularly herniation through the outer edge of the disc, can give rise to various nerve symptoms.

olecranon bursitis (ō-lek'ra-non bur-sī'tis). Inflammation of or in the bursa at the tip of the elbow.

opisthotonos (op-is-thot'o-nos). Exaggerated anterior bowing of the spinal column, generally due to spasm of the back muscles.

osteomalacia (os-tē-ō-mal-ā'sha). OS= bone; MALAC=soft. A condition characterized by softening of the bones due to disease or to Vitamin D deficiency.

paralytic (par-a-lit'ik). A person afflicted with paralysis. (Also used as an adjective.)

paraplegia (pair-a-plē'jē-a *or* –ja). Paralysis involving *both* legs and the lower body. (*adj.* – **paraplegic.**)

paraplegic (pair-a-plē'jik). A person afflicted with paraplegia.

phlebitis (fle-bī'tis). PHLEB=vein. Inflammation of the wall of a vein.

phlebothrombosis (flēb-ō-throm-bō'sis). THROM=clot. Development of an adherent blood clot within a vein, generally secondary to **phlebitis** or following surgery.

physical medicine. *See* introductory paragraphs.

physiatrist (fiz'i-a-trist). *See* introductory paragraphs.

physical therapist (ther'a-pist) *or* **physiotherapist.** *See* introductory paragraphs.

physical therapy (ther'a-pē) — **physiotherapy.** The treatment of disease by physical, nonmedical means.

poultice (pōl'tis). A soft, moist mass applied to the skin surface to improve or increase the circulation in that part of the body.

pronation (prō-nā'shun). The act of rotating the hand palm-backward or palm-downward; or of turning the foot arch-downward at the ankle joint. Also, the resulting position.

proprioception (prō-prē-ō-sep'shun). The sense which gives knowledge of the position or movement of a part of the body without the need for visual observation. (*adj.* – propriocep'tive.)

prosthesis (pros-thē'sis). An artificial part substituting for or replacing one that is absent.

quadriceps femoris (kwad'ri-seps fem'or-is). A combined name for the four muscles of the anterior portion of the thigh.

quadriplegia (kwad-ri-plē'jē-a *or* –ja). A paralysis of all four limbs.

quadriplegic (kwad-ri-plē'jik). A person afflicted with **quadriplegia.**

Raynaud's disease (Rā-nōz'). A chronic disease or condition characterized by constriction of certain terminal **arterioles** of the extremities.

rhizotomy (rī-zot'ō-my). The surgical dividing of certain roots of the spinal nerves, generally done for the relief of incurable pain.

roentgen rays (rent'gen). Electromagnetic radiation of high energy and extremely short wave length which is used for taking x-rays.

sacro-iliac joint (sā-krō-il'ē-ak). The paired slightly mobile joint between the ilium and the sacrum.

Sayre headsling (Sā'er). A halter placed around the neck and secured beneath the chin by means of which traction can be applied to the spinal column, using the body as a counter weight.

sciatica (sī-at′i-ka). A term referring to pain along the course of the sciatic nerve.

scoliosis (skō-lē-ō′sis). A definite abnormal curvature of the spine, always in a lateral direction. *See* **kyphosis** and **lordosis.**

sinusoidal current (sīn-us-oid′al). One type of electric current, frequently employed in physical therapy.

sitz bath (sits). A particular kind of bath technique used for applying heat to the hips and pelvic regions.

skeletal traction (skel′e-tal). A stretching procedure carried out by attaching one end of the traction apparatus directly to a bone of the skeleton.

spasticity (spas-tis′i-ty). Increased reflex excitability of a muscle, particularly that kind caused by a brain or spinal cord lesion.

spondylitis (spon-dil-ī′tis). Inflammation in or of one or more vertebral bodies, generally referring to tuberculous inflammation (**Pott's disease**) or to an **ankylosing** disease of the entire spine.

sternocleidomastoid (stern-ō-klīd-ō-mas′toyd). See **sternomastoid.**

sternomastoid (stern-ō-mas′toyd) *or* **sternocleidomastoid.** A large muscle of the side of the neck.

Stryker frame (Strī′ker). A frame fitted to a bed on which a patient is attached and rotated around his longitudinal axis.

subluxation (sub-lux-ā′shun). An incomplete dislocation.

supination (sūp-in-ā′shun). The act of rotating the hand palm-forward or palm-upward; it also applies to the foot. The term also designates the resulting positions.

synergist (sīn′er-jist). In physical medicine, a muscle which acts with and assists another muscle in producing a movement. (*adj.* –syn′ergistic.)

synovitis (sīn-ō-vī′tis). Inflammation in or of the membrane lining a joint cavity (the **synovial membrane**).

syringomyelia (sir-ing-gō-mī-ē′lē-a). A spinal cord disease. It causes various conditions which are treated by physiotherapy.

talipes (tal′i-pēz). A multi-type foot deformity which results, generally, in the foot's being twisted out of shape. A synonym is **clubfoot.**

tenosynovitis (tēn-ō-sīn-ō-vī′tis). TEN= tendon. Inflammation within the sheath of a tendon.

thermopenetration (ther-mō-pen-e-trā′shun). **Diathermy.**

tolerance test, Master's (tol′er-ans). A standard exercise test used to determine the ability of the cardiovascular system to tolerate physical exertion.

torticollis (tor-ti-kol′is). TORT=twist; COLL=neck. A spastic condition, or shortening, of the neck muscles resulting in a continuous tilting of the head ("wryneck").

traction (trak′shun). TRAC=draw. The application or exerting of pull upon a part of the body by any one of many methods, in order to overcome spasm, tension, or overriding of the fragments of a fractured bone.

ultrasound—ultrasonic. (ul-tra sownd′) A term referring to sound waves which have frequencies beyond the upper limit of sounds audible to human ears. Also, the type of apparatus used for producing such waves, for use in therapy.

ultraviolet rays (ul-tra-vī′ō-let). The short (**hyperemia**-producing) rays of the spectrum, frequently used therapeutically.

varicosity (var-i-kos′i-ty) *or* **varix.** A dilated, stretched vein or a group of such veins. (*adj.* –var′icose *or* var′icosed.)

vertigo (ver′tē-gō). VERT=turn. The type of dizziness associated with the sensation of whirling.

vibrator (vī′brā-tor). A device or apparatus used in massage to produce rapid to-and-fro motion or the sensation of it in a part of the body.

walker. A frame like apparatus used to support or assist the patient in walking.

wavelength. A term applied to the length of the interval between identical phases of two succeeding waves.

20 Preventive Medicine and Public Health

THE FUNCTION OF **Preventive Medicine** and **Public Health** is mainly an administrative one. Unlike other branches of medicine that work largely in a direct one-to-one relationship with individual patients, the public health physician has the community as his patient.

The health officer no longer spends his time tacking up quarantine signs and looking into privies. People know more about medical affairs and, with the increased population all over the world and the belief that everyone is entitled to good health, demands for public health services of all kinds have increased.

Larger and larger portions of all medical practice are focusing on preventive rather than curative care. The public health physician does not compete with the private practice physician — he complements him. By working with private physicians, he strives to maintain for the nation a high level of health and medical care. The health office also works with hospitals, housing officials, educational groups, and labor organizations in setting up programs of disease immunization and control.

The United States Public Health Service offers intensive training in public health, clinical practice, or administration. On an international basis, the World Health Organization carries on a large share of international health programs.

The American Board of Preventive Medicine requires completion of two years of approved residency, one year of study in a School of Public Health, and three years of full time experience in public health work before a candidate is eligible for certification examinations.

CONSULTANT

William H. Aufranc, M.D.
Diplomate, American Board of Preventive Medicine; Former Regional Director, U.S.P.H.S.
San Francisco, California

abattoir (ab′a-twar). A slaughter house, especially one of large capacity.

actinomycosis (ak-tin-ō-mī-kō′sis). A disease primarily of cattle or swine but sometimes transmitted to man.

aerosol (air′ō-sol). AER=air. A means of dispersing insecticides of various types into the atmosphere.

amebiasis (am-e-bī′a-sis). AMEB= ameba. Intestinal infestation with the Entamoeba histolytica. It is important in preventive medicine because of its spread by "carriers."

ancylostomiasis (an-kil-ost-ō-mī′a-sis). An affliction generally called "hookworm disease."

anthrax (an′thraks). A disease sometimes transmitted from animals to man, mostly through the handling of hides, skins, wool, and hair.

antivenin (an-ti-ven′in). VEN=poison. A general term covering serums containing substances protective against the venom of snakes.

ascariasis (ask-a-rī′a-sis). Infestation with the round worm, Ascaris lumbricoides, common in the tropics and also seen in Southeastern United States.

Bang's disease. A disease of cattle. The milk from infected animals may cause **brucellosis** (undulant fever) in humans.

beriberi (ber′i-ber′i). An infrequently seen disease which is due to Vitamin B₁ (thiamine) deficiency.

beryllium (ber-il′ē-um). A metal extensively used in industry, particularly in the manufacture of fluorescent lamps. Extensive exposure may cause lung and skin reactions, a condition known as **berylliosis.**

botulism (botch′ū-lizm). A serious disease contracted by eating food poisoned by infection with the botulinus organism. The toxin may develop in canned infected food since the organism is an **anerobe.**

brucellosis (brū-sel-ō′sis). A serious disease transmitted to humans through infected milk from cattle who have **Bang's disease.** It is also called **undulant fever** or **Malta fever.**

cadmium (kad′mē-um). A metal used industrially, particularly in plating, which may cause lung or gastrointestinal symptoms.

carbon monoxide (mon-oks′īd). A poisonous, asphyxiating gas occurring in high concentration in automobile exhausts. It is also a component of commercial household cooking gas.

carrier (kair′i-er). A person capable of infecting others with a disease which he "carries" but from which he himself may have no symptoms.

chlordane (klōr′dān). A well-known insecticide capable of causing toxic symptoms in humans.

chlorination (klōr-i-nā′shun). A method of disinfection utilizing chlorine gas.

cholera (kol′er-a). A severe, specific gastrointestinal disease spread by infected fecal material. Fortunately it is now seldom seen in America.

communicable (kom-myūn′i-ka-bl). *adj.* Referring to diseases which can be transmitted from one person to another. *See* **contagious.**

contact. *adj.* Referring to contagious or communicable diseases for the transmission of which body or utensil contact is required.

contagious. *adj.* Referring to disease which is communicable. (*noun—*contagion.)

contamination. Pollution by the addition of undesirable substances.

DDT. A well-known synthetic insecticide which has shown many undesirable qualities such as resistance to self-destruction.

dengue (deng′gē). An acute mosquito-borne fever.

disinfection (dis-in-fek′shun). A vague term which implies the killing, by chemical means, of microorganisms or other infectious agents.

echinococcosis (e-kin-ō-kok-kō′sis). A parasite-transmitted disease important in the sheep raising areas of the world. Also called **hydatid disease.**

Echinococcus (E-kin-ō-kok′kus). A genus of tape worms. Its larva, known as the **hydatid,** may form tumors or cysts in man (notably in the liver).

encephalitis (en-sef-a-lī′tis). CEPH= head. Inflammation of the brain sometimes transmitted to man from animals, notably horses.

endemic (end-em′ik). *adj.* Referring to a disease more or less constantly present in an area or community. *See* **epidemic.**

enterobiasis (ent-er-ō-bī′a-sis). ENTER =intestine. Another parasite-transmitted intestinal disease, this one due to Oxyuris vermicularis, better known as "pinworms."

epidemic (ep-i-dem′ik). A sudden increase in the prevalence of a disease in a community.

epidemic parotitis (pair-ō-tī′tis). **Mumps** (inflammation of the parotid gland).

epidemiology (ep-i-dēm-ē-ol′ō-jē). The field of science that investigates various factors possibly involved in the frequency and distribution of diseases.

flagellate (flaj′el-lāt). An intestinal parasite which can cause diarrhea, especially in children.

"flu". A commonly used abbreviation for influenza.

fluke (flūk). A parasite which sometimes causes severe liver or lung damage in the host.

fluorine (flūr′ēn). An industrial source of potential damage to workers who are involved with it.

fomites (fōm′i-tēz). *plural.* Agents other than food that can harbor and transmit infectious organisms. (*sing.* — fom′es.)

formalin (form′a-lin). A 40% solution of formaldehyde sometimes used as an antiseptic and disinfectant.

frambesia (fram-bē′zē-a *or* –zha). Another name for **yaws**; in tropical regions this may be almost epidemic in proportions.

fumigation (fyūm-i-gā′shun). The dispersing of poison gases (notably sulfur fumes) formerly widely used to disinfect utensils or areas. It is still used for antivermin protection.

germicide (germ′i-sīd). GERM=bacteria. A specific kind of disinfectant used for the destruction of a specific organism.

gonorrhea (gon-or-rē′a). A contagious venereal disease.

granuloma inguinale (gran-yūl-ō′ma ing-gwin-al′lē). A mildly infectious ulceration resembling chancroid but differing from it in certain specific ways.

helminthic infections (hel-min′thik). A general term covering intestinal infestations with worms or worm like parasites.

hepatitis (hep-a-tī′tis). An inflammation of the liver, sometimes toxic and sometimes the result of infection transmitted by a virus.

histoplasmosis (hist-ō-plas-mō′sis). A systemic infection with a yeast-like fungus. How it gets into the body is still a mystery.

host. In preventive medicine, a plant or animal in which a parasitic organism resides.

hydatid disease (hī-dat′id). *See* **echinococcosis.**

hydrogen sulfide (hī′drō-jen sul′fīd). An industrially-encountered gas which has irritating effects and which may be harmful.

hydrophobia (hī-drō-fōb′ē-a). Another name for **rabies.**

hygiene (hī'jēn). The branch of medical science which relates to the preservation of health.

immunization (im-myūn-i-zā'shun). The natural or artificially-induced process of rendering a person immune to the effects of certain diseases.

incubation period (in-kyū-bā'shun). The consistent lapse of time which intervenes between the implanting of an infectious agent and the appearance of the first symptom of the associated disease.

industrial hygiene. In its broadest sense, that branch of preventive medicine which concerns itself with everything that influences the health of people at work.

infantile paralysis. A formerly used name for poliomyelitis.

infectious jaundice (jawn'dis). Another name for infectious **hepatitis.**

influenza. A general name for an acute, infectious, epidemic disease responsible for respiratory, gastrointestinal and nervous symptoms of varying degree and duration (generally spoken of as "flu").

insecticide (in-sek'ti-sīd). A general name for a group of materials used to eradicate or control certain insects.

latrine (la-trēn'). A toilet, particularly a public one, used without sewage-system connections.

lead poisoning. A group of symptoms which may be induced by continuous or repeated exposure to lead or lead products.

leprosy (lep'rō-sē). A chronic, specific infection characterized by nodules in the skin and mucous membranes or by a specific skin eruption. Nerve changes and an erratic disease course are common. Also called **Hansen's disease.**

Lysol. A proprietary disinfectant solution which is made from coal tar and has a characteristic odor.

Malta fever. Another name for **brucellosis** or undulant fever.

meningococcal meningitis (men-in-jō-kok'kl men-in-jīt'is). MENIN=meninges. An epidemic type of **meningitis** due to infection with the meningococcus.

meningoencephalitis (men-in'jō-en-sef-al-ī'tis). A relatively uncommon complication following an attack of mumps (**epidemic parotitis**).

mental hygiene. MENT=mind. A branch of public health which concerns itself with the prevention of mental illness, particularly in relation to its effects on employment and general health.

mercury poisoning. A chronic illness sometimes brought on by occupational exposure to mercury and mercury compounds.

Merthiolate (Mer-thī'ō-lāt). A proprietary disinfectant solution primarily used on the skin. Its worth is questioned by many doctors.

methane (meth'ān). The chief constituent of natural gas and an important component of manufactured gas.

mononucleosis (mon-ō-nūk-lē-ō'sis). An acute infectious disease characterized by swelling of lymph glands (particularly those of the neck) and a characteristic blood picture.

morbidity rate. MORB=sick. The percentage relationship of sick to well persons in a community, particularly during an epidemic.

mortality rate. MORT=death. The percentage ratio of the number of deaths resulting from a certain disease or situation to the total number of persons who experience it.

mosquito control. A many-sided public health program aimed at controlling the multiplication of mosquitos.

mumps. An epidemic sickness generally called **epidemic parotitis.** It creates public health problems because of the long and variable incubation period.

mushroom poisoning. A severe, frequently fatal, complication from the eating of poisonous mushrooms.

nutrition. The division of public health which considers the presence or absence of essential food elements available, and eaten, in a community.

occupational dermatosis (derm-a-tō'sis). A skin condition related to or caused by the patient's type of employment. (*plural* – dermatos'es.)

occupational diseases. Those diseases related to or resulting from exposure of workers to causative factors, conditions or materials associated with their work.

pasteurization (pas-tūr-i-zā'shun). A sterilizing process consisting of heating and holding milk at 68°C for thirty minutes, followed by rapid cooling. It is required of all marketed milk in most states; in other states, "certified raw milk" (with a lower bacterial count than pasteurized milk) is marketable.

plague (plāg). An acute, usually fatal infectious disease which is communicable. It is transmitted to man from infected rodents through the bite of fleas.

pneumoconiosis (nūm-ō-kon-ē-ō'sis). A general term referring to the reaction on the lungs of various occupational dusts.

pollution (pol-lū'shun). The introduction of injurious substances into the atmosphere, water or streams; also, their presence in these public locations or situations.

psittacosis (sit-a-kō'sis). A formal name for "parrot fever" which is a disease of birds frequently transmitted to man.

pyrethrum (pī-rēth'rum). A popular insecticide made from certain types of chrysanthemums. It is the active ingredient of most household fly-sprays.

Q fever. A name given to an influenza-like disease transmitted (mostly to livestock handlers) by mites and fleas.

rabies (rāb'ēz). A specific, infectious, almost invariably fatal disease gener-

ally contracted through the bite of an infected animal. Also called **hydrophobia.**

rat-bite fever. A disease transmitted from rats to man through the bite of an infected animal.

relapsing fever. A disease transmitted by lice and ticks, fortunately not common in America.

Rhus poisoning (Rūs). A cutaneous, frequently systemic reaction to the sap of poison ivy, poison oak, sumac, and a few other shrubs.

Rocky Mountain spotted fever. A severe systemic disease transmitted through the bite of a tick.

Salmonella (Sal-mon-el'a). A genus of bacteria responsible for outbreaks of **salmonellosis.**

salmonellosis (sal-mon-el-ō'sis). A severe infection transmitted to man by the meat or intestinal excreta of infected animals.

sanitorium (san-i-tōr'ē-um). A hospital for the care of patients not acutely ill. The term indicates institutions providing special care for tuberculosis, alcoholism, mental illness, and other chronic diseases. (*plural* – sanitor'ia *or* sanitor'iums.)

San Joaquin Valley fever. (San Wah-kēn'). Another name for coccidioidomycosis.

septic tank. A scientifically designed tank for the storage and treatment of sewage in areas where sewage connection is not available. Bacterial decomposition is essential to and responsible for its success.

Shigella (Shig-el'a). A type of intestinal bacteria giving rise to **dysentery** of varying degrees of severity. The disease is also called **bacillary dysentery** or **shigellosis.**

sludge (sludj). In public health, referring to an integral part of sewage treatment. Technically, it is a mixture of well-agitated and separated sewage, and water. The mixture is then aerated thoroughly to allow oxidation to take place by bacterial actions.

"strep" throat. A common term referring to a severe infection of the throat caused by hemolytic streptococci. It has some relationship to **scarlet fever.**

"students' disease". A name sometimes applied to infectious mononucleosis; also sometimes called "kissing disease."

trichinosis (trik-in-ō′sis) *or* **trichiniasis** (trik-in-ī′a-sis.) An illness brought on by the eating of undercooked meat from animals infected with trichina, a parasitic worm. The most commonly infected animals are hogs and bear.

undulant fever (und′ū-lant). See **brucellosis** or Malta fever.

vaccination (vak-sin-ā′shun). The injection of killed or weakened bacteria to induce antibody production and thus prevent contracting the disease.

vaccinia (vak-sin′ē-a). The name of a disease of cattle (cowpox). The infectious material is treated and used as a vaccination to protect humans from smallpox. (The vaccination's reaction is an attenuated local case of cowpox.)

venereal diseases (ven-ēr′ē-al). A general term covering diseases contracted or transmitted by sexual contact.

warfarin (war′far-in). A poison used for the elimination of rodents, particularly rats.

yaws. An infectious disease seen chiefly in moist, tropical areas, among dark-skinned people. The skin of the lower legs generally exhibits the first lesion, a sore from which the infection is transmitted to other areas and to other people. It is nonvenereal.

yellow fever. An acute febrile disease spread by mosquitos. All ages and sexes are susceptible, but vaccination offers protection.

21 Proctology

PROCTOLOGY WAS ORIGINALLY defined as that branch of medicine which dealt with treatment of diseases of the anus (in accordance with the Greek word "proctos" or anus). Later the definition was expanded to include diseases of both the rectum and the anus, and for the past thirty years its scope has included surgical treatment of diseases of the colon as well.

The certifying board is known as the American Board of Colon and Rectal Surgery. It was organized in 1934 and is thus one of the oldest American Boards. Certification by the Board requires – in addition to the usual professional qualifications – three years of a general surgical residency followed by two years of either a specialty residency or an accepted preceptorship (practicing under a recognized specialist in the proctologic field). The demand for specialization in this field is steadily increasing.

CONSULTANT

Walter Birnbaum, M.D., F.A.C.S.
Diplomate, American Board of Surgery; Clinical Professor, University of California Medical Center
San Francisco, California

adenoma (ad-en-ōm′a). ADEN=gland; OMA=tumor. A benign, sometimes precancerous, tumor frequently seen on the inner (mucosal) lining of the rectum and colon; it is sometimes called a polyp. (*adj.* — adenom′atous.)

adenomatosis   (ad-en-ōm-a-tōs′is). OSIS=condition. The condition of having many adenomas. Also called **polypo′sis.**

amebiasis   (am-e-bī′a-sis).   AMEB= ameba; ASIS=condition. Infection of the bowel lining with ameba, one type of intestinal parasite.

ampulla of the rectum (am-pūl′la). The dilated midportion of the rectum. (Fig. 19, below)

anal canal (ān′al ka-nal′). The terminal 4 cm. of the bowel, surrounded by the sphincter muscles and connecting the rectum with the outside world. (Fig. 19, below)

anal papilla (ān′al pa-pil′la). One of several cone shaped surface elevations at the junction of the anal canal with the rectum. (*plural* — papil′lae.) (Fig. 19, below)

anal verge (verj). The external margin of the anus. (Fig. 19, below)

anoplasty (ān-ō-plas′tē). PLASTY= reshape surgically. The surgical correction of a deformity of the anal canal.

anorectum (ān-ō-rek′tum). The region of the junction of the anal canal with the rectum. It corresponds roughly with the **dentate line.** (*adj.* — anorec′tal.) (Fig. 19, below)

anoscope (ān′ō-skōp). SCOPE=instrument to look through. A short instrument used in examining the interior of the anal canal and the lower rectum. Types are: Brinkerhoff, Hirschman, Kelly, Martin, Newman, Otis, and Pratt.

anoscopy (ān-os′kō-pē). Visual examination with the anoscope.

anus (ān′us). The external orifice of the anal canal. (*adj.* — an′al.) (Fig. 19, below; Fig. 20, p. 190)

aperient (a-per′i-ent). The most gentle of a number of drugs given to increase peristalsis and induce bowel

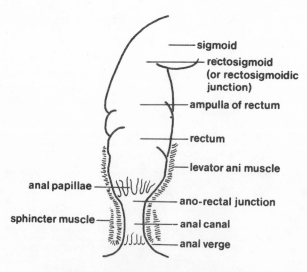

FIG. 19. Rectum and Anus

evacuation. Similar medicines (arranged in increasing degrees of bowel activity produced) are: laxatives, cathartics, physics, and purgatives.

atresia ani (a-trē′zha ān′ē). TRES= hole, opening. Congenital absence or closure of the anus.

Blumer's shelf (Blūm′erz). A characteristic hard mass which can sometimes be felt through the rectal wall. It is usually due to cancer.

cathartic (ka-thar′tik). *See* **aperient.**

cecostomy (sēk-ost′ō-mē). CEC=cecum; STOM=mouth, opening. An opening made into the cecum for purposes of drainage or for relief of distension. *See* **colostomy.**

cecum (sēk′um). The first part of the colon, located in the right lower quadrant of the abdomen. The ileum empties into it and the appendix originates from it. (Fig. 20, p. 190; Fig. 21, p. 212)

coccygodynia (kok-sē-gō-din′ē-a) or **coccydynia** (kok-sē-din′e-ah). DYN= pain. Pain in the **coccyx** (tail bone).

colectomy (kōl-ek′tō-mē). ECTOMY= cut out. The surgical removal of part or of all of the **colon.**

colitis (kōl-ī′tis). Inflammation of the **colon.**

colon (kōl′on). The large intestine, exclusive of the rectum. It includes the cecum and the ascending, transverse, descending, and sigmoid portions of the colon. (*adj.* — colon′ic.) (Fig. 20, p. 190)

colonoscope (kōl-on′ō-skōp). A long flexible tube used for visual examination of the interior of the colon.

colonoscopy (kōl-on-osk′ō-pē). Examination with a **colonoscope.**

colostomy (kōl-ost′ō-mē). An opening made into the colon which has been brought through the abdominal wall to the surface and secured there. A bag attached to the skin collects the intestinal contents. Colostomies are designated by the part of the colon in which they are made, e.g., cecosto-

my, transverse colostomy, sigmoid colostomy, etc.

condyloma (kon-dil-ō′ma). A wart-like growth which may occur near the anus. (*Plural* — condylom′as *or* condylom′ata.)

constipation (kon-sti-pā′shun). A condition in which bowel evacuation is incomplete or infrequent.

cryptitis (kript-ī′tis). Inflammation of the **crypts of Morgagni.**

crypt of Morgagni (mor-gahn′yē). CRYPT=hidden. One of several minute blind pockets or pouches at the junction of the rectum and the anal canal.

defecation (def-e-kā′shun). FEC=feces. The discharge of fecal matter from the bowel; a bowel movement ("B.M.").

dentate line (den′tāt). DENT=tooth. The irregular surface marking of the anorectal junction, so called because of its imagined similarity to a row of teeth. *See* **pectinate line.**

diarrhea (dī-a-rē′a). A condition characterized by frequent discharges of watery bowel movement. (*adj.* — diarrhe′ic.)

dilator (dī′lāt-er). One of a graduated series of tapered instruments. In proctology, dilators are sometimes used for stretching a constriction of the anal canal. Types of dilators are Pratt, Young.

diverticulitis (dī-vert-ik-yū-līt′is). VERT=turn. Inflammation of **diverticula.**

diverticulosis coli (dī-vert-ik-yū-lō′sis kōl′ē). The condition of having **diverticula** of the colon.

diverticulum (dī-vert-ik′yū-lum). A bulge or a pocket of the wall of the colon. (*plural* — divertic′ula *or* divertic′ulums.)

enema (en′e-ma). Liquid introduced into the rectum for one of several purposes; the most common use is to initiate defecation.

fecal incontinence (fēk′l). Inability to control the discharge of feces.

fecalith (fēk′a-lith). LITH=stone. A hardened ball of fecal material within the intestine.

feces (fē′sēz). Waste material excreted from the intestinal tract. (*adj.* —fe′cal.)

fissure in ano (fish′er in ā′nō). A painful split or ulcer in the lining of the anal canal.

fistula (fist′yū-la). An abnormal channel or tube between hollow organs, or between a hollow organ and the skin. (*plural* — fist′ulae.) Protologic types are: **anorectal** (anorectum to skin), **enterocolic** (small intestine to colon), **rectovaginal** (rectum to vagina), and **rectovesical** (rectum to bladder).

fistulectomy (fist-yūl-ek′tō-mē). The surgical removal of a **fistula.**

flatulence (flat′yūl-ens). Distention of the intestinal tract with a collection of air or gas.

flatus (flā′tus). Air or gas in the intestinal canal.

Hartmann's operation (Hart′manz). One of several surgical procedures used in treating carcinoma of the rectum.

hemorrhoid (hem′ōr-royd). HEM=blood. A swelling consisting of one or more dilated blood vessels in the lower rectum or anus ("piles").

hemorrhoidectomy (hem-or-royd-ek′tō-mē). The surgical excision of **hemorrhoids.**

hepatic flexure (hē-pat′ik flek′shur). HEP=liver; FLEX=bend. The abrupt turn made by the colon at the junction of its ascending and transverse portions. It is located near the liver, hence its name. (Fig. 20, p. 190)

Hilton's line (hil′tonz). An encircling surface marking on the lining of the anal canal about halfway between the anal verge and the anorectal junction.

Hirschsprung's disease (Hirsh′sprungz). A congenital condition in which the colon is tremendously enlarged. Also called **meg′acolon.**

Kraske's position (Kras′kēz). A particular position into which a patient is placed, on his side, for carrying out certain proctologic procedures.

laxative (laks′a-tiv). *See* **aperient.**

levator ani (lēv-ā′tor ā′nē). A broad muscle which helps to form the floor of the pelvis. It helps to support the rectum and the vagina. (Fig. 19, p. 186)

megacolon (meg′a-kōl-on). MEG=large. See **Hirschsprung's disease.**

Mikulicz's operation (Mik′ū-litz-ez). A surgical procedure sometimes employed for removing a lesion of the colon.

Miles' abdominoperineal resection (Mīlz ab-dom-i-nō-per-i-nē′al). A procedure used in removing the rectum. It is usually done for cancer.

mucosa (myū-kōz′a). The inside (mucosal) lining of the intestine.

obstipation (ob-sti-pā′shun). An extreme and obstinate form of constipation.

pecten band. PECT=comb. A fibrous band underlying the lining of the anal canal. (Its existence is questioned by some proctologists.)

pectinate line (pik′tin-āt). The irregular junction of the rectum with the anal canal, so called because of its resemblance to a cock's comb. *See* **dentate line.**

pedunculated (pē-dunk′yū-lāt-ed). *adj.* Having a pedicle or stem. *See* **sessile.**

perianal (pair-i-ān′al). *adj.* Around or surrounding the anus.

perineum (pair-i-nē′um). The area between the scrotum (or the vagina) and the anus.

physic (fiz′ik). *See* **aperient.**

"piles". A common name for hemorrhoids.

pilonidal cyst (pīl-ō-nīd′al). PIL=hair. A sealed-over collection of hair follicles near the tip of the coccyx. The follicles may continue to produce hairs and the cavity frequently becomes infected.

polyp (pol'ip). A tumor originating from the rectal or colonic lining. *See* **adenoma**. It may have a stem (**pedunculated**) or no stem (**sessile**).

polyposis (pol-ip-ō'sis). Same as **adenomatosis**.

proctalgia (prokt-alj'ē-a). PROCT= rectum; ALG=pain. Pain in the rectum. *See* **proctodynia**.

proctectomy (prokt-ek'tō-mē). Surgical excision of the rectum.

proctitis (prokt-īt'is). Inflammation of the rectum.

proctoclysis (prokt-ō-klīs'is). The slow introduction of fluid into the rectum for purposes of absorption.

proctodeum (prokt-ō-dē'um). The embryonic forerunner of the anal canal.

proctodynia (prokt-ō-din'ē-a). Pain in or about the rectum; also called **proctal'gia**.

proctologist (prokt-ol'ō-jist). A specialist in proctology.

proctology (prok-tol'ō-jē). *See* introductory paragraphs.

proctoscope (prokt'ō-skōp). A lighted, hollow tube, about 15 cms. in length, used for visual examination of the interior of the rectum.

proctoscopy (prokt-osk'ō-pē). Examination of the interior of the rectum via the **proctoscope**.

proctosigmoiditis (prokt-ō-sig-moyd-īt'-is). Concurrent inflammation of the rectum and the sigmoid.

pruritus ani (prūr-īt-us ā-nē). PRUR= itch. Itching in or about the anus.

purgative (purg'a-tiv). *See* **aperient**.

rectal procidentia (prōs-i-den'shē-a). External protrusion of the full thickness of the rectal wall; commonly called **rectal prolapse**.

"rectal prolapse" (prō'laps). A common name for external protrusion of the rectum or of the rectal mucosa.

rectoscopy (rek-tos'kō-pē). **Proctoscopy**.

rectosigmoid (rek-tō-sig'moyd). The region of the junction of the rectum with the sigmoid colon. (Fig. 19, p. 186)

rectum (rek'tum). The dilated terminal portion of the large intestine between the lower end of the sigmoid colon and the upper end of the anal canal. The rectum is about 13 cms. in length. (Fig. 12, p. 119; Fig. 19, p. 186; Fig. 20, p. 190; Fig. 26, p. 245)

retrorectal (ret-rō-rek'tal). RETRO= behind. *adj*. Pertaining to the region behind the rectum.

"sentinel pile". An elevation of the skin at the anal verge which warns of the probable presence of a fistula just above it.

sessile (ses'il). SES=sit. *adj*. Having a broad base as opposed to having a pedicle or stem, particularly as relating to tumors.

sigmoid (sig'moyd). *adj*. Referring to the S-shaped portion of the colon immediately above the rectum, so called because of its similarity to the Greek letter Sigma (Σ). Sigmoid is also used as a noun. (Fig. 19, p. 186; Fig. 20, p. 190)

sigmoidectomy (sig-moyd-ek'tō-mē). The surgical excision of the sigmoid colon.

sigmoiditis (sig-moyd-īt'is). Inflammation of the sigmoid colon.

sigmoidoscope (sig-moyd'ō-skōp). A hollow tube about 25 cms. in length which is used for visual examination, via the anus, of the lining of the rectum and the distal portion of the sigmoid.

sigmoidoscopy (sig-moyd-os'kō-pē). Examination of the sigmoid colon by use of the **sigmoidoscope**.

sigmoidostomy (sig-moyd-os'tō-mē). The surgical creation of an artificial opening in the sigmoid wall for purposes of fecal diversion. *See* **colostomy**.

Sims' position (simz). A specific position into which a patient is placed, on his side, for carrying out certain proctologic procedures.

sphincter ani (sfink'ter ā'nē). The circular anal muscle which controls the passage of feces.

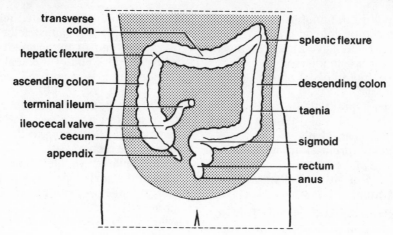

transverse colon
hepatic flexure
ascending colon
terminal ileum
ileocecal valve
cecum
appendix

splenic flexure
descending colon
taenia
sigmoid
rectum
anus

FIG. 20. Colon

splenic flexure (splen'ik flek'shur). The
acute angle of the colon at the junction of its transverse and descending
portions. It is located near the
spleen, hence its name. (Fig. 20,
above)

stricture (strik'tchur). Diminution in
the size of the channel of a tube or a
duct. In proctology it generally refers
to anal, rectal or colonic narrowings.

thrombosed hemorrhoid (throm'bōst).
THROMB=clot. A painful blood
clot under the skin, near the anus,
due to rupture of a vein.

volvulus (vol'vyūl-us). VOLV=twist.
Twisting of the colon.

22 Psychiatry

PSYCHIATRY IS THE medical science that deals with the origin, prevention, diagnosis, and treatment of mental and emotional disorders. It is thus probably the most personal of the medical specialties. It also includes such special fields as mental retardation and the effect of the emotions on physical disorders.

Psychoanalysis is practiced by certain psychiatrists who have had additional training and who employ the techniques of psychoanalytic theory originated by Sigmund Freud. They are also known as "analysts." Freud's theory stipulated that a person's emotions and behavior are influenced by his (unconscious) repressed "instinctual drives" and the (unconscious) emotional conflicts produced by these factors.

The practitioner of psychiatry (a psychiatrist) is a licensed doctor of medicine. The American Board of Psychiatry and Neurology—it also certifies neurologists—requires that the doctor complete three years of accredited postgraduate study and training and practice psychiatry for two years before he is eligible to apply for certification as a psychiatrist.

A psychologist also specializes in the study of mental processes and behavior. He generally holds a Ph.D. degree (or a master's degree) in psychology. Most psychologists are involved in experimental work in association with psychiatrists or other doctors. A smaller number (clinical psychologists) are practitioners who diagnose and treat mental problems. Their field of practice is specified in different ways by various state licenses, none of which includes the prescribing of drugs.

CONSULTANTS

Robert M. Isaac, M.D.
Diplomate, American Board of Psychiatry and Neurology. (Psychiatry) Santa Rosa, California.

Stephen S. Lowe, M.D.
Diplomate, American Board of Psychiatry and Neurology. (Psychiatry) Santa Rosa, California.

addiction (ad-dik′shun). An uncontrollable dependence upon the habitual use of a drug. Increasing doses are generally required because of tolerance, and withdrawal symptoms follow its discontinuance.

aerophagia (air-ō-fāj′ē-a). AER=air; PHAG=eat, swallow. The nervous habit of air-swallowing.

affect. Emotion; a person's state of feeling, or his "emotional feeling tone."

aggression (a-gres′shun). An emotional state characterized by forceful behavior, physical or verbal, toward other persons.

agnosia (ag-nōs′ē-a). GNOS=to know. An organic brain disorder which prevents recognizing and interpreting sensory impressions.

alienist (āl′ē-en-ist). An obsolete legal term for a psychiatrist who testifies in court regarding a person's sanity and/or mental competence.

ambivalence (am-biv′a-lens). AMBI= both. The simultaneous presence of opposing emotions such as love and hate in an individual, directed toward a specific person, object, or goal.

amentia (a-men′shē-a). MEN=mind. Congenital mental retardation. *See* **dementia.**

amnesia (am-nēz′ē-a *or* –zha). Pathological loss of memory of an area of one's past experiences.

analyst (an′a-list). A psychoanalyst.

anxiety (angs-ī′e-tē). In psychiatry, the term refers to apprehension, tension or uneasiness based on the anticipation of vague or imagined danger. By contrast, **fear** stems from consciously recognized threats or dangers.

aphasia (a-fāz′ē-a *or* a-fā′zha). PHAS= speak, speech. A disturbance of speech characterized by inability to pronounce words, particularly those associated with recognized objects. *See* **aphonia.**

ataractic (at-ar-ak′tik). A name given to drugs used to decrease anxiety, allowing minimal use of sedatives. Their function is the same as that of tranquilizers.

aura (awr′a). A warning subjective sensation (flash of light, etc.) which many epileptics receive preceding a convulsion.

behaviorism (bē-hāv′yor-izm). A psychologic theory based on objective data which can be seen or measured, rather than on such unmeasurable subjective factors as ideas and emotions.

borderline intelligence. A term used by the American Association for Mental Deficiency, referring to a person having an I.Q. between 70 and 85.

"brain waves." A graphic recording of minute electrical impulses arising from brain cell activity. The record is called an encephalogram (EEG). Abnormalities of the recording may indicate disease of the brain.

catalepsy (kat-a-lep′sē). Diminished responsiveness in a person, secondary to organic conditions, psychological disorders or hypnotic states. Trancelike behavior is characteristic.

catatonic state (kat-a-ton′ik). A condition characterized by muscular rigidity or inflexibility and sometimes by complete immobility. It may be diagnostic of schizophrenia.

catecholamines (kat-a-kōl′a-mēnz). The end products of some of the secretions of the adrenal glands. Certain of them, notably epinephrine and norepinephrine, influence nervous system activity. They are also the transmitter substances that pass the nerve impulse from one nerve to the next nerve, at the synapse.

causalgia (kawz-alj′ē-a). ALG=pain. In psychiatry, the sensation of burning pain, which may be due to psychic factors.

clinical psychologist (klin'i-kl sīk-ol'ō-jist). A psychologist with a graduate degree (generally a Ph.D.) who has had additional training in medical situations, and who generally works in collaboration with psychiatrists and other physicians, in the diagnosis and the treatment of mental or emotional disorders.

combat fatigue. Physical and emotional fatigue of disabling proportions, brought on by military combat. Also called **combat neurosis.**

compensation. An unconscious defense mechanism which causes the individual to try to make up for real or imagined deficiencies.

complex. A group of associated ideas, generally unconscious, which influence attitudes and behavior. Examples: Oedipus complex, attachment to a parent of the opposite sex; inferiority complex, a feeling of inferiority resulting from real (or imagined) physical or mental or social inadequacies—a common result is either anxiety or attempts at overcompensation.

compulsion. An insistent, undesired urge to perform an act contrary to one's conscious wishes or standards.

confusion. In psychiatry, a disturbance of orientation in regard to time, places, or persons.

delirium. A toxic mental state of psychotic proportions characterized by disorientation and confusion. Delirium may follow high fevers, or sustained alcoholic or drug intoxication.

delusion. A false persistent belief frequently due to unconscious needs. Examples are delusions of grandeur, and delusions of persecution.

dementia (dē-men'sha). MENT=mind. A term used to denote loss of intellectual function. Formerly the term denoted (imprecisely) any "madness or insanity." *See* **amentia.**

depression. In psychiatry, a sad, dejected, slowed, or melancholic state.

deterioration. In psychiatry, progressive loss of intellectual or emotional capacities.

disorientation (dis-ōr-i-en-tā'shun). Mental confusion regarding one's position in time, place, or personal relationships.

Down's syndrome. A type of congenital mental retardation. Along with severe intelligence defects are physical features, including a fold of skin above the inner angles of the eyes giving a "mongoloid" appearance. It is due to abnormality of the chromosomes. Also called **mongolism.**

drive. A basic instinct, urge, or activating factor.

dynamics. In psychiatry, emotional forces which determine the pattern of feelings and behavior. They arise from the interaction of drives and defenses.

ego. The rational function of the mind, particularly in mediating compromises between the id, the superego, and reality.

egomania (ē-gō-mān'ē-a). An extreme degree of preoccupation with self.

electroencephalogram (ē-lek-trō-en-sef'a-lō-gram). CEPH=head; GRAM=record. *See* "**brain waves.**"

emotion. A conscious, or unconscious, feeling such as anger, fear, grief, joy, or love. In psychiatry, a somewhat equivalent word is affect, which relates more to the expression.

empathy (emp'ath-ē). The objective insight into another's feelings, emotions and behavior, obtained by mentally inserting oneself into the other's person and situation.

euphoria (yūf-ōr'ē-a). EU=well. An exaggerated feeling of physical and emotional well-being.

exhibitionism. In psychiatry, body exposure, especially that of the male genitalia, to females.

extrasensory perception. Perception or communication achieved without the apparent conventional use of any of the physical senses.

extrovert (eks'trō-vert). EXTRA=outside; VERT=turn. A person whose attention and energies are largely diverted outward, as opposed to one whose concentration is directed toward himself or his own activities (**introvert**).

fantasy. A dreamed-up mental image of conditions or events.

fetish (fet'ish *or* fēt'ish). In psychiatry, an inanimate object symbolically possessing some special (usually sexual) meaning.

forensic psychiatry (for-en'sik). PSYCH=mind, mental. That branch of psychiatry which deals with the legal aspects of mental disorders.

free association. A term referring to the verbal expression of whatever comes into a psychiatric patient's mind. It is useful in psychoanalysis.

Freud, Sigmund (Froyd). The founder of psychoanalysis.

functional illness. Illness of emotional origin generally without organic evidence of disease.

general paresis (pair'e-sis *or* pair-ē'sis). A psychosis associated with organic brain disease caused by a chronic or late (tertiary) stage of syphilitic infection.

group therapy. A technique of psychotherapy which utilizes the interactions of members of the group to assist the patient in recognizing his problem.

hallucination (hal-lūs-in-ā'shun). A sensation without an external stimulus *See* **illusion.**

homosexuality (hōm-ō-seks-yū-al'i-tē). HOMO=same. A sexual attraction to members of the same sex (male or female).

hyperkinesia (hī-per-kin-ēz'ē-a). HYPER=excessive; KINE=movement. A disorder sometimes seen in children, characterized by increased or excessive muscular activity. (*adj.* — hyperkinet'ic.)

hypesthesia (hīp-es-thēz'ē-a). ESTHE= feeling. Diminished sensitivity to tactile stimuli.

hypnosis (hip-nōs'is). HYPN=sleep. A state of increased receptivity to suggestion or direction, initially induced by the influence of another person. Extreme degrees of hypnosis may include surgical anesthesia.

hypochondria (hīp-ō-kond'rē-a). Excessive concern about possible illnesses.

hysteria (his-ter'ē-a). An illness resulting from emotional conflict, frequently characterized by attention-seeking, impulsive demonstrations.

id. A term which, in the theory of Freud, includes that part of the personality structure which harbors the unconscious instinctive desires and strivings of the individual.

identification. A defense mechanism by which an individual unconsciously endeavors to pattern himself after another person.

idiot. An old term (now abandoned) for a mentally defective person with a mental age of less than three years and an I.Q. of less than 25.

illusion. The misinterpretation of a real, external sensory experience. *See* **hallucination.**

imbecile (im'be-sil). An old term (no longer used) for a mentally defective person, usually with a mental age between three and eight years and an I.Q. between 25 and 50.

impulse. An instinctive urge.

incompetent. A legal term for a person who, because of mental defects, cannot be held responsible in certain legal procedures. These include making a will, entering into a contract, or standing trial.

inhibition. A mental interference with the performance of a specific activity, as the result of an unconscious defense against forbidden instinctual drives.

insanity. A vague, legal term (no longer used in psychiatry) connoting legal incompetence, the inability to distinguish right from wrong, and the presence of a mental condition interfering with the individual's self-care or constituting a danger to himself or to others.

insight. The recognition by the patient that he is ill or the self-understanding of his condition. It is one of the major goals of psychotherapy.

instinct. An inborn drive such as the instinct of self-preservation.

intelligence. The ability to solve problems, to adapt to new situations, to profit from experience, and to learn.

intelligence quotient (I.Q.). A numerical rating, determined through psychological testing, which indicates approximately the relationship of the person's mental age to his chronological age, according to a formula; also, a measurement of an individual's learning ability.

introvert (in'trō-vert). INTR=into; VERT=turn. A person unduly occupied with himself, resulting in decreased interest in the outside world; roughly, the opposite of an extrovert.

involutional psychosis (in-vōl-ū'shun-al sīk-ō'sis). A psychotic reaction occurring in older life, not necessarily related (as formerly thought) to the female menopause or to the male climacteric. It is characterized by an agitated and depressed state.

Jung, Carl Gustav (Yūng). A Swiss psychoanalyst who founded the school of analytic psychology.

lesbian (les'bē-an). A homosexual woman.

libido (lib-ēd'ō *or* lib'i-dō). A psychic drive usually associated with the sexual instinct.

lunacy (lūn'a-sē). A legal term (now seldom used) for a major mental illness.

lunatic (lūn'a-tik). A legal term (now obsolete) for a psychotic person.

malingering (mal-ling'ger-ing *or* mal-inj'er-ing). A false, conscious simulation of illness or disability, for personal gain or attention.

mania (mān'ē-a). A form of mental illness characterized by excessive preoccupation with, or a compulsive need to engage in, some activity. (Also used as a suffix to denote this obsession.)

Examples: **dipsomania**—compulsion to drink alcoholic beverages, DIPS=thirst; **egomania**—pathological preoccupation with self, EGO=self; **kleptomania**—compulsion to steal, KLEP=steal; **megalomania**—excessive preoccupation with delusions of wealth or power, MEG=large; **nymphomania**—abnormal desire, in females, for sexual intercourse; **pyromania**—a compulsion to set fires, PYRO=fire.

maniac (mān'ē-ak). An inaccurate, misleading lay term applied to any person who is emotionally disturbed.

manic depressive psychosis (man'ik dēpres'siv sīk-ō'sis). A psychiatric disorder characterized by conspicuous cyclic swings of mood from elation to deep depression and back, over a period of months.

masochism (mas'ō-kizm). Pleasure derived from pain (physical or psychological) either self-inflicted or imposed by others.

melancholia (mel-an-kōl'ē-a). Severe deep depression.

mental age. The age level of mental ability, determined by intelligence tests.

mental health. The relative state of mental balance which a person has achieved and exhibits.

mental hygiene (hī'jēn). A term designating measures employed to reduce the incidence of mental illness.

mental retardation. A term indicating a lack of intelligence, from birth or early life, to a degree that interferes with reasonable social adjustment.

mentally defective. *adj.* A term applied to anyone having an I.Q. of less than 70. *See* **idiot, imbecile, moron.**

mesmerism (mes'mer-izm). An early name (now seldom used) for hypnotism.

mongolism (mon'gōl-izm). See Down's syndrome.

moron (mōr'on). A term indicating a mentally defective person usually having a mental age of eight to twelve years and an I.Q. of 50 to 70.

narcolepsy (nark'ō-lep-sē). NARC=sleep. A term applied to brief, uncontrolled episodes of sleeping.

negativism (neg'a-tiv-izm). Perverse opposition and resistance to suggestions or advice.

"nervous breakdown." A nonmedical, nonspecific term for emotional illness.

neuropsychiatry (nūr-ō-sīk-ī'a-trē). NEUR=nerve; PSYCH=mind. A combination of the specialties of neurology and psychiatry.

neurosis (nūr-ō'sis). See psychoneurosis.

nymphomania (nimf-fō-mān'ē-a). Exaggerated sexual drive in the female (compare satyriasis).

obsession (ob-ses'shun). A persistent idea, interest, or activity, not necessarily logical or reasonable.

organic psychosis. Any serious psychiatric disorder resulting from a demonstrable physical disturbance of brain function. Common causes are tumors, infections, or brain injuries.

paranoia (pair-an-oy'a). A relatively rare personality disorder which may begin in early adulthood, is progressive, and may become chronic. It is mainly characterized by delusions of persecution and sometimes by those of grandeur. (adj. — par'anoid.)

paresis (pair-ē'sis or pair'e-sis). Incomplete paralysis or weakness of organic origin (brain damage from tertiary syphilis). The term is interchangeable with general paresis.

perception. The brain mechanism which recognizes sensory stimuli and interprets and integrates them in accordance with past experiences.

personality disorder. A general term covering mental conditions in which the basic disorder lies in the personality of the individual.

phobia (fōō'ē-a). A persistent unrealistic fear of some person, animal, condition, or situation. Types: acrophobia — fear of high places; agoraphobia — fear of open places; algophobia — fear of pain; claustrophobia — fear of closed places; mysophobia — fear of dirt and germs; photophobia — fear of light; xenophobia — fear of strangers.

pica (pīk'a). A craving for unnatural food, sometimes seen in hysterical or emotionally disturbed children or in pregnant women.

psychasthenia (sīk-as-thēn'ē-a). ASTHEN=weak. An old term covering anxieties, doubts, fears, or obsessions regarding real or imagined inadequacies.

psyche (sīk'ē). The mind or soul; the result of the mental life of an individual, including both his conscious and unconscious processes.

psychiatric social worker (sīk-ē-at'rik). A social worker with a graduate degree, who confines his activities to psychiatric problems, under the supervision of a psychiatrist.

psychiatrist (sīk-ī'a-trist). A doctor who specializes in psychiatry.

psychiatry (sīk-ī'a-trē). See introductory paragraphs.

psychoanalysis (sīk-ō-an-al'i-sis). A theory of human development and behavior (as well as its treatment) originated by Sigmund Freud.

psychoanalyst (sīk-ō-an'al-ist). A psychiatrist or clinical psychologist with additional training in psychoanalysis, who employs the techniques of psychoanalytic theory.

psychologist (sīk-ol'ō-jist). A person with a graduate degree in the study of behavior.

psychology (sīk-ol'ō-jē). The science and study of behavior.

psychoneurosis (sīk-ō-nūr-ō'sis). One of the two major categories of emotional illness, the other being the psychoses. A neurosis is usually less severe than a psychosis; both are due to unresolved, unconscious conflicts. Common types of neuroses: **anxiety neurosis** — uncontrollable apprehension, out of proportion to any obvious causes; **depressive reaction** — a depressed state resulting from a real or imagined loss. It may progress to psychotic depths; **disassociative reaction** — characterized by such features as amnesia, sleep walking, or dream states; **obsessive compulsive reaction** — characterized by a compelling necessity to carry out certain acts repeatedly; **phobic reaction** — characterized by specific, irrational fears out of proportion to apparent causes.

psychopathic personality. A person whose behavior is predominantly antisocial and characterized by impulsive, irresponsible actions, without regard for obvious social consequences and lacking in evidence of concern or guilt. Such a person is sometimes called "a psychopath."

psychosis (sīk-ō'sis). A severe mental disorder in which the patient departs from the normal pattern of thinking, feeling, and acting. There is generally a loss of contact with reality. Progressive deterioration may occur. (*plural* — psycho'ses; *adj.* — psychot'ic.) *See* **involutional psychosis, manic depressive psychosis, senile psychosis.**

psychosomatic (sīk-ō-sō-mat'ik). *adj.* Referring to the constant interreaction of the mind and the body. It refers particularly to illnesses with physical manifestations, related at least partially to emotional factors.

psychotherapy (sīk-ō-ther'a-pē). A general term referring to any type of treatment based primarily on verbal, or nonverbal, communication with the patient rather than on the use of medicinal, surgical, or other measures.

"psychotic" (sīk-ot'ik). A person afflicted with a **psychosis.**

pyromaniac (pīr-ō-mān'i-ak). A "firebug." *See* **mania.**

rationalization. An unconscious defense mechanism in which the individual attempts to justify his behavior.

sadism (sad'izm). Pleasure derived from the inflicting of physical or psychologic pain on others.

satyriasis (sat-i-rī'a-sis). Exaggerated sexual drive in the male. It corresponds to nymphomania in the female.

schizoid (skiz'oyd). *adj.* Referring to, or describing, traits of excessive shyness, excessive introspection, or introversion.

schizophrenia (skitz-ō-fren'ē-a). A psychosis marked by a retreat from reality and formerly called **dementia praecox.** Delusions, hallucinations, and severe emotional disturbances may be present. Types: **simple** — characterized by withdrawal, apathy, indifference, and impoverished human relationships; **ambulatory** — a schizophrenic who "just stays out of institutions"; **hebephrenic** — characterized by inappropriate, unpredictable, childish behavior and emotions (it tends to be progressive); **paranoid** — see **paranoia; catatonic** — see **catatonic state.**

schizophrenic (skitz-ō-fren'ik). A person afflicted with **schizophrenia.**

senile psychosis. A mental illness of old age characterized by eccentricity, irritability, progressive loss of memory, and deterioration of personality. It is presumably caused by generalized brain atrophy.

shock treatment. A form of psychiatric treatment in which medication or electric stimulation is administered to the patient, producing a convulsive or comatose reaction, in an attempt to influence favorably the course of his mental illness. The application of electric current is the means most commonly employed.

somnambulism (som-nam′būl-izm). SOM=sleep; AMBUL=walk. Sleep walking.

superego (sūp-er-ē′gō). In psychoanalytic theory, that part of the personality associated with ethics, standards, and self-criticism, formed by the infant's identification with important persons in his early life, particularly his parents.

telepathy (tel-ep′ath-ē). TELE=far. The scientifically questioned theory of the possible communication of thought between persons without the intervention of physical means. *See* **extrasensory perception.**

Thorazine (Thōr′a-zēn). A proprietary drug used extensively to relieve agitation, anxiety, and tension without inducing sleep.

tic (tik). An intermittent, uncontrollable muscular twitching. In psychiatry, the term refers to a twitching related to hidden emotional conflicts rather than to organic neurologic disease.

trance (trans). A state of diminished activity and consciousness, resembling sleep. Common types are hypnotic and hysterical states.

tranquilizer (tran′kwil-ī-zer). A popular name applying to any one of the ata-ractic drugs. In psychiatry, it usually refers to anti-psychotic drugs. Tranquilizers never produce general anesthesia, and the patient can always be aroused. Commonly used tranquilizers are: Sparine, Thorazine, Mellaril, Compazine, Phenergan, Milltown, Equanil, Valium, Librium and others.

transference. The unconscious "transfer" to a third person, of the attitudes and feelings which one has formerly felt toward another person with whom he has been closely associated.

transvestism (trans-vest′izm). Pleasure derived from dressing or appearing in clothing of the opposite sex.

traumatic neurosis (traw-mat′ik). A condition in which neurotic reactions follow, or are attributed to, an event or a series of events.

voyeurism (voy′yūr-izm). A nice name for the emotional—probably sexual—impulse that activates the "peeping Tom."

withdrawal. In psychiatry, a pathological retreat or attempted escape from people and the world of reality, or both. It is a characteristic sometimes exhibited by **schizophrenics.**

23 Radiology

RADIOLOGY IS THAT medical specialty which primarily uses ionizing radiation in the diagnosis and treatment of disease. The most commonly involved modalities are x-rays and gamma rays; alpha rays, beta rays and other types of radiation are used to a lesser extent. A radiologist is a physician who has specialized in the study, use and application of these ionizing radiations.

This specialty is being subdivided into three general categories: Diagnostic Radiology, Therapeutic Radiology and Nuclear Medicine.

Diagnostic Radiology encompasses fluoroscopy, the consultative interpretation of x-ray "pictures" (radiograms), and the conducting of examinations using radiopaque contrast media injected into the vascular system or body cavities. The major emphasis is on the application of medical knowledge and specialty training in the interpretation of radiographic findings to determine their significance in the diagnosis and treatment of the patient's illness.

Therapeutic radiology relates to the treatment of disease with ionizing radiation. This disease is most frequently cancer, but other inflammatory and benign conditions are also treated. The ionizing radiations may be derived from a variety of sources including units of varying kilovoltage capacity, radium, radiocobalt therapy units, linear accelerators, betatrons, etc. Accurate dosimetry, careful beam planning, and knowledge of radiobiology are of utmost importance.

Nuclear medicine involves the use of radioactive isotopes for organ imaging, vascular flow studies, blood chemistry studies and metabolic studies, and for the treatment of certain disease entities. These studies are performed with a variety of sophisticated instruments including scintillation probes, body and organ scanning devices, gamma cameras, well counters, and similar instruments.

After completing internship, an applicant is first required by the American Board of Radiology to devote three to five years to the study of radiology before applying for certification. The various organizations and associations of radiologists are presently considering the formation of additional boards to cover the activities of therapeutic radiologists and nuclear medicine specialists.

Diagnostic Radiology

CONSULTANTS

Robert H. Butler, M.D.
Diplomate, American Board of Radiology; Associate Professor, Clinical and Ambulatory Medicine, University of California Medical Center
Santa Rosa, California

Sydney M. Miller, M.D.
Diplomate, American Board of Radiology
Santa Rosa, California

achondroplasia (ā-kon-drō-plā′zha *or –* zē-a). A disease which prevents proper early development of bones because of poor cartilage formation.

agenesis (ā-jen′e-sis). GEN=origin. The congenital failure of a part of the body to develop.

air contrast enema. A means for studying the lower bowel by utilizing air distention following introduction (and expulsion) of a **barium enema.**

air cystogram — air cystography (air sist′ ō-gram — air sistog′ra-fē). CYST= bladder. Radiologic visualization of the urinary bladder after distending it with air (causing a "negative" bladder shadow).

angiocardiogram — angiocardiography (anj-ē-ō-kard′ē-ō-gram – anj-ē-ō-kard-ē-og′ra-fē) ANG=blood vessel; CARD=heart. Radiologic visualization of the heart and its large vessels, using an opaque substance previously released into the blood stream within or near the heart.

angiogram — angiography (anj′ē-ō-gram – anj-ē-og′ra-fē). X-ray visualization of one or more blood vessels, using an opaque substance previously released into the blood.

anteroposterior (an-tēr-ō-pōs-tēr′yor). *adj.* Referring to an x-ray exposure made with the patient facing the x-ray tube.

anthracosis (an-thra-kō′sis). ANTHRAC=coal. A lung condition caused by prolonged inhalation of fine particles of coal dust. It is frequently demonstrated by x-ray.

aortogram — aortography (ā-ort′ō-gram –ā-or-tog′ra-fē). X-ray visualization of the aorta and its branches utilizing the localized release of opaque material into the abdominal aorta.

arteriogram — arteriography (ar-tēr′ē-ō-gram – ar-tēr-ē-og′ra-fē). X-ray visualization of an artery or arteries, generally utilizing the localized release of opaque material into the thoracic or abdominal aorta.

artifact (art′i-fakt). A false image on an x-ray film caused by mechanical factors in equipment or processing.

asymmetry (ā-sim′e-trē). The lack of similarity between paired organs or between paired parts of the body.

barium enema (bair′ē-um). A mixture of barium and water given as an enema during the radiologic visualization of the lower bowel.

barium meal. A mixture of barium and water swallowed by the patient during radiologic examination of the upper gastrointestinal tract.

barium swallow. Radiologic examination of the throat and the esophagus during the swallowing of a thin or thick barium mixture.

bronchogram — bronchography (brong′ kō-gram – brong′kog′ra-fē). X-ray visualization of the bronchial tree, outlined by the use of an opaque material previously introduced into it.

Bucky diaphragm (dī′a-fram). A part of every modern radiographic table. It improves the quality of the picture and was invented by Dr. Gustav Bucky. It is also sometimes called a Bucky grid.

Bucky film (Buk′ē). An x-ray film made with the help of the Bucky diaphragm.

calcinosis (kal-sin-o′sis). CALC=stone, calcium. A condition in which calcium is demonstrated in soft tissues which do not normally contain calcium, notably the kidneys and the skin.

cardia (kard'ē-a). The first portion of the body of the stomach, into which the esophagus empties. (Fig. 5, p. 51)

cardiac catheterization (kard'ē-ak kathe-ter-i-zā'shun). CARD=heart. The passing of a catheter into the heart (usually by way of a vein) for releasing **contrast medium** within the heart to improve its radiologic visualization, or to obtain blood samples.

cardiac diameters. The measures utilized in determining and recording the size of the heart. They are obtained from x-ray films.

cardiac fluoroscopy (flūr-os'kō-pē). The examination, using a **fluoroscope,** of the heart and its action.

cardiac silhouette (sil'ū-et). The outline of the heart as seen on a chest film.

cardiospasm (kard'ē-ō-spazm). Spasm of the distal esophagus at its junction with the cardia of the stomach.

cassette (kas-set'). A holder for the unexposed film when making an x-ray picture. It generally contains two intensifying screens for decreasing exposure factors.

cathode (kath'ōd). The negative terminal of an electrical apparatus, especially of an x-ray tube.

cervical rib (serv'i-kl). CERV=neck. An extra rib arising from the seventh cervical vertebra. It is usually detectable only by x-ray.

cholangiogram — cholangiography (kol-anj'ē-ō-gram — kol-anj'ē-og'ra-fē). CHOL=bile. Radiologic visualization of the bile ducts.

cholecystogram — cholecystography (kōl-ē-sist'ō-gram — kōl-ē-sist-og'ra-fē). CHOL=bile; CYST=bladder. Radiologic visualization of the gallbladder following introduction of an opacifying substance by mouth or intravenously.

Cholografin (kōl-ō-graf'in). A proprietary solution commonly used intravenously for visualizing the gallbladder and the bile ducts.

cinefluorography — cineradiography (sin-e-flūr-og'ra-fē *or* sin-e-rād-ē-og'ra-fē). CINE=moving picture. A diagnostic procedure employing the simultaneous use of a **fluoroscope** and a moving picture camera. The camera records an amplified picture by using image intensification.

collimator (kol'im-ā-tor). A type of **cone** which utilizes an adjustable diaphragm. *See* **cone.**

cone (kōn). In radiology, a metallic tube interposed between the x-ray source and the patient to properly limit the x-ray exposure to the desired area. A **collimator** is one type.

contrast. In radiology, the differences in density between the lighter and darker shadows seen on an x-ray film.

contrast media. *plural.* Various radiopaque chemical substances introduced into the body by one of several means to improve radiologic visualization of a part.

Coolidge tube. The father of x-ray tubes.

costophrenic angle (kost-ō-fren'ik). COST=rib; PHREN=diaphragm. The intrathoracic space limited by the acute angle between the ribs and the dome of the diaphragm. Its shape changes with respiration. (Fig. 24, p. 232)

density. A term referring to heavier shadows on an x-ray film which are cast by structures which are more radiopaque.

developer. A chemical used in the processing of x-ray film.

encephalogram — encephalography (en-sef'a-lō-gram — en-sef-a-log'ra-fē). CEPH=head. Radiologic visualization of portions of the brain after introducing air into the brain ventricles and subarachnoid spaces or into the spinal canal.

esophageal varices (ē-sof-a-jē'al vair'i-sēz). *plural.* VARIX=dilated vessel. Dilated veins at the lower end of the esophagus which are frequently demonstrated radiologically.

extravasation (eks-trav-a-sā′shun). In radiology this generally refers to the escape of intravenously injected material from a vessel or from a hollow **viscus.**

fecalith (fēk′a-lith). FEC=feces; LITH=stone. A small collection of intestinal content which has become partially infiltrated with calcium.

filament (fil′a-ment). An essential part of the apparatus used in producing x-rays.

filling defect. The "negative" shadow caused by a normal or abnormal mass projecting into a hollow organ which has been filled with an opaque material or with air for radiologic visualization.

filter. Sheets of varying thickness used to absorb or "filter out" certain undesirable rays. Aluminum is the material most commonly used. Also used as a verb.

fixer. A chemical used in the processing of x-ray films.

fluorography (flūr-og′ra-fē). An arrangement and process used for producing a permanent record of the image seen during **fluoroscopy.**

fluoroscope (flūr′ō-skōp). SCOP=see. A part of x-ray equipment which allows immediate visualization on a fluoroscopic screen, without the use of x-ray films.

fluoroscopic intensifier (flūr-ō-skop′ik) — **image intensifier.** An apparatus which amplifies and intensifies the image seen on the fluoroscopic screen.

fluoroscopy (flūr-os′kō-pē). The process of conducting an examination which utilizes the fluoroscope.

fogging. Blurring of an x-ray film resulting from its unintentional exposure to light or to the action of chemicals.

GB Series. An abbreviation for a series of films used in radiologic examination of the gallbladder.

Ghon complex (Gōn). A particular kind of radiologic image sometimes seen in connection with pulmonary **tuberculosis.**

GI Series. An abbreviation for a series of films used in radiologic examination of the intestinal tract. They are commonly divided into "upper GI" and "lower GI" series.

grid. A part of the equipment used in producing and controlling x-ray films.

grid marks. Linear shadows sometimes produced on an x-ray film by improper functioning of the **Bucky diaphragm.**

hydronephrosis (hī-drō-nef-rō′sis). HYDR=water; NEPH=kidney. Co-existing **dilatation** of the pelvis and the **calyces** of the same kidney.

hydropneumothorax (hī-drō-nūm-ō-thōr′aks). PNEUM=air. A collection of air and fluid in the pleural cavity.

Hypaque Sodium (Hī′pāk). Another proprietary drug given intravenously to demonstrate kidney function radiologically (usually called simply "Hypaque").

hypovitaminosis D (hī-pō-vīt-a-min-ō′sis). A deficiency disease sometimes resulting in rickets and frequently diagnosed radiologically.

ileus (il′ē-us). Cessation of normal intestinal progression resulting from either mechanical or physiological causes.

image amplifier. Equipment used to increase the brightness of the image seen on the **fluoroscopic** screen.

intervertebral space (in-ter-vert-ē′bral). The space between two adjoining vertebrae which is occupied by the intervertebral disk. Significant changes of this space are frequently demonstrable radiologically.

"joint mouse". A detached fragment of cartilage or bone which is loose within a joint cavity.

kilovoltage (KV) (kil-ō-vōlt′āj). A factor in radiography which determines x-ray penetration and influences the quality of the x-ray record produced.

laminogram (lam'in-ō-gram). LAMIN= layer. One of a series of radiographic films made with only one plane (**lamina**) of the part in clear focus. Also called a **tomogram.**

lateral decubitus (dē-kyūb'i-tus). A particular position of the patient used in radiography to demonstrate certain features and organs.

linitis plastica (lin-ī'tis plast'i-ka). A disease in which the stomach wall is thickened and becomes abnormally inflexible.

Lipiodol (Lip-pī'a-dawl). A proprietary radiopaque oil used to outline certain cavities before x-ray examination.

lipping. Bony overgrowths at the margins of joint surfaces which are sometimes seen in arthritis.

mammography   (mam-mog'ra-fē). MAMM=breast; GRAPH=record. Radiologic examination of the breasts which is generally done to demonstrate abnormal masses of tissue.

mask. A lead shield used to protect the surrounding area during x-ray examination or therapy.

metastasis (met-tas'ta-sis). A secondary growth of cancer in a remote site, transferred either by the lymph or the blood systems. (*plural* – metastases.)

milliampere (mil-lē-amp'ēr). One of the units of measurement used in designating the specifications of an x-ray exposure (1/1000 of an ampere).

milliampere seconds. A radiologist's term for indicating the intensity of an x-ray exposure – the seconds (length of time) multipled by the number of milliamperes used.

motor meal. A meal given with accompanying barium and used to demonstrate the progress of food through the intestinal tract.

multiple myeloma (mī-el-ōm'a). MYEL=bone marrow. A malignant tumor of bone frequently diagnosed by x-ray.

myelogram – **ography** (mī'el-ō-gram – og'ra-fē). Radiologic visualization of the spinal canal.

myositis ossificans (mī-ō-sīt'is os-sif'i-kanz). MYO=muscle. The infiltration of certain muscles with calcium, which sometimes goes on to **ossification** of the muscle.

nephrocalcinosis (nef-rō-kal-sin-ō'sis). NEPH=kidney; CALC=stone. Calcification scattered throughout the kidney. It is frequently discovered by x-ray examination.

nonopaque (non ō-pāk'). *adj.* The opposite of **opaque.**

nonvisualization. Failure of an organ to become **radiopaque** after the administration of a drug which normally accomplishes this result.

opaque (ō-pāk') – **radiopaque** (rād'ē-ō-pāk). *adj.* In radiology, referring to anything relatively impervious to the passage of x-rays.

osteogenesis (os-tē-ō-jen'e-sis). The process of bone development. It is particularly adaptable to radiologic observation.

osteolysis (os-tē-ō-lī'sis). LYS=soften or destroy. A condition in which there is softening and destruction of bone; also, the process.

osteosclerosis   (os-tē-ō-sklēr-ō'sis). SCLER=hard. An increase in the **radiopacity** of bone which may be due to a number of causes.

overexposure. Too heavy an exposure of a film to x-rays, resulting in too "black" a film to have the best diagnostic quality.

overpenetration. The use of excessive kilovoltage, resulting in too dark a film for easy interpretation.

Pantopaque (Pan'tō-pāk). A proprietary compound used in **myelography.**

pelvimetry (pelvim'e-trē). In radiology, the taking of measurements of the pelvis from an x-ray film made to exact specifications. It is generally done late in pregnancy to determine possible disproportion between the fetal head and the mother's pelvis.

phlebolith (fleb'ō-lith). PHLEB=vein; LITH=stone. A **calculus** formed in a vein. Phleboliths are sometimes difficult to differentiate from urinary calculi.

photofluorography (fō-tō-flūr-og'ra-fē). The process of producing miniature condensed x-ray films, generally of the chest.

photofluororoentgenography (fō-tō-flūr-ō-rent-gen-og'ra-fē). The process of making miniature films of the image seen on the fluoroscopic screen.

planigram (plăn'i-gram). Another name for a **laminogram; tomogram.**

pneumocystogram—pneumocystography (nūm-ō-sist'ō-gram – nūm-ō-sist'og' ra-fē). PNEUM=air; CYST=bladder. Other names for **air cystogram—air cystography.**

pneumoencephalogram – pneumoencephalography (nūm-ō-en-sef'a-lō-gram – nūm-ō-en-sef'a-log'ra-fē). PNEUM=air; CEPH=head. Other names for **encephalogram—encephalography.**

pneumogram—pneumography (nūm'ō-gram—nūm'og'ra-fe). A general term relating to the process of producing x-ray films of the chest and lungs with the help of air artificially introduced into the chest cavity.

pneumoperitoneum (nūm-ō-per-i-tōn-ē' um). Air in the peritoneal cavity which has either escaped through the injured wall of the gastrointestinal tract or has been introduced as an aid to radiologic diagnosis.

posteroanterior (pōst-ĕr-ō-an-tēr'yor). *adj.* A term referring to x-ray films taken with the patient facing away from the x-ray tube.

Potter-Bucky diaphragm. Another name for a **Bucky diaphragm.**

prepylorus (prē-pī-lōr'us). The portion of the stomach just before the pylorus.

psoas shadow (sō'as). The radiologic image of the psoas muscles, often important diagnostically.

pulmonary emphysema (pul'mon-air-ē em-fi-sēm'a). PULM=lung. Enlargement and overdistention of the terminal air spaces of the lungs.

pyelectasis — pyelectasia (pī-el-ek'ta-sis – pī-el-ek'tā'zē-a). Dilatation of the kidney pelvis.

pyelocaliectasis (pī-el-ō-kāl-i-ck'ta-sis). PYEL=pelvis. Dilatation of the **calices** (as well as of the pelvis) of a kidney. Also called **hydronephrosis.**

pyelogram — pyelography (pī'el-ō-gram – pī'el-og'ra-fē). Radiologic visualization of the pelvis of the kidney. Types are excretory (opaque material introduced intravenously and excreted by the kidneys) and retrograde (opaque material introduced from below, by way of the ureter).

pyelolymphatic backflow (pī-el-ō-limfat'ik). A feature sometimes observed in retrograde **pyelography.** Also called "pyelovenous backflow."

radiogram — radiography (rād'ē-ō-gram – rād'ē-og'ra-fē). General terms used to designate radiologic visualization.

radiologist (rād-ē-ol'ō-jist). A doctor who specializes in radiology.

radiology (rād-ē-ol'ō-jē). *See* introductory paragraphs.

radiolucent (rād-ē-ō-lūs'ent). *adj.* Referring to the property of certain tissues to allow x-rays to pass through them; nonopaque.

radiopaque (rād-ē-ō-pāk'). *adj.* The opposite of **radiolucent.**

rarefaction (rair-e-fak'shun). The condition of abnormally decreased density of a part, resulting in greater **radiolucency.**

rectifier (rek'ti-fī-er). A specific part of x-ray equipment.

retrocaval (ret-rō-kāv'al). *adj.* Referring to a position behind the vena cava.

retrocecal (ret-rō-sēk'al). *adj.* Referring to a position behind the cecum.

retrograde (ret'rō-grād). *adj.* Referring to something introduced against the normal current, or up from below, as in retrograde **pyelography.** (The word is also used as an adverb.)

retroperitoneal (ret-rō-per-i-ton-ē'al). *adj.* Referring to a position behind the peritoneal cavity.

Roentgen, Wilhelm Conrad (Rent'gen). The physicist who discovered x-rays.

roentgen (rent'gen). A primary unit of measure used in describing x-ray production.

roentgen rays. X-rays.

roentgenogram — roentgenography (rent-gen'ō-gram — rent-gen-og'ra-fē). Other terms ˙synonomous with **radiogram — radiography.**

roentgenologist (rent-gen-ol'ō-jist). Another name for a radiologist.

roentgenology (rent-gen-ol'ō-jē). Another name for radiology.

rotating anode tube (an'ōd). One kind of x-ray tube.

Skiodan (Skē'ō-dan). A proprietary drug sometimes used in the production of excretory or retrograde **urograms.**

sodium iodide (ī'ō-dīd). A radiopaque solution sometimes used for distending the bladder in making cystograms.

soft tissue shadows. The darker shadows seen on x-ray films which are cast by radiolucent body tissues as opposed to lighter ones cast by bones. (Bones contain calcium and therefore impede the passage of x-rays.)

Telepaque (Tel'a-pāk). A proprietary drug used in visualizing the gallbladder.

tenting of the diaphragm. An angular tent like elevation of the dome of the diaphragm, generally indicating a pleural adhesion.

tomogram — tomography (tōm'ō-gram — tōm-og'ra-fē). *See* **laminogram.**

urogram — urography (yūr'ō-gram — yūr-og'ra-fē). UR=urine. Radiologic visualization of the entire urinary tract, generally accomplished by the intravenous injection of drugs which are radiopaque when excreted by the kidneys. This process is called excretory urography.

Therapeutic Radiology and Nuclear Medicine

CONSULTANT

Robert H. Butler, M.D.
*Diplomate, American Board of Radiology; Associate Professor, Clinical and Ambulatory Medicine, University of California Medical Center
Santa Rosa, California*

activity. Radiologists' abbreviation for radioactivity.

alpha particles (alf'a). Positively charged particles given off when certain radioactive material disintegrates. The alpha rays produced penetrate poorly.

atom. The smallest part of any element which can exist alone. It contains a central nucleus and surrounding electrons.

beta particles (bāt'a). Some of the electrons are negatively charged particles given off by radioactive substances when they disintegrate. *See* **alpha particles.**

betatron (bāt'a-tron). A device for accelerating electrons.

cobalt unit (kō'bawlt). A commonly used therapy unit which utilizes cobalt (^{60}Co) as the source of gamma rays.

"cow". A common name for the mother source of radioactive molybdenum, from which radioactive technetium is derived.

cross firing. The concentrating of x-rays at a certain desired internal point by directing them from different positions in order to avoid excessive skin exposure in any area.

curie (kyūr'ē). The unit used in measuring the activity of all radioactive substances.

dosage. A term used in therapeutic radiology to designate a specified amount of radiation desired by the radiologist, or given to a patient.

dosimetry. The measuring and mapping of treatment dosages to different parts of the body.

electrons (ē-lek'tronz). Negatively charged particles which revolve around the nucleus of an atom.

epilation (e-pil-ā'shun). PIL=hair. Temporary or permanent loss of hair sometimes occurring as the result of radiation. It may also be caused by a number of diseases.

fission (fish'un). The "splitting of an atom" into fragments.

gamma camera. A sophisticated electronic device for producing images of radioisotope distribution in an organ. The **gamma** emission from these radioisotopes produces "pictures" of a particular type which are interpretable by radiologists.

gamma rays. Certain specific radiations spontaneously given off by radioactive material. Gamma rays are more penetrating than **alpha** or **beta rays.**

Geiger counter. An instrument that measures or detects radioactivity.

half-life. The time required for the natural loss of one-half of the effective value of a specified amount of radioactive material.

intracavitary therapy (in-tra-kav'i-tair-ē). Radiation applied inside a body cavity by means of various types of radioisotopes which have been introduced into the cavity.

ion (ī'on). An atom or a group of atoms carrying a charge of electricity.

ionization (ī-on-īz-ā'shun). The process which separates the ions of a substance, changing it into an **electrolyte** (electricity conductor).

ionizing radiation (ī'on-īz-ing). Any radiation which reacts with an atom, leaving it with an electrical charge.

irradiation. A general term referring to the process of administering radiation.

isotope (īs'ō-tōp). An element in which all atoms have the same atomic number but differ in atomic weights.

linear accelerator (lin'e-ar ak-sel'er-a-tor). An extensive, refined piece of equipment designed to improve the efficiency of the radiotherapy of certain diseases. (LINAC is a commonly used abbreviation.)

nuclear medicine. The application of nuclear energy to medical practice, particularly the use of radioisotopes either diagnostically or therapeutically. *See* introductory paragraphs.

nucleus (nūk'lē-us). In nuclear medicine, the central, positively charged portion of the atom.

rad (rad). Abbreviation for "radiation absorbed dose" (the unit used in measuring the amount of radiation energy employed in the treatment of an area or mass to be irradiated).

radiation. The electromagnetic waves or "particulate energy" emanating from any source of electromagnetic energy.

radiation sickness. A reaction to exposure to electromagnetic waves, often resulting in gastrointestinal and other symptoms.

radiation therapy. *See* introductory paragraphs.

radioactive. *adj.* Having the property of diffusing spontaneously emanated electromagnetic waves or particles.

radioactive contamination. The unintended spread of radioactivity to persons or equipment where it can cause damage.

radioactive decontamination. The removal of harmful radioactive material from persons, areas or gear.

radioactive tracers. Radioisotopes used in very small amounts to obtain diagnostic information radiologically.

radiobiology (rād-ē-ō-bī-ol'ō-jē). The reaction of tissues to ionizing radiation.

radioisotope (rād-ē-ō-īs'ō-tōp). A chemical element which has been made

radioactive; some radioisotopes do occur naturally. Radioisotopes are:

radioarsenic (^{74}As) (rād-ē-ō-ars'en-ik). A radioisotope used in diagnostic studies of brain tumors and in therapy.

radiochromium (^{51}Cr) (rād-ē-ō-krōm'-ē-um). Another radioisotope used in diagnostic studies of the blood.

radiocobalt (^{60}Co) (rād-ē-ō-kō'bawlt). A radioisotope used in the diagnosis of certain anemias, but mostly as a source of radiation in radiotherapy.

radiofluorine (^{18}Fl) (rād-ē-ō-flōr'ēn). A radioisotope used in skeletal surveys to detect malignant metastases.

radiogold (^{198}Au). A radioisotope used diagnostically, principally in the detection of liver tumors.

radioiodine (^{131}I) (rād-ē-ō-ī'ō-dīn). A radioisotope used principally in testing thyroid function, but also in therapy.

radioiron (^{59}Fe). A radioisotope used in bone marrow and blood cell studies.

radiopotassium (^{42}K) (rād-ē-ō-pō-tas'-ē-um). A radioisotope used in some brain tumor studies.

radiotechnetium (^{99}Tc) (rād-ē-ō-tek-nē'shē-um). A radioisotope currently in common usage.

radioresistant (rād-ē-ō-rē-sis'tant). *adj.* Referring to the resistance of certain tissues to the effects of radiation.

radiosensitive. *adj.* The opposite of radioresistant.

radium (rād'ē-um). A radioactive element which occurs naturally and is used in the treatment of certain diseases.

radium implants. Containers of radium or radon which are left in tissues to provide a source of radiation for varying lengths of time.

radon (rād'on). A gas which emanates from radium and which has radioactive properties.

rectilinear scanner (rek-ti-lin'e-ar skan'-er). Another device for recording radioisotope distribution in an organ—in this case, either by mechanically printing (via a ribbon like a typewriter ribbon) or by exposing x-ray film to variable-intensity light beams.

roentgenotherapy (rent-gen-ō-ther'a-pē). Another name for the use of x-rays in the treatment of disease.

scan—scanning. The radiologic visualization of the concentration of a radioisotope in certain tissues follow-ing its administration (generally intravenously). Valuable information is sometimes afforded by "scanning," particularly data relative to malignant tumor cell concentration and to thyroid and liver functions.

scintillation probe (sin-til-lā'shun prōb). A detector which converts ionizing radiation into visible light energy.

well counter. A sophisticated **radioisotope** counting device.

24 General Surgery

THE FIELD OF general surgery is overlapped and encroached upon by many special branches of surgery. In the days when there were only three branches of medicine – medicine, surgery and obstetrics – the surgeon did everything that wasn't medical or obstetrical. Nowadays, several subbranches of surgery overlap with the activities of the general surgeon. There are cardiac surgeons, gynecologic surgeons, hand surgeons, neurosurgeons, ophthalmic surgeons, otolaryngologic surgeons, orthopedic surgeons, pediatric surgeons, plastic surgeons, proctologic surgeons, thoracic surgeons, vascular surgeons and urologic surgeons. Not all of these specialties have their own boards and those which do, base their requirements for certification on the amount of training required by the American Board of Surgery.

In general, most general surgeons restrict their practice to surgery of abdominal conditions, traumatic situations and tumor conditions. However, there is no restriction on his activities, and many general surgeons take on additional fields as their training, interest and capabilities dictate. The limits a general surgeon sets for himself depends to some extent on where he received his post-graduate training and the usual customs in that area, as well as on his own special interests. One surgeon may choose to add vascular surgery, another may elect to do hand surgery or pediatric surgery, and so on.

A surgeon is not merely a doctor who operates. A Board surgeon is a highly trained physician who deals with diseases and injuries which generally, in their normal course, require some sort of surgical treatment. He must have special diagnostic ability, possess keen judgment, and understand normal and abnormal physiology, to enable him to prevent complications and properly care for patients after surgery.

The American Board of Surgery requires four years of specialized surgical residency training before an applicant can be examined for certification by the Board.

CONSULTANTS

H. Edward Raitano, M.D.
Diplomate, American Board of Surgery
Santa Rosa, California

John M. Olney, Jr. M.D.
Diplomate, American Board of Surgery
Santa Rosa, California

"abdominoperineal" (ab-dom'in-ō-per-i-nē'al). Surgical abbreviation for an abdominal-perineal resection, a procedure used for the relief of malignancy of the lower bowel. In the procedure both the abdominal and perineal approaches are used.

abscess (ab'ses). A localized collection of pus. (Also used as an adjective.)

adenitis (ad-en-ī'tis). ADEN=gland; ITIS=inflammation. Inflammation of, or in, a lymphatic gland.

adenopathy (ad-en-op'a-thē). A general term for any disease of the lymphatic glands; it generally also implies gland enlargement.

adhesion (ad-hē'zhun). Abnormal sticking together of organs or tissues, frequently resulting in obstructions which require surgical relief.

adrenalectomy (ad-rēn-al-ek'tō-mē). ECTOMY=remove surgically. Surgical removal of one or both adrenal glands (when both are re-moved, their vital secretions must be supplied artificially to sustain life).

amputate (am'pyū-tāt). *verb.* To remove surgically all or part of a limb or other structure. (*noun*—amputa'-tion.)

amputee (am-pyū-tē'). A person who has lost one or more limbs by **amputation.**

anastomosis (an-as-tōm-ō'sis). The joining together of two passages or two hollow organs, such as the intestine, arteries, ureters and so forth. (*adj.*—anastomot'ic; *plural*—anastomos'es; *verb*—anastomose'.)

appendectomy (ap-pend-ek'tō-mē). Surgical removal of the **appendix.**

appendicitis (ap-pend-i-sīt'is). Inflammation of the **appendix.**

appendix (ap-pend'iks). A common name for the vermiform appendix, a semihollow structure arising from the cecum. (*plural*—append'ices; *adj.*—appendice'al.) (Fig. 20, p. 191; Fig. 21, below)

ascites (as-sīt'ez). An abnormal accumulation of fluid in the abdominal cavity. (*adj.*—ascit'ic.)

asepsis (ā-sep'sis). The prevention or exclusion of infection by the use of sterile techniques. (*adj.*—asep'tic.)

atresia (a-trē'zha). The absence or closure of a normal body opening or passage, such as the intestine, ducts, and so forth. (*adj.*—atret'ic.)

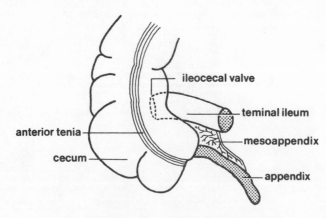

FIG. 21. Appendix

avulsion (ā-vul′shun). VULS=tear. In surgery, the forcible separation and removal of a part or a structure from an imbedded position. Avulsion may also occur during accidents. (*verb* — avulse.)

Bard-Parker blade. A commonly used, disposable scalpel blade which can be attached to or detached from a suitable handle. The blades are made in various sizes, types, and patterns for surgical use.

Billroth's operations I and II. Operation for the relief of ulcer in which a portion of the stomach is removed. Billroth I and II differ in the manner in which the stomach and intestines are rejoined.

biopsy (bī′op-sē). The removal of a small segment of tissue for microscopic examination. Also used as a *verb* (to excise a biopsy specimen) and as a *noun* (the specimen).

"bleeder" (blēd′er). Medical jargon for a blood vessel cut in the course of surgery which requires **ligation** or **cauterization**. It may also refer to a patient with an abnormal tendency to bleed.

"Bovie" (Bō′vē). An electrical apparatus which, by means of electric current, can **cauterize** or cut tissues.

carbuncle (kar′bung-kl). A specific, extensive, deep, pus-forming infection which is generally limited to the skin and subcutaneous tissues.

cardiospasm (kard′ē-ō-spazm). Spasm of the terminal esophagus at its juncture with the stomach.

case. A medical term referring to a specific incidence of a specific disease but *not* to the patient afflicted with the disease.

"clean case." Operating room parlance for a surgical case in which there is a minimum of obvious infection present, and in which the presence of infection is not the reason for the surgery.

"dirty case." Operating room jargon for a surgical case in which pus or ob-vious infection is present, particularly of a communicable type. Following the completion of a "dirty case," to avoid possible contamination, all of the instruments and non-disposable linens are cleaned and sterilized separately, before being re-added to the general supply for further sterilization and reuse.

cauterization (kaw-ter-i-zā′shun). The application of heat or corrosive chemicals for searing or destroying tissue. Cauterization is used to control bleeding or for the total destruction of tissue, as in the treatment of some malignant tumors.

cecostomy (sē-kos′tō-mē). A procedure in which the cecum is attached to the abdominal wall and opened for the collection of intestinal contents. A suitable receptacle is attached to the abdominal wall over the opening.

cellulitis (sel-yūl-ī′tis). Inflammation of cellular or connective tissue. It generally results from infection, but sometimes follows injury.

cholangitis (kōl-anj-ī′tis). CHOL=bile; ANG=vessel. Inflammation of the bile ducts.

cholecystectomy (kōl-e-sist-ek′tō-mē). CYST=bladder, hollow structure. Surgical removal of the gallbladder.

cholecystitis (kōl-e-sist-ī′tis). Inflammation of the gallbladder.

cholecystostomy (kōle-sist-ost′ō-mē). STOM=opening. Surgical incision of the gallbladder with establishment of drainage to the outside.

choledochotomy (kōl-e-dō-kot′ō-mē). Surgically opening the common bile duct for purposes of examination or to remove stones.

cholelithiasis (kōl-e-lith-ī′a-sis). The condition of having or forming stones in the gallbladder.

clamp. A general name for a two-ringed, sturdy, self-locking forceps. It is generally used for compression of tissue to stop bleeding. Types are Crile, Judd, Kocher, Mayo, Ochsner, and others.

coarctation (kō-ark-tā′shun). Narrowing or constricting of the opening in a tube, particularly an artery.

colostomy (kōl-ost′ō-mē). An opening made into the colon which has been brought through the abdominal wall to the surface, and secured there. A suitable receptacle is attached over the opening and collects the intestinal contents. Types are divided, double-barrel loop, transverse, and sigmoid.

common duct. The main bile duct, formed by the union of the cystic and hepatic ducts. (Fig. 10, p. 93)

conjoined tendon (kon′joynd ten′don). The fused tendons of the transversalis and the internal oblique muscles on each side of the lower abdomen. The conjoined tendon is often involved in the repair of inguinal **hernias.**

contaminated (kon-tam′in-āt-ed). adj. In surgery, this term refers to clothing, equipment, instruments, materials and utensils which have been made potentially infectious by contact with an unsterile surface or with unsterile materials. (noun – contamination; verb – contaminate.)

cryosurgery (krī-ō-surj′er-ē). CRYO= cold. The exposure of tissues to extreme degrees of cold in order to accomplish their destruction.

"cut-down." Medical lingo for the procedure of surgically exposing an inaccessible vein for use in intravenous injection. (Also used as a verb, to do a "cut-down.")

cyst (sist). A hollow, sac-like tumor having a definite wall and generally containing some sort of fluid. Most cysts are benign. Types are pancreatic, echinococcus, dermoid, ovarian, pilonidal, branchial, inclusion, sebaceous, multilocular, urachal, and chocolate.

decompression (dē-kom-presh′un). Lowering the pressure in an organ or a part, generally by removal of some of the contents.

dermatome (derm′a-tōm). A specialized instrument employed in removing thin layers of skin to be used as grafts in some other skin area.

dermoid cyst (derm′oyd sist). DERM= skin. A congenital cyst containing embryonic elements which have developed outside of their normal position. A dermoid cyst of the ovary may contain hair, teeth, and so forth.

dilatation (dil-a-tā′shun). A stretched or dilated condition.

dilation (dī-lā′shun). The procedure of stretching or enlarging the opening in a tube or duct. See **mydriatic.**

distention (dis-ten′shun). Stretching or enlargement of an organ due to increase in pressure, or content, within its lumen.

diverticulectomy (dī-vert-ik-yūl-ek′tō-mē). The surgical removal of one or more **diverticula.**

diverticulitis (dī-vert-ik-yūl-ī′tis). Inflammation of one or more **diverticula,** usually occurring in the sigmoid colon.

duodenum (dū-ō-dēn′um or dū-od′e-num). The first 30 cm of the small intestine located immediately downstream from the pylorus. (Fig. 5, p. 51; Fig. 10, p. 93; Fig. 22, p. 217)

elective surgery. Nonemergency surgery – surgery which can be safely postponed until a convenient time.

endotracheal tube (end-ō-trāk′ē-al). A tube placed in the trachea to facilitate respiration.

enterolysis (ent-er-ō-lī′sis). The surgical freeing of adhesions which interfere with or obstruct intestinal progression.

enucleate (e-nūk′lē-at). verb. NUK= center, core. To remove an organ or a part by a "shelling" process along the natural lines of cleavage, so that it comes out whole without being cut into. (noun–enuclea′tion.)

Esmarch's tourniquet (Es′marks turn′i-ket). A flat rubber bandage used for driving the blood out of an extremity in order to provide a blood-less field for surgery.

excise (eks-sīz′). *verb.* CIS=cut. To cut out or remove surgically. (*noun* — excision.)

explore (eks-plōr′). *verb.* In surgery, to perform an operation in order to examine by visual, manipulative, or other physical means. (*noun* — explora′tion; *adj.* — explor′a-tory.)

"exploratory" (eks-plōr′a-tō-rē). Medical name for a surgical procedure carried out when the exact diagnosis is not apparent and relief is required.

exteriorize. *verb.* To connect an organ or a part within the body with the outer surface of the body, generally done to accomplish drainage. (*noun* — exterioriza′tion.)

extraperitoneal (eks-tra-per-i-tōn-ē′al). *adj.* EXTRA=outside of. Referring to a position outside of the peritoneal cavity but adjacent to it.

extravasation (eks-trav-a-sā′shun *or* eks-trav-a-zā′shun). The escape of fluid or semi-fluid material from the organ or space it normally occupies, into adjacent tissues.

fascia (fash′ya). Any one of the many sheaths of fibrous connective tissue which function by surrounding, supporting or separating the various organs and parts of the body.

felon (fel′on). A painful, pus-forming infection involving the terminal phalanx of a finger or a thumb. Happily their occurrence is decreasing (since the advent of antibiotics) as a felon is one of man's most painful afflictions.

fibrosis (fib-rō′sis). OSIS=condition. The process of replacement of damaged or diseased tissue by fibrous or "scar" tissue, particularly following infection.

foramen of Winslow (for-a′men). A normal opening which connects the greater and lesser peritoneal cavities. It is of great importance to surgeons. Also called the **epiploic foramen.**

forceps (for′seps). In surgery, an instrument having two blades and two handles, used for grasping, handling, or compressing tissue or other material. Some forceps have teeth, some do not; some have ring-handles, others do not; some are self-locking; some are smooth-tipped, and some have teeth which intermesh; some have sharp, penetrating points. (*plural* — forceps.) Types include alligator, bullet, bone-holding, clamp, clip, dressing, hemostatic, tenaculum, thumb, tissue, towel, and others.

gas gangrene (gang-grēn′). A very bad form of gangrene resulting from infection of tissues with a gas-producing organism.

Gelfoam (jel′fōm). A spongy, absorbable, medicated proprietary product used to control venous bleeding (by packing in places where ligating or coagulating is not feasible).

granulation (gran-yūl-ā′shun). A stage in the process of the healing of wounds characterized by the appearing of soft, reddish, fleshy mounds of tissue (granulation tissue, colloquially called "proud flesh").

hemostasis (hē-mō-stā′sis). The stopping of escaping blood; the spontaneous (or intentional) stoppage of the flow of blood to a part.

hemostat (hēm′ō-stat). A two-ringed, self-locking forceps used mostly for grasping bleeding vessels prior to ligating or coagulating them. Types are Crile, Halsted, Mayo, Ochsner, Pean, and others.

hepatomegaly (hē-pat-ō-meg′a-lē). HEP=liver; MEG=large. Enlargement of the liver.

hernia (hern′ē-a). A general term referring to any abnormal protrusion of part of an organ through a weakened confining structure, or through a stretched, normally present opening. An *incarcerated hernia* is one in which the protruding part is stuck and the hernia is therefore "irreducible"; a *strangulated hernia* is an incarcerated hernia in which the blood supply of the protruding part is cut off by the pressure of the constricting opening. (*Plural* — hern′ias *or* hern′iae; *adj.* — hern′ial.) Types of hernias are: diaphragmatic, direct, indirect, inguinal, hiatal, umbilical, sliding, ventral, and omental.

hernial sac. The membrane which precedes and encloses the protruding part in most hernias.

herniorrhaphy (hern-ē-or′ra-fē). ORRHAPHY=reshape. Surgical correction of a hernial condition.

hydatid cyst (hī-dat′id sist). A cyst formed by the larvae of the Echinococcus; also called echinococcal cyst.

ileocecal valve (il-ē-ō-sēk′al). The circular muscle which surrounds the junction of the terminal end of the ileum with the cecum. (Fig. 20, p. 190; Fig. 21, p. 212)

ileostomy (il-ē-os′tō-mē). A loop of ileum brought out through the abdominal wall where it is secured and opened. A suitable container collects the intestinal contents. *See* colostomy.

ileum (il′ē-um). The thin-walled distal one-half of the small intestine which ends at the ileocecal valve.

ileus (il′ē-us). Lack of bowel peristalsis. It may have any one of several causes, most notable of which is peritonitis. Temporary ileus often follows abdominal operations.

imbrication (im-bri-kā′shun). In surgery, the intentional overlapping of successive, contiguous layers of tissue, generally done to insure additional strength.

incision (in-sizh′un). The surgical cut made in any tissue or part of the body but generally referring to the initial cut made in the skin when beginning an operation. Typical incisions are: classical, hockey-stick, median (or midline), McBurney, muscle-splitting, Pfannenstiel, rectus, semilunar, transverse, and many others.

infarction (in-fark′shun). The development of a devitalized segment of tissue, resulting from interruption or obstruction of its blood supply.

inoperable (in-op′er-a-bl). *adj.* A term used to refer to a condition or disease in which surgery or operation would be of no value. It usually applies to advanced stages of cancer.

intussusception (in-tus-sus-sep′shun). The infolding (telescoping) of a part of the intestine within itself. Most frequently it occurs in children.

ischemia (is-kēm′ē-a). A condition in which there is diminished or insufficient blood supply to a region of the body. It is of particular interest to surgeons because of its adverse effect on healing or regeneration of tissue.

ischiorectal (is-kē-ō-rek′tl). *adj.* Referring to the space between the ischium and the rectum, in which abscesses sometimes form.

jejunum (je-jūn′um). The 8-foot long, relatively heavy-walled, segment of the small intestine between the duodenum and the ileum.

laparotomy (lap-ar-ot′ō-mē). LAPAR= flank, abdomen. Any operation in which the peritoneal cavity is opened.

Levin tube (Lev-ēn′). A small tube passed into the stomach by way of the nose, throat, and esophagus. It is often used to remove gas and fluids and to avoid their accumulation.

ligation (lī-gā′shun). The closing or tying off of a channel with an encircling ligature. (*verb* — li′gate.)

ligature (lig′a-tchūr). The material used to accomplish **ligation.** Ligature materials are cotton, catgut, dacron, nylon, silk, and others.

lithotomy (lith-ot′ō-mē). LITH=stone. A broad term used to designate any procedure carried out to accomplish the removal of a stone.

lobe (lōb). A term designating a more or less well-separated portion of an organ, particularly referring to the lungs, the thyroid, the adrenals, the liver, the ear, and the brain.

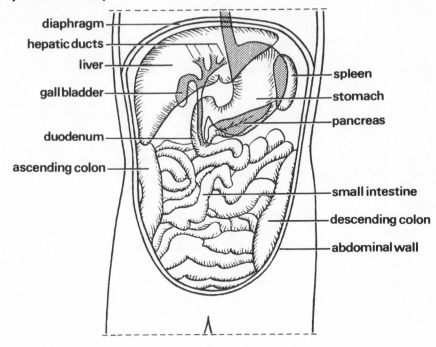

diaphragm
hepatic ducts
liver
gall bladder
duodenum
ascending colon

spleen
stomach
pancreas

small intestine
descending colon
abdominal wall

FIG. 22. Abdominal Organs

The ribs, transverse colon, and omentum have been omitted. Underlying parts of organs are shaded.

lymphadenectomy (limf-ad-en-ek′tō-mē). The surgical excision of one or more lymph glands.

mastectomy, simple (mas-tek′tō-mē). The surgical removal of the breast.

mastectomy, radical. The removal of all of the breast, together with its underlying muscles and the axillary lymph vessels and glands which drain the area. It is done in cases of malignancy or suspected malignancy.

mesentery (mes′en-tair-ē). The fold of posterior peritoneum which suspends most of the abdominal organs, and through which the blood vessels, lymph vessels, and nerves reach the organ. The term mesentery usually refers to the fan shaped structure by which the small intestine is suspended from the posterior wall of the abdominal cavity.

mesoappendix (mē-zō-ap-pen′diks). The mesentery by which the appendix is attached. (Fig. 21, p. 212)

mesocolon (mē-zō-kōl′on). That part of the mesentery which supports the colon and keeps it in position.

Metzenbaum scissors (Mets′en-bom). A specific type of scissors commonly used in abdominal surgery.

Miller-Abbott tube. A tube similar to a Levin tube except that it has an inflatable bag at or near the end to allow the intestine to move it "downstream" by **peristalsis.**

neoplasm (nē′ō-plazm.) NEO═new. A general term which includes any new or abnormal growth, either benign or malignant.

omentopexy (ō-ment-ō-peks′ē). Surgical fixation, with sutures, of the omentum, to other abdominal tissues. It may be done for one of several reasons.

omentum (ō-ment'um). The "apron" of fatty tissue suspended principally from the stomach, in the anterior part of the abdominal cavity. Favorably, it may assist in walling off infections; unfavorably, it often makes up the mass within hernial protrusions.

paracentesis (par-a-sen-tē'sis). The removal of fluid from a body cavity (usually the abdominal cavity) through a needle or a tube.

paronychia (pair-ō-nik'ē-a). Inflammation around the edges of a finger nail or a toe nail.

Penrose drain (Pen'rōz). Tubing made of very thin, very flexible rubber. It is made in various sizes and is sometimes temporarily left in wounds to keep them open for drainage.

peristalsis (per-i-stal'sis). The rhythmic, progressive contraction of the muscular walls of the intestinal tract which results in the forward propulsion of its contents.

peritoneal cavity (per-i-ton-ē'al). The largest of the body cavities. It is lined by the peritoneum and is sometimes called the abdominal cavity.

peritoneoscope (per-i-ten-ē'ō-skōp). A lighted instrument allowing visual examination of the interior of the abdomen through a small opening.

peritoneum (per-i-ton-ē'um). The smooth, thin, serous membrane which both lines the abdominal cavity and covers the surfaces of the abdominal organs.

peritonitis (per-i-ton-ī'tis). Inflammation or infection of the **peritoneum.**

phlebitis (fleb-ī'tis). PHLEB=vein. Inflammation in or irritation of the wall of a vein. It sometimes results in thrombus formation.

phlebotomy (fleb-ot'ō-mē). An incision into or a large puncture of a vein for the purpose of withdrawing blood. *See* **venesection.**

plegmon (fleg'mon). Inflammation of the subcutaneous connective tissue. It may result in fibrosis and induration, or go on to abscess formation requiring surgical drainage. It is rare since the advent of antibiotics.

pilonidal cyst (pīl-ō-nī'dl). A cyst under the skin overlying the tail bone.

plicate (plī'kāt). *verb.* To surgically shorten a structure or to reduce the size of a cavity by putting in a permanent fold or tuck. (*noun* — plica'tion).

"prep". Hospital name for the preoperative preparation of the part of a patient's body on which surgery is contemplated. It generally consists of thorough cleansing, shaving, and the application of antiseptic solutions the evening before surgery.

psuedocyst (sūd'ō-sist). PSEUD=false. An abnormal or dilated, unfilled space resembling a cyst but having no definite cyst wall.

pustule (pust'yūl). A small circumscribed elevation of the skin containing pus and having an inflamed base.

pyloroplasty (pī-lōr-ō-plas'tē). Surgical revision of the pylorus, generally done to increase the caliber of its contracted opening.

Ramstedt's operation (Ram'steds). An operation performed on the hypertrophied pyloric muscle in infants to relieve obstruction at the outlet of the stomach.

rebound tenderness. A diagnostic sign which is valuable to surgeons in certain abdominal conditions. It is characterized by pain elicited when pressure exerted over or adjacent to an inflamed region is suddenly removed.

rectus abdominis (rek'tus ab-dom'i-nis). A very important (paired) muscle in the middle portion of the anterior abdominal wall.

retractor (rē-trak'tor). An instrument for drawing back the edges of a surgical incision, or for restraining parts of organs which have been intentionally displaced away from the operative site. Typical retractors are Crile, Deaver, Army, Balfour, Mayo, Richardson, and many others.

retroperitoneal (ret-rō-per-i-ton-ē'al). *adj.* Referring to the region behind the peritoneal cavity and in front of the muscular posterior wall of the abdomen.

sarcoma (sark-ōm'a). A malignant tumor arising from connective tissue.

"scrub". A name given to the thorough cleansing (with brush and antiseptic soap) of the hands and forearms before doing a surgical procedure.

sebaceous cyst (sēb-ā'shus). A dilated, sebaceous gland whose opening has become obstructed. Its common name is "wen."

serosanguineous (sēr-ō-sang'gwin-us). *adj.* Referring to a liquid, generally a discharge, which is a mixture of blood and serum.

serous (sēr'us). *adj.* In surgery, generally referring to the serous membrane (**serosa**) or to the clear, yellowish fluid which exudes from injured or inflamed tissues.

sigmoidoscopy (sig-moyd-os'kō-pē). Examination of the interior of the sigmoid with the sigmoidoscope. It is done prior to lower bowel surgery and to subsequently check on the result, particularly in the case of tumors.

Silverman needle (Sil'ver-man). A hollow needle used for obtaining biopsy specimens without the need for surgically exposing the part to be biopsied.

sphincter (sfink'ter). A cutoff or puckering muscle which closes a normal opening or passageway.

sphincterotomy (sfink-ter-ot'omy). Surgically dividing a sphincter muscle. It generally refers to the sphincter of Oddi, which can prevent bile from entering the intestine.

splenectomy (splen-ek'tō-me). Surgical removal of the spleen.

sterile (ster'il). In surgery this term refers to the operating room clothing, equipment, instruments, materials and utensils which have been sterilized and subsequently handled only by sterile techniques. It also refers to an area of skin which has been rendered relatively free of bacteria by special treatment preparatory to surgical incision. (*noun* — steril'ity *or* asep'sis.)

sterile technique (tek-nek'). A special method developed for packaging, unpacking, and using sterilized instruments, equipment and clothing without danger of their becoming contaminated.

subphrenic abscess (sub-fren'ik). An abscess located immediately beneath the diaphragm.

supernumerary (sup-er-nūm'er-air-ē). *adj.* Referring to a structure or structures in excess of the usual normal number, such as an eleventh toe or a third nipple.

suppuration (sup-pyūr-ā'shun). The presence, formation or discharge of pus.

surgical "draping." The covering of the patient, instrument tables and necessary surgical equipment (exclusive of the surgically prepared incision area) with sterilized "drapes" handled by "sterile techniques" in order to avoid possible contamination.

surgical "prep". Preoperative operating room preparation of the incision site by the use of various means, techniques, and materials, to render it as bacteria-free as possible.

suture (sūt'cher). *verb.* To approximate tissues or bring together the edges of a wound or incision by sewing. Also *noun,* the material used in the sewing.

suture material. Any one of several kinds of material used in suturing. Classifications are absorbable (catgut, etc.) and nonabsorbable (cotton, silk, nylon, wire, etc.).

taenia (tēn′ē-a). A flat band of connective tissue extending down the length of the colon. It may be multiple.

tenaculum (ten-ak-′yūl-um). A two-ringed, toothed, self-locking forceps with long teeth, used for obtaining traction or for holding. Types are towel-clip, uterine, vulsellum (*plural* — vulsella), and others.

thumb forceps. A straight handled, spring forceps (like tweezers) held between the thumb and index finger. The tips may be smooth or toothed. Types are angle, bayonet, bulldog, dressing, mouse-tooth and others.

thyroidectomy (thī-royd-ek′tō-mē). Surgical removal of part or all of the thyroid gland.

thyrotoxicosis   (thī-rō-toks-i-kō′sis). TOX=poison. A condition in which there is "poisoning" of the system by the overproduction of thyroid gland secretions.

tourniquet (tūr′ni-ket). A constricting, elastic band which is applied tightly about an extremity to temporarily interrupt the flow of blood to or from that extremity.

trocar (trō′kar). A two-piece instrument consisting of a cannula and a sharp pointed, tightly fitting, removable steel core. It is used for withdrawing fluid from cavities.

tympanites (tim-pan-īt′ēz). The presence of gas or air in the intestine or in the peritoneal cavity, causing distention of the abdomen.

tympany (timp′an-ē). A hollow sound elicited when the abdominal wall is tapped over the air-distended intestines or stomach. (*adj.* — tympanit′ic.)

varicose veins (vair′i-kōs). Veins which are stretched, elongated, and folded upon themselves because of non-function of their valves. They occur most frequently in the legs where the weight of the blood is a producing factor.

varicosity (vair-i-kos′i-tē). A dilated, stretched vein or a group of such veins. (*adj.* — var′icose *or* var′icosed.) It is also called a varix. (*plural* — varices′.)

varix (vair′iks). *See* varicosity.

vascular (vas′kyūl-ar). *adj.* Referring to the blood or to the circulatory system.

vasculature (vas′kyūl-a-tyūr). The vascular system of the body or of any part of it.

vein stripping. A technique for surgically removing varicose veins.

venesection (vēn-e-sek′shun). The opening of a vein for the purpose of withdrawing blood. Also called a phlebotomy.

viscus (vis′kus). Any one of the large interior organs of the body, but particularly those contained in the abdominal cavity. (*plural* — vis′cera; *adj.* — vis′ceral.) (Differentiated, in spelling, from viscous!)

volvulus (volv′yūl-us). VOLV=turn. The twisting of a part of the intestines, usually the colon, tightly enough to cause obstruction.

wound. In operating room parlance this refers to the incisional opening, whether superficial or deep, incident to the performing of a surgical procedure.

"clean wound." An operative incision — as well as an accidental laceration — in a case in which no apparent infection is involved.

"dirty wound." The operative incision — or traumatic laceration — in a case in which there is probable, or apparent, infection present.

25 Plastic and Reconstructive Surgery

PLASTIC SURGERY SEEMS to overlap with almost every other surgical specialty. This is inevitable since its scope is the correction of congenital and acquired defects. Its broad aim is to improve both the function and the cosmetic appearance of the affected body part.

Performing the feats of plastic surgery — including the transplantation of tissue — requires not only the most meticulous skill and techniques, but also the most patient and careful postoperative care — care which is often tedious and very protracted. The results, many of which continue to be constantly visible, can be either most rewarding or most disappointing — nature often exhibits apparently misdirected but extremely stubborn whims. No surgeon tries harder.

Prior to examination for certification by the American Board of Plastic Surgery, a candidate is required to have completed three years of a General Surgery residency. He must also have practiced plastic surgery exclusively for two years and have submitted complete, detailed case histories (with photographs) of a large number of patients, thereby demonstrating his competence.

CONSULTANTS

Albert M. Trucker, M.D.
Diplomate, American Board of Plastic Surgery
Santa Rosa, California

Leo H. LaDage, M.D., F.A.C.S.*
Diplomate, American Board of Plastic Surgery
Long Beach, California

*deceased

Abbé operation (Ab-bā′). A name applied to any one of several reconstructive procedures devised by Dr. Abbé, but usually applied to a specific method of repairing defects of the upper lip.

Abbé-Estlander operation (Est′lander). A modification of the Abbé lip procedure.

acrobrachycephaly (ak-rō-brak-ē-sef′a-lē). ACRO=peak; BRACHY=short; CEPH=head. A congenital malformation of the head, due to developmental errors resulting in an anteroposteriorly shortened skull.

acrocephalosyndactyly (ak-rō-sef-al-ō-sin-dak′til-ē). DACTYL=fingers or toes. **Acrobrachycephaly** plus webbed fingers or toes.

acrocephaly (ak-rō-sef′a-lē). Another congenital malformation of the head sometimes called "turret skull."

ankylosis (ang-kil-ō′sis). The stiffening or fixation of a joint, sometimes intentionally produced surgically. *See* **arthrodesis.**

anthropometric points (an-thrō-pō-met′rik). ANTHRO=man; METR=measure. Specific points from which measurements are made for recording physical characteristics of the face. They include gnathion (nāth′ē-on), nasion (nāz′ē-on), subnasale (sub-nāz-al′), and trichion (trik′ē-on).

antihelix (an-ti-hēl′iks). The inner curved ridge of the external ear. Also called **anthel′ix.**

arthrodesis (arth-rō-dē′sis). ARTH=joint. A surgical procedure used for solidifying or stiffening a joint by removal of the cartilaginous joint surface. (*plural*—arthrode′ses.)

arthroplasty (arth-rō-plas′tē). Any one of various surgical procedures used to restore or increase the mobility of a joint.

autogenous (aw-toj′e-nus). AUTO=self; GEN=origin. *adj.* Originating within or produced by the patient himself. In this specialty the term generally refers to **grafts.**

autotransplant (aw-tō-trans′plant). A term applied to tissue moved to another part of the same person.

avulsion (a-vul′shun). VULS=draw. A tearing away, traumatically or surgically, of a part or structure.

"baseball finger." A deformity at the distal interphalangeal joint sometimes resulting from a sharp blow to the end of an extended finger (a frequent baseball injury).

Biesenberger operation (Bēs′en-berger). A surgical procedure sometimes used to reduce the size of female breasts.

bifid (bī-fid). *adj.* Split or divided into two parts.

blepharophimosis (blef-a-rō-fī-mō′sis). BLEPH=eyelid. A condition in which there is inability to separate the eyelids to the normal extent.

blepharoplasty (blef-a-rō-plas′tē). A general term denoting any plastic operation performed on the eyelid.

branchial arch syndrome (brang′kē-al). A group of congenital defects due to nonclosure of the (embryological) branchial clefts. Types are cysts, fis′tulae, and si′nuses.

canaliculodacryocystostomy (kan-al-ik-yū-lō-dak-rē-ō-sist-ost′ō-mē). DACRY=tears. A plastic procedure sometimes used on the lacrimal system of the eye to improve the drainage of tears.

canaliculorhinostomy (kan-al-ik-yū-lō-rīn-ost′ō-mē). RHIN=nose. A surgical procedure sometimes employed in plastic surgery on the lacrimal duct, particularly its opening into the nose.

canthoplasty (kan'thō-plas-tē). The surgical correction of a deformity or injury of the canthus.

canthotomy (kan-thot'ō-me). An incision made into the canthus, used to enlarge the eyelid opening.

carpal tunnel syndrome (kar'pal). A group of symptoms in one or both hands associated with compression of the median nerve at the wrist.

"cauliflower ear." The well-known "boxers' ear" or "wrestlers' ear" characterized by a distorted and thickened helix and antihelix.

cephalometric roentgenography (sef-a-lō-met'rik rent-gen-og'ra-fē). METR=measure; GRAPH=record. An x-ray procedure used for measuring and recording facial dimensions.

chemabrasion (kem-a-brā'zhun). The application of a cauterizing agent to the skin to cause destruction of the superficial layers.

chemosurgery (kēm-ō-sur'jer-ē). A specific method and procedure employed in removing skin cancers.

chondroma (kond-rō'ma). CHONDR= cartilage. A benign tumor of cartilaginous origin.

cicatrix (sik-ā'triks *or* sik'a-triks). A scar. (*adj.*—cicatricial; *plural.*—cicat'rices.)

cleft palate. A congenital fissure in or near the midline of the palate.

clinodactyly (klīn-ō-dak'til-ē). DACTYL=fingers or toes. A general term referring to a number of deformities of the fingers.

columella nasi (kol-um-el'a nā'zē). The fleshy external portion of the nasal septum.

conjunctivodacryocystostomy (kon-junk-tī-vō-dak-rē-ō-sist-ost'ō-mē). Another surgical procedure sometimes used on the lacrimal system of the eye.

conjunctivorhinostomy (kon-junk-tī-vō-rīn-ost'ō-mē). Another name for **conjunctivodacryocystostomy.**

craniofacial dysostosis (krān-ē-ō-fā'shal dis-os-tō'sis). CRAN=skull; DYS= bad; OS=bone. A term referring to a particular group of congenital facial defects.

cranioplasty (krān'ē-ō-plas-tē). Surgical correction of congenital or accidental defects in the skull.

"crow's feet." Lines of expression extending outward from the eyes; also called "laugh lines."

decubitus ulcer (dē-kyū'bit-us ul'ser). An ulceration caused by prolonged external pressure, frequently over the hip or lower back, in patients confined to bed for long periods of time.

dermabrasion (derm-a-brā'zhun). DERM=skin. Surgical removal of the superficial layers of the skin.

dermatome (derm'a-tōm). An instrument employed in the removal of partial or full thickness of skin to be used as a graft. Types are Padgett, Brown, and Reese-Padgett.

dermomuscular suspension (derm'ō-mus'kyū-lar). One of the surgical methods of correcting a drooped eyelid.

dyschondroplasia (dis-kon-drō-plā'zē-a *or* –zha). DYS=bad; CHONDR= cartilage. A condition characterized by abnormal cartilage growth along the shafts of long bones, sometimes causing deformities.

ectrodactyly (ek-trō-dak'til-ē). A shortness of the fingers due to the absence of one or more bones.

ectropion (ek-trōp'ē-on). A turning outward **(eversion)** of the edge of the eyelid.

electrodiagnosis (ē-lek-trō-dī-ag-nō'sis). The evaluation of nerve and muscle disorders by using measured amounts of electrical currents for stimulation.

electrolysis (ē-lek-trol'e-sis). LYS=destroy. An electrical process sometimes used to destroy the roots of unwanted hairs. (*adj.* — electrolyt′ic.)

electromyography (ē-lek-trō-mī-og′ra-fē). MYO=muscle; GRAPH=write, record. One of the most important forms of electrodiagnosis, demonstrating muscle function.

epicanthus (ep-i-kan′thus). A congenital deformity consisting of a skin fold alongside the nose. It conceals the inner corner of the eye and occurs in many Oriental faces. Types are invers′us, palpebral′is, superciliar′is, tarsal′is.

epicranium (ep-i-krān′ē-um). The muscular and cutaneous coverings of the top of the skull.

epidermis (ep-i-derm′is). The outer layer of the skin. (*adj.* — epider′mal.)

eschar (es′kar). A hard slough sometimes induced surgically by the application of electricity or corrosives.

face-lifting. A surgical procedure sometimes employed to accomplish a younger appearance.

face-peeling. One form of **chemabrasion.**

facial clefts. Congenital defects in the face caused by noncompletion of embryonic closures.

facial landmarks, anatomic. Another name for anthropometric points.

facial palsy. Sagging of one side of the face due to varying degrees of muscle or nerve paralysis.

fascial slings (fash′ē-al *or* fash′al). Bands of fascia employed surgically to support or stabilize structures.

flap. A partially detached segment of skin-covered tissue used to repair a defect elsewhere on the body. Types are Abbe, advancement, a′lar, derm′al, Est′lander, ped′icle, fan, perios′teal, rotation, and transposition.

"funnel chest." A colloquial name for **pectus excavatum.**

genotype (jen′ō-tīp). GEN=origin. Genetic makeup of an individual, particularly regarding his suitability to donate or receive skin grafts.

graft. A segment of skin or other tissue transplanted from another part of the same or another person, or from an animal, to overcome a defect. Types are: *autograft* (from the same person), *homograft* (from another person), and *heterograft* (from a different species).

harelip. A congenital defect of the upper lip, sometimes accompanied by a **cleft palate.** It is also sometimes called "cleft lip."

helix (hēl′iks). The cartilaginous rim of the outer ear.

hemangioma (hēm-an-jē-ō′ma). HEM=blood; ANG=blood vessel. A benign tumor, generally of the skin, consisting of tissues which tend to form blood vessels.

homotransplant (hōm-ō-trans′plant). HOMO=man. Transplanted skin or tissue obtained from another person.

immune serum (im-mūn′). Serum in which a specific antibody content is high, due to recovery of the donor from a particular infection.

Imuran (im′yūr-an). A proprietary drug sometimes used to decrease the tendency toward rejection.

integument (in-teg′yū-ment). A fancy name for the skin.

intermaxillary fixation (in-ter-maks′il-air-ē). The wiring together of the jaws to correct fractures or dental malocclusions.

intraoral (in-tra-or′al). *adj.* Within the mouth.

irradiation dermatosis (derm-a-tōs′is). RAD=ray. Changes produced in the skin by exposure to x-rays or similar agents. Also called **radio dermatitis.**

keloid (kēl′oyd). A specific type of abnormal, heavy, raised scar formation. The cause is unknown.

lipectomy (līp′ek-tō-mē *or* lip′ek-tō-mē). LIP=fat. The surgical removal of excessive fatty tissue.

lipoma (līp-ō′ma). A benign, generally subcutaneous, fatty tumor found in many regions of the body.

lymphedema (limf-e-dēm'a). Retention of fluid in the subcutaneous tissues due to blocking of the lymph vessels.

macroglossia (mak-rō-glos'sē-a). GLOSS=tongue. Excessive enlargement of the tongue.

macromastia (mak-rō-mast'ē-a). Abnormal size or shape of the female breasts.

macrostomia (mak-rō-stōm'ē-a). STOM=mouth. A congenital deforming enlargement of the mouth.

macrotia (mak-rō'shē-a *or* –sha). OT= ear. Abnormal enlargement of the protruding portion of the ear.

malocclusion (mal-ok-klū'zhun). Failure of the opposing teeth of the two jaws to meet properly.

mammoplasty (mam'mō-plas-tē). MAMM=breast. A general term covering any surgical operation designed to overcome deformity or excessive size of one or both breasts.

maxillectomy (maks-il-lek'tō-mē). A surgical procedure used in an attempt to remove cancer of the upper jaw.

melanoma (mel-a-nōm'a). A tumor, generally superficially located, consisting principally of cells containing black pigment.

nevus (nēv'us). A sharply limited, congenital skin lesion of any one of many kinds. (*plural* – nev'i).

omphalocele (om-fal'ō-sēl). A fancy name for an umbilical **hernia.**

otohematoma (ōt-ō-hēm-a-tōm'a). OTO=ear; HEM=blood. A silly name for a "cauliflower ear."

palatoplasty (pal'a-tō-plas-tē). The general name covering any operation which repairs a cleft palate.

pectus carinatum (pekt'us kair-in-at' um). PECT=breast. A congenital protrusion of the upper chest ("pigeon breast").

pectus excavatum (pekt'us eks-ka-vat' um). The opposite (hollowed) type of deformity of the upper chest ("funnel chest").

pedicle (ped'i-kl). In plastic surgery, the temporarily retained connecting structure which carries its original blood supply to an implanted autograft in order to to insure its viability.

"pigeon breast." A coloquial name for **pectus carinatum.**

planing (plān'ing). The removal of superficial layers of skin by mechanical or hand sanding.

plantar wart. A painful localized area of skin change occurring at one of the pressure points on the sole of the foot.

polydactylism (pol-ē-dak'til-izm). A deformity characterized by the presence of additional fingers or toes.

polyester (pol-ē-es'ter). A material sometimes used as a prosthetic implant for improving female breast contour.

polyether sponge (pol-ē-ēth'er). Another type of material sometimes implanted for the same purpose as **polyester.**

prolabium (prō-lāb'ē-um). LAB=lip. A specific part of the upper lip which is important in some cases of cleft lip.

pterygium colli (ter-ij'ē-um kol'lē). Congenital "webbing" of the skin of the side or back of the neck.

reinnervation (rē-in-ner-vā'shun). The reestablishment of sensation in a grafted area.

rhinophyma (rīn-ō-fīm'a). RHIN=nose. A bulbous swelling of the tip of the nose, sometimes seen in cases of advanced **rosacea.**

rhytidoplasty (rit-i-dō'plas-tē). Plastic surgery performed on the face and/or neck for the removal of wrinkles.

Romberg's disease (Rom'bergz). A progressive unilateral facial deformity caused by atrophy or lack of development on one side of the face.

scaphocephaly (skaf-ō-sef'a-lē). A congenital skull malformation resulting in a narrow, elongated head, with bulging forehead.

Silastic (sil-ast'ik). The trade name of a form of silicone rubber sometimes used in plastic surgery.

silicone (sil'a-kōn). A substance sometimes injected, or implanted, to improve facial or female breast contours.

spina bifida (spīn'a bif'i-da). A congenital deformity of the lower spine characterized by incomplete closure of the roof of the spinal canal.

staphylorrhaphy (staf-fil-or'ra-fē). Surgical closure of a cleft in the soft palate.

Strombeck operation. A surgical procedure used to reduce the size of enlarged female breasts.

supernumerary (sū-per-nūm'er-air-ē). *adj.* Referring to duplicated parts varying in range from doubling of a single phalanx to duplication of an entire extremity.

suture (sūtch'er). A method of bringing together the edges of a wound; also the material used. Types used in plastic surgery include continuous locking mattress, everted, figure of eight, hemostatic, horizontal mattress, intradermal buried, intradermal mattress, interrupted, interrupted intradermal, subdermal horizontal mattress, traction, and vertical mattress.

symblepharon (sim-blef'ar-on). An adhesion between the eyeball and one of the eyelids.

syndactylia (sin-dak-til'ē-a). Webbing of the fingers or toes.

synovectomy (sīn-ōv-ek'tō-mē). The surgical removal of all or part of the synovial membrane lining a joint.

"tongue-tie." A condition in which tongue movement is abnormally restricted by a membrane which "ties" it to the floor of the mouth.

torticollis (tort-i-kol'lis). TORT=twist; COLL=neck. A spastic condition causing shortening of the neck muscles resulting in a continuous tilting of the head ("wryneck").

transplantation. The surgical moving of bone, cartilage, fat, organs, etc. from one location (or person) to another.

"trigger finger." A condition in which there is partial adhesion of a finger tendon to its sheath, causing a snapping noise when the finger is bent inward.

urethroplasty (yū-rēth'rō-plas-tē). URETH=urethra. The surgical reconstruction of an abnormal urethra.

vascularization (vas-kyū-lar-i-zā'shun). In plastic surgery, the development of adequate blood supply within a graft or a flap, to insure its life.

Z-plasty. A widely used surgical technique for obtaining additional length by "advancing" opposing triangular flaps.

26 Thoracic, Vascular, and Cardiac Surgery

FOR THE MOST part, the practice of thoracic surgery was initially concerned with procedures on the lungs, the esophagus and the chest wall. As newer techniques (bypass), newer instruments (vascular clamps), and newer apparatus (heart-lung machines) developed, the scope of surgery in the thorax extended to the major blood vessels (the aorta and its branches), and to the heart (its walls, valves, and blood supply). It was natural, therefore, for the surgical techniques used on the vascular system within the thorax to be extended to the peripheral vascular system, and vice versa. Thoracic surgeons have been classified according to their particular field of practice as thoracic, cardiothoracic, cardiovascular, thoracic and cardiovascular, cardiac, or peripheral vascular surgeons.

Tuberculosis was once the major disease process for which thoracic surgical techniques had to be developed — viz., drainage procedures, thoracoplasty, and finally resection (segmental resection, lobectomy and pneumonectomy). More recently, bronchogenic carcinoma, trauma, and congenital and degenerative heart disease have occasioned most of the surgical procedures within the thorax.

The fascinating field of cardiovascular surgery is probably the most rapidly developing in the practice of surgery. Abnormal communications between the chambers of the heart can now be closed and patched. Narrowed channels can be widened and blood flow to vital organs can be reestablished. Various types of prostheses can be utilized in the replacement of diseased tissues. It is even now possible to accomplish cardiac excision and replacement.

The American Board of Thoracic Surgery is still reviewing its requirements for certification. It previously required certification by the American Board of Surgery and an additional two years of residency in an approved training program in cardiothoracic surgery. Because many thoracic programs do not now offer training in cardiovascular surgery, the applicant's training is individually reviewed before he is allowed to sit for examination by the board.

CONSULTANT

Douglas W. Cardozo, M.D., F.A.C.S.
Diplomate, American Board of Surgery
Santa Rosa, California

achalasia (ak-a-lā'zha). In thoracic surgery, a functional obstruction at the esophagogastric junction. It is sometimes incorrectly referred to as **cardiospasm.**

agenesis of lung (ā-jen'esis). GEN=origin. Complete absence of a lung.

aneurysm (an'yūr-izm). A dilated or stretched portion of a blood vessel forming an expansion or sac which is continuous with the lumen of the vessel. Common types are: abdominal, arteriovenous, diffuse, dissecting, fusiform, intramural, popliteal, pulsating, and thoracic.

aortic stenosis (ā-ort'ik sten-ō'sis). STEN=narrow. Varying degrees of obstruction to aortic blood flow, generally occurring in or near the aortic valve.

aortic valve prosthesis (pros-thē'sis). A substitute device or mechanism surgically implanted to function in place of a removed diseased aortic valve.

aortoiliac bypass (ā-ort-ō-il'ē-ak). A substitute blood shunt from the aorta to the iliac arteries to bypass obstruction in and near the bifurcation of the aorta.

apnea (ap'nē-a *or* ap-nē'a). The temporary cessation of respiration which may be brought on by deep, forceful breathing.

arteriotomy (ar-tēr-ē-ot'ō-mē). TOM= cut. The surgical opening of an artery, generally done for the purpose of removing clots or atheromatous plaques, or for inserting a canula.

aspergillosis (as-per'gil-ō-sis). A destructive lung disease due to a fungus.

atelectasis (at-a-lek'ta-sis). The collapse or incomplete expansion of a lung or of part of a lung.

atheromatosis (ath-er-ō-ma-tō'sis). Fatty degeneration of the inner wall of an artery which may occur in advanced **arteriosclerotic** hardening. The condition occurs in **plaques** and often produces obstruction to blood flow.

autogenous vein graft (aw-toj'e-nus). A segment of a patient's own healthy vein taken out and used as a replacement for a nonfunctioning portion of another vein or artery in his own body.

bifurcation (bī-fur-kā'shun). A branching or splitting into two parts.

Blalock procedure (Blā'lok). A surgical procedure for the relief of a congenital heart defect. Sometimes called the "blue baby operation."

bronchiogenic carcinoma (brong-kē-ō-jen'ik kar-sin-ōm'a). A primary malignant tumor originating in the bronchus of a lung.

bronchogram — bronchography (brong' kō-gram — brong-kog'ra-fē). Radiologic visualization of a bronchus after the instillation of **radiopaque** material into it.

bronchopleural fistula (brong-kō-plūr' al). A fistulous communication originating in a lung or in a bronchus and opening into the pleural cavity. It may be either infectious or traumatic in origin.

bronchoscope (brong'kō-skōp). SCOP= see. A distally lighted tube and lens system allowing visual examination of the inner lining surface of the bronchial tubes. Types included Jackson, and Negus, among others.

bronchoscopy (brong-kos'kō-pē). A visual examination, from within, of the bronchial tubes, utilizing the **bronchoscope.**

bypass. A tubular **prosthesis** sutured into the opened sides of two blood vessels to allow blood to bypass diseased or injured structures. It is sometimes called a "shunt."

cardiac tamponade (tam-pon-ahd'). The presence of enough blood or fluid within the pericardial sac, outside of the heart, to interfere with heart action. It is generally the result of heart injuries or infections.

carina (kar-ēn'a). A ridge forming the point of division of the trachea into the two main bronchi.

cavitation (kav-i-tā'shun). In pulmonary medicine, the formation of an air-containing space in the lung tissue, generally caused by slough from infection (abscess) or injury, and frequently communicating with a bronchial tube.

cervical rib (serv'i-kl). CERVIC=neck. An accessory rib (above the first rib) articulating with the 7th cervical vertebra, occurring generally on the left side but sometimes bilaterally.

chorda tendinea (kor'da ten-din'ē-a). Any one of the many tendinous strings which connect the edges of the two atrioventricular valves to the walls of the ventricles. (*plural* — chord'ae tendin'eae.) (Fig. 9, p. 88)

coarctation (kō-ark-tā'shun). Narrowing or constriction of a blood vessel.

decortication (dē-kort-i-kā'shun). CORT=covering. Surgical removal of thickened peel of tissue from the visceral pleura, a procedure utilized in the treatment of a nonexpanding lung.

diaphragmatic hernia (dī-a-frag-mat'ik hern'ē-a). A defect in the diaphragmatic musculature allowing abdominal contents (generally the stomach) to protrude into the pleural cavity. It may be congenital or acquired. (Fig. 23, below)

emphysema (em-fis-ēm'a). A condition in which there is overinflation and destruction of the terminal air spaces of the lungs. The loss of elasticity of the connective tissue elements results in poor air exchange and difficult breathing.

empyema (em-pī-ēm'a). PY=pus. A collection of pus or pus-containing fluid in the pleural cavity.

endarterectomy (end-art-er-ek'tō-mē). A surgical procedure in which an artery is opened and the thickened, obstructing inner wall of the vessel is removed or "reamed out," reestablishing the channel.

esophageal atresia (ē-sof-a-jē'al a-trē'zha). A developmental defect occurring usually at or near the **upper end**

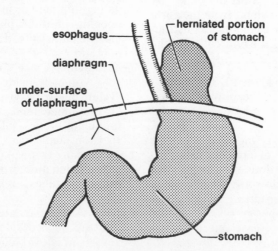

esophagus
diaphragm
under-surface of diaphragm
herniated portion of stomach
stomach

FIG. 23. Diaphragmatic Hernia

of the esophagus in which there is closure of the normal passageway in the esophagus.

esophagoscope (ē-sof'a-gō-skōp). A lighted tubular instrument through which the interior of the esophagus can be visually examined.

esophagoscopy (ē-sof-a-gos'kō-pē). Visual examination of the interior of the esophagus with the **esophagoscope.**

external carotid ligation (kar-ot'id). Tying off of the external carotid artery, sometimes done for control of **intracranial** bleeding.

extrapulmonary (eks-tra-pul'mon-air-ē). *adj.* Outside of the main body of the lung or lungs, generally referring to location within the pleural cavity.

femoropopliteal bypass (fem-o-rō-pop-lit-ē'al). A surgically created new channel for the passage of blood from the femoral artery to the popliteal artery. Either artificial material or autogenous veins are used.

fistula (fist'yūl-a). An abnormal, tube like canal, tract, or connection permitting drainage from one organ to another, or to the exterior. Thoracic fistulae generally originate from congenital defects, infections, or injuries. (*plural* – fist'ulae.)

heart valves. Leaflike structures suspended across the exits from the four heart chambers. Some valves "close" at the *end* of the contractile (systolic) phase of the heart cycle, preventing reflux flow of the blood back into the heart; others "close" at the *beginning* of the contractile (systolic) phase, thus providing unidirectional blood flow.

hemopericardium (hēm-ō-per-i-card'ē-um). HEM=blood; CARD=heart. Blood within the pericardial space.

hemopneumothorax (hēm-ō-nū-mō-thōr'aks). PNEUM=air, hence lungs. An abnormal collection of both blood and air within the pleural cavity.

hemothorax (hēm-ō-thōr'aks). A collection of blood within the pleural cavity.

hiatus hernia (hī-ā'tus hern'ē-a). A type of diaphragmatic hernia allowing abnormal protrusion of the stomach into the pleural cavity.

hilus – hilum (hīl'us – hīl'um). The root or central portion of each lung before its division into separate lobes.

histoplasmosis (hist-ō-plaz-mō'sis). An infrequent cause of chronic cavity formation in the lungs due to a fungal infection.

homograft (hōm'ō-graft). HOMO=the same. A piece of tissue for transplanting, which is obtained from the body of a donor of the *same species* as that of the recipient.

hydrothorax (hī-drō-thōr'aks). HYDRO=water. A collection of serous fluid within the pleural cavity, generally associated with cardiac or circulatory failure.

lingula (ling'gyū-la). A name given to the tongue-like lower portion of the left upper pulmonary lobe. It is the counterpart of the right middle lobe.

lobe (lōb). In chest medicine, any one of the more or less well-separated divisions of each lung. (Fig. 24, p. 232)

lobectomy (lōb-ek'tō-mē). The surgical excision of a lobe of a lung.

mediastinum (mēd-ē-as-tīn'um). The mass of tissue in the middle of the chest. It separates the two halves of the thoracic cavity and contains the heart, the esophagus, and many other vital structures. (*adj.* – mediastin'al.) (Fig. 24, p. 232)

myocardium (mī-ō-kard'ē-um). MYO= muscle; CARD=heart. The muscular tissue making up the bulk of the outer walls of the heart cavities, particularly the ventricles.

orthopnea (or-thop-nē'a). Inability to breathe comfortably when the subject is lying flat in the supine position.

papillary muscle (pap'i-lair-ē). One of several muscular projections originating from the ventricular walls, to which the chordae tendineae attach. (Fig. 9, p. 88)

pectus carinatum (pek'tus kar-in-ā'tum). PECT=chest. A bulging deformity of the chest wall at the sternum, frequently called "pigeon chest."

pectus excavatum (eks-ka-vā'tum). A depressed deformity of the anterior chest wall at the sternum, frequently called "funnel chest."

pericardiocentesis (per-ē-kard-ē-ō-sen-tē'sis). The withdrawal of fluid from the pericardial sac by needle aspiration.

pericardiotomy (per-ē-kard-ē-ot'ō-mē). Surgically entering the pericardial sac in order to treat the heart or the pericardium.

pericarditis (per-i-kard-ī'tis). Inflammation of the **pericardium.**

pericardium (per-i-kard'ē-um). The fibrous sac in which the heart is enclosed. Its inner layer (parietal pericardium) is continuous with the layer which covers the heart proper (visceral pericardium).

pleura (plūr'a). The membranous lining of the thoracic cavity. The parietal pleura lines the inner surface of the chest wall, and the visceral pleura covers the outer surface of the lungs. (Fig. 24, p. 232)

pleuritis (plūr-ī'tis). Inflammation of the **pleura.**

plombage (plom-bazh'). A surgical collapse procedure utilizing inert material in tissue spaces for the obliteration of cavities in the lung.

pneumoconiosis (nū-mō-kōn-ē-ō'sis). A general term referring to a chronic condition caused by long-continued inhalation of dust, generally in connection with an occupation. (Sometimes called **pneumo'noconiosis.**)

pneumolysis (nu-mō-lī'sis). LYS=destroy. The surgical freeing of adhesions between the lungs and the thoracic wall. (Sometimes called **pneumon'olysis.**)

pneumonectomy (nū-mō-nek'tō-mē). The surgical removal of a lung.

pneumothorax (nū-mō-thōr'aks). The abnormal presence of air inside the pleural cavity, surrounding the lungs, and thus interfering with their normal operation by destroying the partial vacuum naturally present there.

Pott's disease. Destruction of a vertebral body by disease, notably tuberculous disease. The result was formerly a frequent cause of **kyphosis.**

Potts' procedure. A surgical procedure designed to overcome a congenital narrowing of the pulmonary artery.

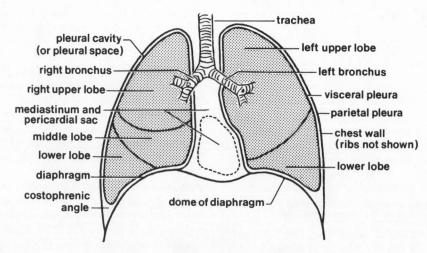

FIG. 24. Respiratory Apparatus

pulmonary fibrosis (pul'mon-air-ē fĭb-rō'sis). PULM=lung. Loss of elasticity of a lung due to proliferation of the connective tissue in the lung.

pulmonary function tests. Tests utilized to assist in determining, measuring, and recording the ability of the lungs to function normally.

pulmonic valve (pul-mon'ik). The three-leafed valve between the right ventricle and the pulmonary artery. It prevents return of blood into the ventricle during diastole. (Fig. 9, p. 88)

pyopneumothorax (pī-ō-nū-mō-thōr'aks). A combination of air and pus in the pleural cavity.

respiratory cripple (resp'er-a-tō-rē). A term applied to a patient who is unable to carry out normal activities because of impaired pulmonary function.

rhonchus (rong'kus). A dry, coarse sound originating in the bronchial tubes and heard through a stethoscope.

saphenous ligation (saf'e-nus lī-gā'-shun). Ligation of the saphenous vein, a surgical procedure frequently done for the relief of varicose veins. The varicose veins are stripped out in the same operation.

shunt. *verb.* To reroute blood or fluid from one course to another by surgical means; also, *noun* – the procedure itself or the material used.

thoracentesis (thōr-a-sen-tē'sis). Removal of fluid or air from the pleural cavity, generally done by needle aspiration.

thoracic duct (thōr-as'ik). A terminal canal located in the upper chest through which lymph, collected from a major portion of the body, passes before entering the blood stream.

thoracoplasty (thōr-a-kō-plas'tē). Surgical removal of a portion of the bony framework of the thoracic cage to effect pressure collapse of cavities in certain parts of the lungs. Types are apical, extrapleural, and thoracoplasty with **plombage.**

thoracoscope (thor'a-cō-skōp). An instrument which allows visual examination of the contents of the thoracic cavity.

thoracostomy (thōr-a-kos'tō-mē). The surgical establishment of an opening (generally for drainage) in the chest wall for temporary use during convalescence.

thoracotomy (thōr-a-kot'ō-mē). Any surgical incision made into or through the chest wall.

thromboendarterectomy (throm-bō-end-art-er-ek'tō-mē). Surgical removal of a **thrombus** and the underlying, thickened, inner obstructing lining of an artery.

thymectomy (thī-mek'tō-mē). Surgical removal of a persistent thymus gland. (The thymus normally disappears at an early age.)

thymoma (thīm-ōm'a). A general term applying to any tumor of the thymus gland.

tidal volume. A term representing the amount of air moved in or out of the lungs with each normal quiet respiratory cycle.

tracheo-esophageal fistula (trāk-ē-ō-ē-sof-a-jē'al fist'yūl-a). An uncommon congenital anomaly: a fistula between the esophagus and the trachea.

tracheostomy — tracheotomy (trāk-ē-ost'ō-mē — trāk-ē-ot'ō-mē). The surgical establishment of an external opening into the trachea to facilitate breathing.

vagotomy (vāg-ot'ō-mē). The surgical cutting or partial removal of the vagus nerve.

vascular (vas'kyūl-er). *adj.* Referring to the blood system; also used to describe tissue heavily supplied with blood vessels.

vascular prostheses (vas'kyūl-er pros-thēs'ēz). *plural.* Various artificial, mechanical, autogenous, or homogenous material used as substitutes for vascular channels. Types are autogenous grafts, dacron, frozen homografts, knitted, nylon, and teflon. (*Sing.* — prosthesis.)

vascular transplant. Any part of the circulatory organs or vessels taken from one area of the body and grafted into another area, either in the same or in another individual.

vein stripping. A term referring to the surgical removal of a vein or a section of a vein by a specific method. It is generally performed in the treatment of varicose veins of the lower extremity. By removing the superficial veins the venous flow is directed to the deeper, more competent circulation.

vital capacity. The maximum amount of air that a patient can exhale after taking the deepest possible breath.

27 Urology

THE TERM UROLOGY implies the study and treatment of diseases of the urinary tract, (the kidneys, which form the urine; the ureters, which convey it to the bladder for temporary storage; the urethra or voiding canal). In actual practice, however, urology does not confine itself to the urinary system. For several reasons, most logical among which is the fact that the male reproductive system connects with and makes use of the urethra, the scope of urological practice also includes the *male* genital system. The *female* genital system has long been the province of the gynecologist; in fact, gynecologists formerly handled female urological problems as well. Nowadays urologists treat the urinary systems of both sexes.

Because urology is a surgical specialty, the problems of actual urine formation are generally referred to an internist. It is the interference with free downstream drainage—stones, tumors, congenital conditions, or injuries may produce stagnation and invite infection—that produces most of the situations for which mechanical (surgical) intervention is required. About one-third of a urologist's patients are women; another third are elderly men (most of whom have prostate gland problems). The recent spectacular advances in kidney transplantation have required the collaboration of physiologists, internists, vascular surgeons and urologists.

Certification by the American Board of Urology requires three years of approved postgraduate training followed by two years of urological practice; written and interview examinations are given by members of the Board.

CONSULTANTS

Frank Hinman, Jr., M.D., F.A.C.S.
*Diplomate, American Board of
Urology; Associate Professor,
University of California Medical
Center
San Francisco, California*

Franklin P. Jeppesen, M.D., F.A.C.S.
*Diplomate, American Board of
Urology
Boise, Idaho*

aberrant (ab-er'ant). *adj.* Away from its normal position, particularly referring to blood vessels.

acid phosphatase (as'id fos'fa-tās). A blood enzyme which is sometimes increased in patients with prostatic cancer.

air cystogram (air sist'ō-gram) — **aerocystogram.** CYST=bladder; GRAM= record. X-ray visualization of the bladder while it is filled with air.

albumin (al-byūm'in). A protein sometimes found in urine. Its presence generally indicates some type of kidney malfunction.

albuminuria (al-byūm-in-ūr'ē-a). The presence of albumin and other proteins in the urine — now usually called proteinuria.

anastomosis (an-ast-ō-mō'sis). STOM= opening. A surgical joining together of two passages, tubes, or hollow organs. (*adj.* — anastomot'ic.)

androgen (and'rō-jen). Any masculinizing hormone. (*adj.* — androgenic.)

anuria (an-ūr'ē-a). The absence or failure of urine to be excreted from the body, generally referring to the nonproduction of urine by the kidneys. (*adj.* — anur'ic.)

azoospermia (a-zō-ō-sperm'ē-a). A condition in which the seminal fluid contains no spermatozoa. (*adj.* — azoosper'mic.)

bacilluria (bas-il-lūr'ē-a). The presence of bacilli in the urine.

bacteriuria (bak-ter-ē-yūr'ē-a). The presence of any kind of bacteria in the urine.

balanitis (bal-an-ī'tis). Superficial inflammation involving the glans penis.

balanoposthitis (bal-an-ō-pōs-thīt'is). Simultaneous inflammation of both the glans and the foreskin of the penis.

bas-fond (bah-faw'). An abnormal conformation of the bladder floor which encourages retention of residual urine. It is generally secondary to bladder neck obstruction.

benign prostatic hyperplasia (bē-nīn' pros-tat'ik hī-per-plāz'ē-a). A specific benign type of enlargement of the prostate gland (vernacular abbreviation, "B.P.H.").

bladder (blad'er). The elastic reservoir where urine is collected and stored before it is voided. (*adj.* — ves'ical.) (Fig. 12, p. 119; Fig. 25, p. 241)

bougie (bū'zhē). A surgical instrument, generally flexible, used for dilating or exploring canals or channels.

Bowman's capsule (Bō'manz kap'sul). The capsule surrounding the glomerulus, where the first stage of urine formation takes place.

Bricker's pouch (Brik'erz). A surgically isolated segment of small bowel which is sometimes used as a urine collector, substituting for the bladder.

bubo (byūb'ō). A name given to a swollen inguinal gland of a particular type.

bulbocavernosus (bul-bō-kav-ern-ō'sus). A paired muscle of the perineum which forms part of the penis.

calcium oxalate (kals'ē-um oks'a-lāt). A compound normally occurring in the urine in small quantities. When present in excessive concentration it may be precipitated as **calculi.**

calculus (kalk'yūl-us). CALC=stone. In urology, a urinary stone. (*adj.* — cal'culous; *plural* — cal'culi.)

calycectomy (kāl-i-sek'tō-mē). The surgical removal of one or more of the **calices** (calyces) of a kidney.

calyx — calix (kāl'iks). One of the several projections of the kidney pelvis which receive urine from the tubules. (*adj.*—calyce′al *or* calice′al; *plural*—cal′yces *or* cal′ices.) (Fig. 25, p. 241)

caput (kap′ut). The upper part or head of the epididymis.

caruncle (kar′ung-kl). A type of benign urethral tumor which is only seen in females.

castration (kast-rā′shun). Surgical removal of the testicles (or ovaries).

catecholamines (kat-a-kōl′a-mēnz). *plural.* Certain end products of adrenal secretions which are sometimes found in the urine. They are important in nerve impulse transfer. *See* **synapse.**

catheter (kath′e-ter). A hollow tube for draining urine from the bladder or the kidneys. Common types of urethral catheters are Coudé, Foley, French, Emmet, Malecot, Pezzer, regular, Robinson, and Tiemann. Common types of ureteral catheters are Blasucchi, Garceau, olive-tip, spiral-tip, whistle-tip, Wishard, and others.

catheterization (kath-e-ter-i-zā′shun). The inserting of a **catheter,** generally done for purposes of drainage.

chancre (shang′ker). The primary lesion of **syphilis.**

chancroid (shang′kroyd). A venereal, genital infection which is not syphilitic.

chordee (kord′ē). Downward curvature of the penis from congenital or inflammatory urethral shortening.

chyluria (kīl-lūr′ē-a). CHY=lymph. The presence of lymph in the urine.

circumcision (ser-kum-sizh′un). CIS= cut. Surgical removal of the foreskin of the penis.

cloaca (klō-ā′ka). A transient embryonic structure which is replaced before birth.

coitus (kō′it-us). Sexual intercourse.

colliculus (kol-lik′yūl-us). A depression in the verumontanum near which the ejaculatory ducts empty into the urethra.

concretion (kon-krē′shun). A stone or **calculus.**

convoluted tubule (kon′vōl-ūt-ed tūb′yūl). A part of the cortex of the kidney in which urine concentration takes place.

corpora amylacea (korp′or-a am-i-lā′sē-a *or* am-i-lā′shē-a). *plural.* Microscopic bodies normally found in prostatic fluid.

corpus cavernosum (korp′us kav-ern-ō′sum). A paired erectile part of the penis. (*plural*—corp′ora caverno′sa.)

cortex (renal) (kort′eks). The solid "working part" of the kidney, sometimes called the **paren′chyma.** (*plural*—cort′ices.) (Fig. 25, p. 241)

Cowper's glands (Kūp′erz). Paired glands emptying into the male urethra.

cremaster (krēm-ast′er). The scrotal muscle which elevates the testicles by contracting.

cryptorchid (kript-ork′id). A name applied to a testicle whose normal prenatal descent into the scrotum has been interrupted. (Also used as an adjective.)

cryptorchism—cryptorchidism (kriptor′kizm—kript-or′kid-izm). CRYPT =hidden; ORCH=testicle. A congenital condition in which a testis failed to descend into the scrotum before birth.

cystectomy (sist-ek′to-me). CYST= bladder. The surgical removal of the urinary bladder.

cystitis (sist-īt′is). Inflammation of the bladder lining.

"cysto" (sist′ō). Medical jargon for **cystoscopy,** or for the cystoscopy room.

cystocele (sist′ō-sēl). **Hernia** of the bladder floor into the anterior part of the vagina.

cystogram—cystography (sist′ō-gram— sist-og′ra-fē). GRAPH=record. Radiologic visualization of the urinary bladder while it is distended with air (**aerocystogram**) or with a radiopaque liquid.

cystogram, voiding. A cystogram made while urine (or radiopaque liquid) is being voided from the bladder.

cystoscope (sist'ō-skōp). A surgical instrument for visually examining and treating the interior of the bladder. Types are: Brown-Buerger, McCarthy ("panendoscope"), Young, and others. Lens systems which are used are: direct, foroblique, right-angle, and retrograde.

cystoscopy (sist-osk'ō-pē). The examination of the bladder through a **cystoscope.**

cystostomy (sist-ost'ō-mē). A surgically made new channel by which urine is drained from the bladder; also, the surgical process of making the new channel.

cystotomy (sist-ot'ō-mē). The making of a temporary incision or opening into the bladder cavity.

cystourethrogram — cystourethrography (sist-ō-yūr-ēth'ro-gram — sist-ō-yūr-ēth-rog'ra-fē). Simultaneous composite radiologic visualization of both the bladder and the urethra.

dartos (dar'tōs). The scrotal muscle which assists in shortening and elevating the scrotum.

Denonvilliers' fascia (Den-awn-vē'yāz fash'ya). The rectovesical **fascia** covering the posterior surface of the prostate.

detrusor vesicae (dē-trūz'or ves'i-kē). A name given to the entire thickness of the muscular coat of the bladder. It is generally called simply "the detrusor."

dilatation (dil-a-tā'shun). A stretched or dilated condition.

dilation (dī-lā'shun). An enlarging, by stretching, from within.

diplococcus (dip-lō-kok'us). A type of bacteria (cocci) occurring in pairs — in urology, usually the gonococcus.

diuresis (dī-yūr-ē'sis). Increased excretion of urine by the kidneys.

diuretic (dī-yūr-et'ik). A drug which causes **diuresis.** (Also an adjective.)

diverticulectomy (dī-vert-ik-yūl-ek'tō-mē). The surgical removal of a **diverticulum** (generally referring to a diverticulum of the bladder).

diverticulum (dī-vert-ik'yūl-um). A sac-like outward projection, or outpouching, generally from the bladder but also from the kidney calices, the ureters or the urethra. (*adj.* — divertic'ulous; *plural* — divertic'ula.)

dysuria (dis-yūr'ē-a). Painful or difficult urination.

ectopia (ek-tōp'ē-a). TOP=position. Congenital displacement of a part or organ. The urinary tract is particularly vulnerable to ectopias throughout its length because of its formation and development. (*adj.* — ectop'ic.)

electrocoagulation (ē-lek-trō-kō-ag-yū-lā'shun). The destruction of tissue by contact with a controlled high-frequency electric current. **Fulguration** is one type of electrocoagulation.

ejaculation (ē-jak-yūl-ā'shun). The emission of seminal fluid. (*adj.* — ejac'ulatory.)

ejaculatory ducts (ē-jak'yūl-a-tō-rē dukts). Paired tubes which convey the seminal fluid from the seminal vesicles to the urethra. (Fig. 26, p. 245)

emasculation (ē-mask-yūl-ā'shun). Removal or loss of the male external genitalia either by surgery or by accident.

endoscope (end'ō-skōp). A surgical instrument for visually examining the interior of a cavity or tube, particularly the bladder or the urethra.

endoscopy (end-osk'ō-pē). Visual examination through an **endoscope.**

enuresis (en-yūr-ē'sis). Uncontrolled voiding of urine, particularly that occurring at night.

epididymectomy (ep-i-did-im-ek'tō-mē). The surgical removal of an **epididymis.**

epididymis (ep-i-did'im-is). A structure attached to each testicle, which collects and conveys spermatozoa to the vas into which it merges. (*plural* — epidid'ymides.) (Fig. 26, p. 245)

epididymitis (ep-i-did-im-ī'tis). Inflammation of the **epididymis.**

epispadias (ep-i-spād'ē-us). A congenital condition in which the urethra opens on the upper side of the penis. (*adj.* – epispad'iac *or* epispad'ic.)

estrogen (es'trō-jen). ESTR=woman; GEN=origin. A feminizing ovarian hormone, commonly called the "female hormone." It is used by urologists in treating cancer of the prostate.

evacuation (ē-vak-yū-ā'shun). The removal of fluid or contents either naturally or surgically from a cavity or hollow organ.

evacuator (ē-vak'yū-ā-tor). A surgical instrument sometimes used to empty the bladder during surgery.

eversion (ē-verzh'un). The turning outward of the edges of an opening. It is either naturally present or brought about by surgery.

excretory urograms (eks'krē-tō-rē yūr'ō-gramz). A series of x-ray films of the urinary tract taken following intravenous injection of radiopaque material which is excreted through the kidneys; also called "I.V. pyelograms."

exstrophy (eks'strof-ē). A congenital malformation of the bladder and urethra in which the bladder opens directly on the pubic region without an intermediate urethra.

extractor (eks-trak'tor). A surgical instrument generally used for removing stones from the ureter. Common types are Councill, Davis, Dormia, Ellik, Howard, Johnson, and others.

extraperitoneal (eks-tra-per-i-ton-ē'al). *adj.* Outside of, and usually behind, the peritoneal cavity.

extravasation (eks-trav-a-sā'shun). The escape of fluids (generally urine or blood) from their normal channel or cavity.

filiform (fil'i-form). A flexible surgical instrument used for following or exploring passages. (also adjective, referring to a narrow tortuous channel.)

follower. A flexible tapered instrument, detachably attached behind the fili-

form, for dilating contracted or narrowed channels.

frenum (frē'num) – frenulum. The thin fold of tissue that connects the under surface of the glans with the prepuce.

fulguration (ful-gūr-ā'shun). Tissue destruction by controlled high frequency electrocoagulation.

fundus (fund'us). In urology, the top portion of the bladder. (*adj.* – fund'al; *plural* – fund'i.)

"G.C." Vernacular name for gonorrhea.

genitalia (jen-i-tāl'ē-a *or* – ya). The reproductive organs, particularly the external genital organs – "The genitals."

Gerota's capsule (Ger-ōt'az kap'sūl). The fibrous capsule surrounding each kidney.

glans penis (glans pēn'is). The head of the penis.

globus major (glōb'us māj'or). The head or beginning portion of the epididymis.

globus minor (mīn'or). The return loop formed by the epididymis opposite the lower end of the testicle.

glomerulus (glō-mer'yūl-us). One of the many capillary tufts in the renal cortex which is involved in the first stage of urine formation. (*plural* – glomer'uli)

glycosuria (glī-kō-syūr'ē-a). GLYCO= sugar. The presence of excessive sugar in the urine.

gonococcus (gon-ō-kok'kus). The specific organism (a diplococcus) responsible for gonorrhea.

gonorrhea (gon-or-rē'a). The commonest of the venereal diseases. Although inflammation of the urethra generally causes the first symptom, progression and/or complications may involve other organs. (*adj.* – gonorrhe'al.)

hematuria (hēm-a-tūr'ē-a). HEM= blood. The presence of blood in the urine.

hemospermia (hēm-ō-sperm'ē-a). The presence of blood in the seminal fluid.

Henle's loop (Hen'lēz). The looped-back part of each kidney tubule.

hermaphroditism *or* **hermaph'rodism** (herm-af'rō-dit-izm *or* herm-af'rō-dizm). Bisexuality.

hilus (hīl'us) — **hilum** (hīl'um). The large opening in the medial edge of the kidney by which the blood vessels enter and leave the organ. The side of the kidney pelvis also generally protrudes out from it.

"Hunner's ulcer" (Hun'erz). A vernacular name for a bladder condition (**submucous fibrosis** or **interstitial cystitis**).

hyaline casts (hī'a-lin kasts). Elements frequently found in the urine of a patient with nephritis.

hydrocele (hī'drō-sēl). HYDR=water. An excessive accumulation of serous fluid within the cavity enclosed by the **tunica vaginalis.**

hydronephrosis (hī-drō-nef-rō'sis). NEPH=kidney. An advanced stage of dilatation of the pelvis of the kidney. It is generally due to obstruction and infection.

hypernephroma (hī-per-nef-rōm'a). A type of malignant kidney tumor.

hyperparathyroidism (hī-per-pair-a-thī'royd-izm). Overactivity of the parathyroid glands which is sometimes the cause of excessive urinary calculi formation.

hyperplasia (hī-per-plā'zha). An increased amount of normal tissue, resulting in benign enlargement. In urology it generally represents the commonest type of prostatic enlargement. *See* **hypertrophy.**

hypospadias (hī-pō-spād'ē-us). A congenital condition in which the urethra opens on the under side of the penis instead of at the end. The accompanying scarring generally imparts a downward curvature to the penis. (*adj.* — hypospad'iac *or* hypospad'-ic.)

impotence (im'pō-tens). The lack of sexual power in males. (*adj.* — im'potent.)

incontinence (in-kon'ti-nens). Inability to control the escape of urine. (*adj.* — incon'tinent.)

indigo carmine (in-di-gō kar'min). A blue dye which appears in the urine when injected intravenously. It is used for determining kidney function or to visualize an ectopic or poorly visualized ureteral orifice.

infundibulum (in-fun-dib'yūl-um). The funnel like part of each major kidney calyx.

interureteric ridge (in-ter-yūr-e-ter'ik). The slightly raised part of the floor of the bladder located between the two ureteral openings.

intramural (in-tra-myūr'al). *adj.* MUR=wall. Referring to a position between the layers of a wall. In urology, the bladder wall is generally inferred.

intravesical (in-tra-ves'i-kl). *adj.* Situated within the bladder.

irreducible phimosis (ir-re-dūs'i-bl fīm-ō'sis). A condition in which swelling and edema of the prepuce, retracted behind the glans penis, prevent its return over the glans.

kidney (kid'nē). One of the paired organs which form urine. (*adj.* — ren'al.) (Fig. 25, p. 241)

"K.U.B." A common name for a composite x-ray film showing the kidneys and the ureteral and bladder regions before opacifying media is used; actually, a plain film of the abdomen.

lavage (la-vazh'). The cleansing irrigation of a cavity. (Also a *verb.*)

lecithin (les'i-thin). A component of prostatic fluid.

leukoplakia (lūk-ō-plāk'ē-a). A particular whitish condition of the bladder lining, notably that covering the base of the bladder. It is sometimes said to be precancerous.

litholapaxy (lith'ō-la-paks-ē). LITH=stone. The surgical procedure of

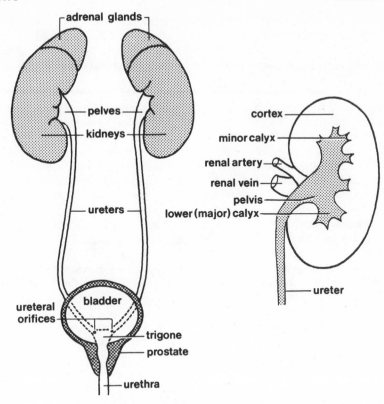

FIG. 25. Urinary System

crushing bladder stones. (Also called **lith′opaxy** or **lithotrip′sy.**)

lithotrite (lith′ō-trīt). The instrument used to accomplish **litholapaxy.** Types include Bigelow, Keyes, Kirwin, Ravich and others. (Also called **lith′olotrite.**)

Marshall-Marchetti operation (Mar′shal-Mark-ket′ē). A surgical procedure sometimes used to correct urinary incontinence.

marsupialization (mar-sūp-ē-al-i-zā′shun). The surgical forming of a wide connection between an internal cavity and the other surface of the body.

meatotomy (mē-a-tot′ō-mē). The surgical enlarging of the opening of the ureter or the urethra.

meatus (mē-āt′us). Any opening; in urology, particularly those at the ends of the ureters and the urethra. (*plural*—meatuses, *not* mea′ti.)

medulla (med-ul′la). A name given to a part of the kidney cortex.

megaloureter (meg-a-lō-yūr′e-ter). A term describing an enlarged, dilated ureter.

micturition (mik-tūr-ish′un *or* mik-tyūr-ish′un). The act of voiding urine.

"Mosenthal" (Mōz′en-thawl). A specific test using multiple urine specimens for determining renal function. Mostly variations in the **specific gravity** of the individual specimens (among other features) are noted.

multilocular (mult-i-lok′yūl-ar). *adj.* Consisting of many cysts or cyst like compartments.

needle biopsy (bī′op-sē). A surgical procedure sometimes used for acquiring a biopsy specimen from the prostrate or from the kidney. Types of needles are Higgins and Silverman, and others.

Neisserian infection (Nī-sēr′ē-an). Gonorrheal **urethritis** (vernacular, "G.C."). Named after Dr. Neisser.

nephrectomy (nef-rek′tō-mē). NEPH= kidney. The surgical removal of a kidney.

nephritis (nef-rīt′is). Urologically speaking, this refers to infection of the kidney parenchyma (sometimes called **pyelonephritis**), as opposed to the noninflammatory degenerative kidney changes commonly called **Bright's disease,** which are generally treated by internists.

nephrocalcinosis (nef-rō-kal-sin-ō′sis). A condition in which calculi are precipitated in the renal tubules.

nephrogram (nef′rō-gram). The x-ray demonstration of a semiopaque (dye-filled) renal cortex.

nephrolithiasis (nef-rō-lith-ī′a-sis). The presence of one or more stones in the kidney pelvis.

nephrolithotomy (nef-rō-lith-ot′ō-mē). The surgical removal of a stone from the kidney by way of an incision through the kidney cortex.

nephron (nef′ron). One of the many functioning units which make up the kidney parenchyma and deliver urine into the pelvis. Each nephron consists of a glomerulus and its attached (urine-concentrating) tubule.

nephropexy (nef′rō-peks-ē). The surgical raising and suspending of a "dropped kidney" to improve its drainage.

nephroptosis (nef-rop-tō′sis). PTOS= drop, fall. A term referring to a pathologically low position of a kidney.

nephrosis (nef-rō′sis). A general term referring to any disease of the kidney tubules. (*plural*—nephro′ses.)

nephrostomy (nef-rost′ō-mē). A surgically-produced new route (temporary or permanent) directly through the cortex of the kidney. Urine can leave the pelvis by this new route rather than by going down the ureter. The

term may also refer to the surgical procedure. *See* **pyelostomy.**

nephrotomy (nef-rot′ō-mē). The making of a temporary incision through kidney tissue for any purpose.

nephroureterectomy (nef-rō-yūr-ē-ter-ek′tō-mē). The surgical removal of a kidney and its ureter.

neurogenic bladder (nūr-ō-jen′ik). NEUR=nerve; GEN=origin. A bladder whose functioning is disturbed by lesions of the brain or spinal cord ("cord bladder").

nocturia (nok-tūr′ē-a). NOCT=night. The voiding of urine during the night.

oliguria (ol-i-gūr′ē-a). Scanty urine formation.

orchid (ork′id). Another name for a **testicle.** (*adj.*—orch′ic.)

orchiectomy (ork-ē-ek′tō-mē). —**orchidectomy** (or-kid-ek′tō-mē). The surgical removal of a testicle.

orchiopexy (ork′ē-ō-peks-ē). —**orchidopexy** (or′kid-ō-pex-ē). The surgical placing and anchoring of a cryptorchid testicle within the scrotum.

orchitis (ork-ī′tis). Inflammation of a testicle.

osteitis pubis (ost-ē-ī′tis pyūb′is). OS= bone. Inflammation or infection of one of the pubic bones, sometimes brought on by operative trauma.

pampiniform plexus (pam-pin′i-form pleks′us). The mesh of veins originating from the testicle which makes up much of the spermatic cord.

papilla (pa-pil′a). One of several mounds on the wall of the kidney pelvis, each marking the openings of tubules through which urine formed in the cortex drains into the pelvis. (*adj.*—pap′illary).

papillitis (pap-i-lī′tis). In urology, inflammation of renal **papillae.**

parenchyma (par-eng′kim-a). The solid functioning portion of each kidney made up of its cortex and medulla (*adj.*—paren′chymal.)

pedicle (ped′i-kl). In urology, the stem or stalk of tissue by which the main blood vessels reach the body of the kidney. (*adj.* — pedic'ular.)

penis (pēn'is). The male sexual organ (*adj.* — pēn'īle.) (Fig. 26, p. 245)

perineal prostatectomy (per-i-nē'al pros-ta-tek'tō-mē). The surgical removal of the prostate gland via the perineal route.

perineum (per-i-nē'um). The region between the external genitalia and the anus.

Peyronie's disease (Pā-rōn'ēz). An abnormal condition (**fibrosis**) affecting the penis. Its cause is unknown.

phallus (fal'lus). The penis. (*adj.* — phal'lic.)

phlebolith (fleb'ō-lith). A **calculus** formed in a vein. In urology, generally referring to those frequently seen in x-rays of the bony pelvis.

"phthalein" (thāl'ēn). Medical abbreviation for the phenolsulfonphthalein test for determining kidney function.

polycystic (pol-e-sist'ik). *adj.* CYST= hollow space. Made up of many cysts. In urology, generally referring to polycystic kidneys, a congenital bilateral condition.

polyuria (pol-ē-yūr'ē-a). Excessive voiding of urine.

prepuce (prep'yūs *or* prēp'yūs). The foreskin of the penis.

priapism (prī'a-pizm). An abnormal state of constant penile erection. The cause is generally obscure.

prostate (pros'tāt). A glandular secondary part of the main sexual system. It surrounds the urethra at the neck of the bladder and produces prostatic secretion which is discharged into the urethra and dilutes the seminal fluid.

prostatectomy (pros-ta-tek'tō-mē). Surgical removal of part or of all of the prostate gland. Bladder neck obstruction due to enlargement of the glandular elements is the usual reason for this frequently done procedure.

prostatism (pros'ta-tizm). The complex of symptoms and conditions resulting

from urinary obstruction due to an enlarged prostate gland at the bladder neck.

prostatitis (pros-ta-tīt'is). Inflammation in the spaces of the prostate gland.

prostatovesiculitis (pros-ta-tō-ves-ik-yūl-ī'tis). Prostatitis with extension of the infection into the seminal vesicles.

proteinuria (prō-ten-ūr'ē-a). The presence of albumin and other proteins in the urine. *See* **albuminuria.**

Proteus (Prō'tē-us). A common name for Proteus vulgaris, a species of bacteria sometimes responsible for persistent urinary infection.

Pseudomonas (sūd-ō-mōn'as). A common name for Pseudomonas aeruginosa, a species of bacteria sometimes found in urinary infections.

"P.S.P." Medical lingo for the phenolsulphonphthalein test. *See* **"phthalein."**

pyelitis (pī-el-ī'tis). PYELO=pelvis. Inflammation of or in the renal pelvis.

pyelogram (pī'-el-ō-gram). An x-ray film of the renal pelvis (excretory, retrograde).

pyelolithotomy (pī-el-ō-lith-ot'ō-mē). The surgical removal of a stone from the kidney pelvis through an incision in the wall of the pelvis. *See* **nephrolithotomy.**

pyelonephritis (pī-el-ō-nef-rī'tis). Inflammation of the pelvis and calices of one or of both kidneys. *See* **nephritis.**

pyeloplasty (pī'-el-ō-plas-tē). The surgical reshaping of the pelvis of a kidney to improve its drainage.

pyelostomy (pī-el-ost'ō-mē). A surgically produced, temporary or permanent new route by which urine may leave the body directly from the kidney pelvis. Also the surgical procedure. *See* **nephrostomy.**

pyelotomy (pī-el-ot'ō-mē). The making of a temporary incision into the kidney pelvis for any purpose.

pyeloureteral junction (pī-el-ō-yūr-ēt′er-al). As it says, the junction of the renal pelvis and the ureter.

pyeloureterectasis — pyeloureterectasia (pī-el-ō-yūr-ē-ter-ek′ta-sis) — (pī-el-ō-yūr-ē-ter-ek-tā′zē-a). Dilatation of both the renal pelvis and the ureter.

pyeloureterogram (pī-el-ō-yūr-ē′ter-ō-gram). An x-ray film showing the renal pelvis and its ureter simultaneously.

pyramid (pir′a-mid). One of the several cone shaped collections of renal tubules found in the cortex of the kidney.

pyramidalis (pir-a-mid-al′is). A muscle of the lower abdominal wall, exterior to the bladder.

pyuria (pī-yūr′ē-a). "Pus in the urine."

raphe (rā′fē). The ridge in the median line of the scrotum.

reanastomosis (rē-an-as-tōm-ō′sis). The surgical rejoining of two parts of the same passage or tube previously separated or divided.

reflux (rē′fluks). Backward flowing of urine up the ureter from the bladder, especially during the act of voiding.

renal (rēn′al). *adj.* REN=kidney. Relating to the kidney.

renal arteriogram (ar-tēr′ē-ō-gram). The x-ray visualization of the renal blood supply, accomplished by suddenly filling the renal arteries with radiopaque material, by way of the aorta.

renal scan (skan). A diagnostic isotope procedure sometimes used in cases of possible or suspected renal tumor.

renal tubule (tūb′yūl). One of the many tubular structures of the kidney cortex in which urine concentration takes place.

resectoscope (rē-sekt′ō-skōp). SECT= cut. A surgical instrument for electric cutting, under water, while under cystoscopic vision. With its use the prostate, or bladder tumors can be removed through the urethra. Types

are McCarthy, Thompson, Iglasias, Nesbit, Gibson, and others.

residual urine (rē-zid′yū-al). Any urine remaining in the bladder after urination has been completed. Normally the bladder is empty after voiding.

retrigonization (rē-trī-gōn-i-zā′shun). Surgical refashioning of the bladder floor, generally following **prostatectomy.**

retrograde (ret′rō-grād). *adj.—adv.* In urology, referring to the progression of fluid, bacteria or instruments up the urinary tract from a lower segment of it, either spontaneously or by definite intent.

retropubic prostatectomy (ret-rō-pyūb′ik prost-a-tek′tō-mē). Surgical removal of the prostate gland via the retropubic space (in front of the bladder). (Vernacular, used as a noun — "a retropubic.")

rongeur (ron-zhūr′). A biting or nipping forceps.

scrotum (skrōt′um). The pouch containing the testicles and their connected structures. (*adj.*—scrot′al.) (Fig. 26, p. 245)

semen (sēm′en). The male sexual fluid carrying the spermatozoa. (*adj.*—sem′inal.)

seminal fluid (sem′i-nal). The male sexual fluid carrying the spermatozoa.

seminal vesicles (sem′i-nal ves′i-kls). *plural.* Paired pockets for the storage of spermatic fluid, located beneath the base of the bladder. (*adj.*—vesic′ular.) (Fig. 26, p. 245)

seminoma (sem-in-ō′ma). A type of testicular tumor.

Sertoli cells (Ser-tō′lē). Certain supporting cells in the testicle which are related to the spermatozoa.

Skene's glands (Skēnz). Paired paraurethral glands discharging alongside the urethral **meatus** (in females only).

sound. One of a graduated set of solid instruments used for dilating narrowings in the urethra. (Sometimes used as a verb, to pass a sound.)

space of Retzius (Ret'zē-us). The space between the bladder and the inner surface of the pubic bone.

sperm. Short form (both singular and plural) for **spermatozoa**. (*adj.* — spermat'ic.)

spermatocele (sperm-at'ō-sēl). An encysted collection of fluid originating from the epididymis and containing spermatozoa.

spermatozoon (sperm-a-tō-zō'on). The male seed. (*plural* — spermatozo'a.)

sphincter (sfink'ter). One of the many cutoff muscles (external, internal, voluntary, involuntary).

"staghorn" calculus (stag'horn kalk'yūl-us). A type of kidney stone, so called from its shape.

stoma (stōm'a). STOM=mouth. The end or opening of a duct or channel. In urology, this generally refers to a urine-carrying structure which is generally surgically created.

strangury (strang'gyūr-ē). Painful urination, with spasms.

stricture (strik'tchur). A region of diminished size of the channel of a tube or duct, especially one due to scar tissue.

stylet (stī-let'). A wire guide sometimes used within a catheter to stiffen it; also called a **mand'rin.**

sulcus, median (sulk'us). In urology, the posterior groove between the two lateral prostatic lobes.

suprapubic prostatectomy (sū-pra-pyūb'ik prost-a-tek'tō-mē). Surgical removal of the prostate gland through the inside of the bladder (which has been opened from a lower abdominal incision). (Vernacular, used as a noun, "a suprapubic.")

teratoma testis (ter-a-tōm'a tes'tis). A type of testicular tumor.

testicle (tes'ti-kl) — **testis.** The paired male genital organ which produces spermatozoa and male sex hormone.

testosterone (tes-tos'ter-ōn). A hormone produced by the testes, generally called "the male sex hormone." It is also made synthetically for therapeutic use.

torsion (tor'shun). TORS=twist. A twisting. In urology the term generally refers to torsion of the spermatic cord.

trabeculation (tra-bek-yūl-ā'shun). A thickening of the bladder wall with

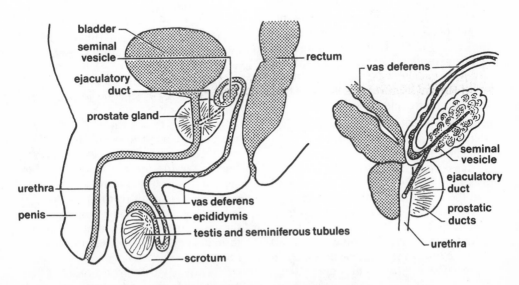

FIG. 26. Male Reproductive System

pocket formation due to bladder outlet obstruction.

tractor (trak'tor). A surgical instrument sometimes used in performing **prostatectomy** by the perineal route.

transurethral resection (trans-yūr-ēth'ral rē-sek'shun). Removal of the prostate gland via the urethra using a **resectoscope** and electric cutting. (Vernacular, "T.U.R." or "resection.")

trigone (trī'gōn). A triangular portion of the bladder floor: the three limiting points are the bladder openings of the two ureters, above, and the urethra, below. (Fig. 25, p. 241)

trilobed (trī'lōbd). *adj.* Three-lobed, generally referring to a particular conformation of an enlarged prostate gland.

trocar (trō'kar). A sharp-pointed, two-piece, hollow instrument sometimes used for draining the bladder through the abdominal wall.

tubule (tūb'yūl). The structure which receives the urine filtrate from the glomerulus and conveys it to the pelvis while concentrating it. *See* **nephron.**

tunica albuginea (tūn'ik-a alb-ū-jin'ē-a). The smooth membrane which intimately covers the testicle proper.

tunica vaginalis (tūn'ik-a vaj-in-al'is). The smooth scrotal lining which also covers each testicle and its epididymis. The cavity formed sometimes encloses hydrocele accumulations.

urachus (yūr-āk'us). A rudimentary structure attached to the top of the bladder. It sometimes persists and occasionally causes trouble.

urea (yūr-ē'a). A waste product found in the blood and in the urine. Excessive amounts indicate renal malfunction.

ureter (yūr'e-ter). The tube (bilateral) conveying urine from each kidney *to* the bladder. (*adj.*—uret'eral.) (Fig. 25, p. 241)

ureteral peristalsis (yūr-ēt'er-al per-i-stal'sis). The rhythmic, wave-like contraction of the ureteral walls, which propels urine from the kidneys down the ureters to the bladder.

ureterocele (yūr-ēt'er-ō-sēl). An abnormal (everted) protrusion of the end of the ureter into the bladder.

ureterolithotomy (yūr-ēt-er-ō-lith-ot'ō-mē). The surgical removal of a calculus from the ureter, through an incision made in the wall of the ureter.

ureteropelvic (yūr-ēt-er-ō-pel'vik). *adj.* Referring to the region of the funnel-like termination of the kidney pelvis into the ureter.

ureterostomy (yūr-ēt-er-ost'ō-mē). A temporary or permanent surgically-produced new route for the urine to leave the body directly from the ureter.

ureterotomy (yūr-ēt-er-ot'ō-mē). The making of a temporary incision through the wall of the ureter, generally for removing a stone.

ureterovesical (yūr-ēt-er-ō-ves'i-kl). *adj.* Referring to the junction of the ureter with the bladder.

urethra (yūr-ēth'ra). The tube conveying urine outward *from* the bladder. (*adj.*—ureth'ral.) (Fig. 12, p. 119; Fig. 25, p. 241, Fig. 26, p. 245)

urethritis (yūr-e-thrīt'is). Inflammation of the lining of the urethra.

urethrogram (yūr-ēth'rō-gram). An x-ray film showing the urethra distended with an x-ray opaque jelly or liquid.

urethrostomy (yūr-e-thros'tō-mē). A temporary or permanent surgically-produced new route by which urine may leave the urethra instead of by way of the urethral **meatus.**

urethrotome (yūr-ēth'rō-tōm). A surgical instrument used for cutting urethral strictures from within the urethral channel. *See* internal urethrotomy.

urethrotomy (yūr-ē-throt'ō-mē). The making of a temporary incision through the wall of the urethra, generally to relieve a strictured condition.

internal urethrotomy. An incision made from within, with special instruments.

external urethrotomy. An incision made from the outside.

urinalysis (yūr-in-al'is-is). The chemical and microscopic examination of urine.

urine (yūr'in). The fluid which contains body waste products and is formed in the kidneys for excretion from the body.

urogenital (yūr-ō-jen'i-tal). *adj.* Pertaining to both the urinary and the genital tracts. Also **genitourinary.**

urogram (yūr'ō-gram). An x-ray film showing the entire urinary tract following the use of intravenous or retrograde opacifying material.

urologist (yūr-ol'ō-jist). A doctor who specializes in urology.

urology (yūr-ol'ō-jē). *See* introductory paragraphs.

varicocele (vair'i-kō-sēl). A collection of varicosed spermatic veins within the scrotum. Varicoceles are generally left-sided.

vas deferens (vas def'er-enz). The tube conveying spermatozoa from each testicle to the bilateral seminal vesicles. (*plural* — vas'a deferen'tia.) (Fig. 26, p. 245)

vasectomy (vas-ek'tō-mē). The surgical procedure of removing a part of the **vas deferens.**

verumontanum (vēr-ū-mont-an'um). A mound in the floor of the prostatic urethra which marks the location of the ejaculatory duct orifices.

vesical (ves'i-kl). *adj.* Pertaining to the bladder. *See* **vesicle** and **seminal vesicles.**

vesicoureteral (ves-i-kō-yūr-ēt'er-al). *adj.* Same as **ureterovesical.**

vesicular (ves-ik'yul-ar). *adj.* In urology, pertaining to the seminal vesicles.

vesiculogram (ves-ik'yūl-ō-gram). An x-ray film showing the seminal vesicles distended with an opaque liquid.

void (voyd). *verb.* To pass urine.

Wilms tumor (vilms). A malignant kidney tumor, usually occurring during childhood.

Y-plasty (wī'plas-tē). A particular type of surgical reconstruction of an outlet, generally performed on the bladder neck.

*

IV ADDENDA

Medical Abbreviations

THE FUNCTION OF an abbreviation is to shorten and simplify. In the case of medical abbreviations this includes the shortening of the names of organizations and of commonly understood medical conditions. It also includes listing the common expressions used by doctors and by paramedical personnel in referring to certain well-known medical situations and procedures. Here is a list of some of the commonly accepted formal abbreviations and other "medical jargon" equivalents. Abbreviations are not listed in the INDEX.

a.c. Before meals.

A.C. Alternating current (a characteristic of some electric power).

A.C.S. The American Cancer Society.

A.C.P. The American College of Physicians.

    F.A.C.P. A Fellow of the American College of Physicians.

A.C.S. The American College of Surgeons.

    F.A.C.S. A Fellow of the American College of Surgeons.

ACTH The adrenocorticotropic hormone.

ad lib As often as desired (by the patient).

AEC The Atomic Energy Commission (which controls the isotope program).

A.F.B. Acid-fast bacillus (generally refers to the tubercle bacillus).

Ag. Silver (chemical symbol).

A/G ratio Albumin-globulin ratio.

AgNo$_3$ Silver nitrate (chemical symbol).

A.H.A. The American Hospital Association.

A.M.A. The American Medical Association.

anes. Anesthesia.

ant. Anterior.

A.P. Anteroposterior (generally referring to the patient's position in relation to the x-ray tube — in this case the tube in front of the patient).

A&P Auscultation and percussion (procedures used in chest examinations).

A.P.H.A. The American Public Health Association.

aq. dest. Distilled water.

A-V Arteriovenous; atrioventricular.

Ba. Barium (chemical symbol).

B.I.D. — bid Twice a day.

B.M. A bowel movement.

B.M.R. The basal metabolic rate.

B.P. The blood pressure level.

B.P.H. Benign prostatic hyperplasia.

B.U.N. The urea nitrogen level (in the blood).

C. Centigrade (one of the temperature scales).

c̄ With.

C₁–C₇ The cervical vertebrae identified by number.

"**C.A.**"–**CA**–**ca** Medical jargon for cancer.

cap. Capsule.

C.B.C.–**CBC**–**cbc** A complete blood count.

cc.–**ccm.** A cubic centimeter (a measure of volume in the metric system).

CHO Carbohydrate.

cm. Centimeter (a measure of length in the metric system).

C.N.S. The central nervous system.

CO₂ Carbon dioxide (chemical symbol).

"**C.P.C.**" Medical jargon for Clinical Pathological Conference.

C.S.F. Cerebrospinal fluid.

C.V.A. Medical abbreviation for a cerebrovascular accident, or "stroke."

D.C. Direct current (a characteristic of some electric power).

D & C Dilation of the cervix and curettage of the uterus.

D.D.S. Doctor of Dental Surgery.

Derm. Dermatology.

D.O.A. Dead on arrival at the hospital.

"**D.T.'s**" Medical lingo for delirium tremens.

E.E.G. An electroencephalogram.

E.K.G.–**E.C.G.** An electrocardiogram.

"**E.N.T.**" Medical jargon for Ear, Nose and Throat.

Etiol. Etiology.

F. Fahrenheit (one of the temperature scales).

F.D.A. Federal Drug Administration.

F.H. Family history.

G.B. Gallbladder.

"**G.C.**" Medical lingo for gonorrheal urethritis (gonorrhea).

"**G.I.**" *adj.* Medical lingo for gastrointestinal.

gm.–**G.** Gram (a measure of weight in the metric system).

"**G.P.**" Medical lingo for a general practitioner.

gr. Grain (a measure of weight in the apothecary system).

gt. A drop (*plural*–gtt.).

"**G.U.**" *adj.* Medical jargon for genitourinary or urological.

GYN Gynecology.

"**Gyn-e**" (gīn'ē) Medical lingo for Gynecology.

Hb.–**hb** Hemoglobin.

HCl Hydrochloric acid (chemical symbol).

Hct. The hematocrit of the blood (same as P.C.V.–the packed cell volume).

Hg. Mercury (chemical symbol).

/HPF The number, per high-power microscopic field.

H.S.–**h.s.** At bedtime. (Actually "hour of slumber"–how soothing!)

"**hypo**" Medical lingo for a hypodermic injection (or for a small syringe).

"**I.M.**" *adv.* Given intramuscularly (hospital term).

"**I.C.U.**" Hospital name for the Intensive Care Unit of a hospital.

in extremis At the point of death.

I.Q. Intelligence quotient.

"**I.V.**" *adv.* Given intravenously (hospital term).

"**I.V.P.'s**" Hospital name for "intravenous" (excretory) pyelograms.

J.A.M.A. The Journal of the American Medical Association.

K Potassium (chemical symbol).

Kg. Kilogram (a weight measurement of the metric system–2.2 pounds).

KI Potassium iodide (chemical symbol).

17 KS 17 ketosteroids.

K.U.B. A film covering the area of kidneys, ureters and bladder.

kv Kilovolt (a measure of electric power).

kw Kilowatt (a measure of electric power).

L₁–L₅ The lumbar vertebrae, identified by number.

lat. Lateral.

LINAC Radiologic lingo for linear accelerator.

L.L.Q. The left lower quadrant of the abdomen.

L.O.A. The left occipito*anterior* position (of the fetus during labor).

L.O.P. The left occipito*posterior* position (of the fetus during labor).

L.P. A lumbar puncture.

L.U.Q. The left upper quadrant of the abdomen.

m. Minim (a drop—apothecary system).

ma. Milliampere (measure of electric power—vernacular "millies").

mg. Milligram (a measure of weight in the metric system).

ml. Milliliter (a measure of volume in the metric system—equivalent to a cubic centimeter).

mm. Millimeter (a measure of length in the metric system).

mm. Hg Millimeters of mercury (a measure of the height of the blood pressure).

NaCl Sodium chloride (chemical symbol for common salt).

N.F. The National Formulary (one of the drug indexes).

N₂O Nitrous oxide (chemical symbol for an anesthetic gas).

noc. Night.

N.P.N. Nonprotein nitrogen level (in the blood).

N.P.O. Nothing by mouth.

Obs. Obstetrics.

"**O.B.**" Medical jargon for Obstetrics.

Opth. Opthalmology.

"**O.R.**" Medical lingo for the operating room.

"**Osteo**" Medical jargon for osteomyelitis.

O.T. Old tuberculin (a particular kind of tuberculin).

oz. An ounce.

"**P.A.**" Medical jargon for pernicious anemia; also, posteroanterior—the patient's back toward the x-ray tube.

para An obstetrical term indicating the number of previous pregnancies completed.

para I A woman who has borne one child.

para II A woman who has borne two children, etc.

p.c. After meals.

P.C.V.—p.c.v. Packed cell volume (same as hematocrit).

P.E. Physical examination.

Ped. Pediatrics.

"**Pent.**" Medical lingo for Pentothal.

P.H. Past history.

P.I. Present illness.

"**P.I.D.**" Medical lingo for pelvic inflammatory disease.

P.M. A postmortem examination.

p.o. By mouth.

post. Posterior.

"**post**" Medical jargon for an autopsy.

"**post-op**" Postoperative—the number of days since surgery.

"**prep**" Hospital term for preparation for surgery, particularly of the operative area. Also used as a verb.

p.r.n. Allowable whenever necessity demands.

P.S.P. The phenolsulfonphthalein test (of kidney function).

pt. The patient.

Px Physical examination.

q. Every, each.

q.d. Every day.

q.h. Every hour.

q. 2h. Every two hours, etc.

Q.I.D.—qid Four times a day.

q.n.s. Insufficient quantity.

q.s. Sufficient quantity.

rad Abbreviation for "radiation absorbed dose."

RBC's Red blood cells.

RH neg. Rh negative (blood type).

Rh pos. Rh positive (blood type).

R.L.Q. The right lower quadrant of the abdomen.

R.N. Registered nurse.

R.O.A. The right occipito*anterior* diameter of the pelvic outlet (obstetrical).

R.O.P. The right occipito*posterior* diameter of the pelvic outlet (obstetrical).

R.U.Q. The right upper quadrant of the abdomen.

"R-X" Medical lingo referring to a prescription (Rx).

s̄ Without.

"sed. rate" Medical lingo for sedimentation rate, a laboratory procedure.

S.G. The specific gravity.

"S.M.R." Vernacular name for a submucous resection (nasal operation).

S.M.W.D.Sep. Single, married, widowed, divorced, separated.

"Staph" Medical lingo for staphylococcus or staphylococcic.

stat At once.

"Strep" Medical lingo for streptococcus or streptococcic.

"subcu." Medical lingo referring to a subcutaneous injection (also adverb, given subcutaneously).

T_1-T_{12} The thoracic vertebrae, identified by number.

T.&A. Tonsils and adenoids.

"T.&.A." Medical lingo referring to the removal of the tonsils and adenoids.

"T.A." Medical jargon for the toxin-antitoxin mixture used for the prevention of tetanus.

"tb" Medical lingo for a tubercular infection.

tbc. Tuberculosis, or tubercle bacillus.

T.I.D.—tid Three times a day.

T.P.R. Temperature, pulse, respiration.

"T.U.R." Vernacular term for the transurethral resection of the prostate.

umb. The umbilicus or navel (also adjective, umbilical).

ung. An ointment.

"U.R.I." Medical jargon for an upper respiratory infection.

Urol. Urology.

U.S.P. United States Pharmacopoeia (a listing of accepted drugs).

U.S.P.H.S. The United States Public Health Service.

v. Volt (a measure of electric current).

"V.D." Medical lingo for venereal disease.

V.N.A. The Visiting Nurse Association.

w. Watt (a measure of electric current).

WBC's White blood cells.

W.H.O. The World Health Organization.

wt. Weight.

✺

Index

A

H

L

sling (*see* fascial slings; head sling)
slit lamp, 133
slough, 36, 79
sludge, 183
smallpox, 102
Smith-Peterson nail, 141
Smithwick procedure, 113
snare, 149
Snellen's chart, 133
social worker (*see* psychiatric social worker)
sodium iodide, 206
soft palate, 49, 70, 149
soft-tissue shadows, 206
solardermatitis, 79
somnambulism, 198
soporific, 36
souffle, 122
sound, 244
space (*see* interdental space; intervertebral space; subarachnoid space; subdural space)
space of Retzius, 245
space maintainer, 70
spasm (*see* laryngospasm; pylorospasm; bronchiospasm; blepharospasm)
spastic, 36
spasticity, 177
spatulation, 70
specific terms, 22
specific gravity, 163
specimen, 36
speculum, 36
see also anoscope; proctoscope; sigmoidoscope
speech areas, 113
sperm, 245
spermatocele, 157, 245
spermatozoon, 49, 245
sphenoid sinus, 149
sphincter, 49, 219, 245
sphincter ani, 189
sphincterotomy, 219
sphygmomanometer, 102
spina bifida, 113, 226
"spinal," 62

spinal accessory nerve, 113
spinal cord, 49
spinal fluid, 108
spinous process, 141
spirochete, 163
splanchnic, 49
spleen, 49, *217*
splenectomy, 219
splenic flexure, 190, *190*
splenomegaly, 157, 170
see also hepatosplenomegaly
splint, 37, 141
spondylitis, 141, 170, 177
spondylitis deformans, 157
spondylolisthesis, 142
spondylolysis, 142
sporotrichosis, 102, 157
sprain, 142
sprue, 102
sputum, 37
squamous cell carcinoma, 80
squamous cells, 49, 79
squint, 133
"staghorn" calculus, 245
Stanford-Binet test, 170
stapedectomy, 150
stapes, 150
Staphylococcus, 102, 163
staphylorrhaphy, 226
stasis, 102
stasis dermatitis, 80
State Board of Medical Examiners, 10
status angina, 102
status asthmaticus, 102
status epilepticus, 102
steatorrhea, 102
Steinmann's pin, 142
Stellwag's sign, 133
stems, 15
stenosis, 37
see also aortic stenosis; mitral stenosis; pyloric stenosis
Stensen's duct, 150
stereoscopic vision, 133
sterile, 219
see also asepsis
sterile technique, 219

xerophthalmia, 133
xerosis, 80
xiphoid process, *50*, 143
x-rays, 199
Xylocaine (*see* lidocaine)

Y

yaws, 184
yellow fever, 184
Y-plasty, 247

Z

Zenker's diverticulum, 105
Z-plasty, 226
zygoma, 143

†